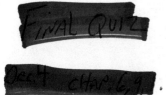

FINAL QUIZ

Oct 4 CHAP. 6, 9.

FOCUS ON NUTRITION

Patricia J. Long

Society for Nutrition Education
Oakland, California

Barbara Shannon

Pennsylvania State University
College of Human Development
University Park, Pennsylvania

PRENTICE-HALL, INC., Englewood Cliffs, New Jersey 07632

Library of Congress Cataloging in Publication Data

LONG, PATRICIA J.
   Focus on nutrition.

   Selections from the author's Nutrition, an inquiry
into the issues.
   Includes bibliographical references and index.
   1. Nutrition. I. Shannon, Barbara. II. Title.
TX354.L6625   1983   641.1   82-15109
ISBN 0-13-322800-2

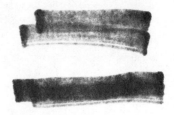

Editorial/production supervision and interior design: Fred Bernardi
Cover design: Zimmerman/Foyster Design
Manufacturing buyer: Harry P. Baisley

Printed in the United States of America

10 9 8 7 6 5 4 3 2 1

ISBN: 0-13-322800-2

PRENTICE-HALL INTERNATIONAL, INC., *London*
PRENTICE-HALL OF AUSTRALIA PTY. LIMITED, *Sydney*
EDITORA PRENTICE-HALL DO BRASIL, LTDA., *Rio de Janeiro*
PRENTICE-HALL CANADA INC., *Toronto*
PRENTICE-HALL OF INDIA PRIVATE LIMITED, *New Delhi*
PRENTICE-HALL OF JAPAN, INC., *Tokyo*
PRENTICE-HALL OF SOUTHEAST ASIA PTE. LTD., *Singapore*
WHITEHALL BOOKS LIMITED, *Wellington, New Zealand*

Contents

Chapter 4
FATS   78

Preface

In today's classroom it is not enough to learn nutrition principles without also discussing current nutrition issues and controversies. This is especially true for those of you who are not majoring in nutrition because, at best, you will be able to take only one nutrition course during your entire college program. So it is important that you have the knowledge to evaluate future nutrition controversies that will confront you once the course has ended.

The emphasis of this book is on all three areas: principles, issues, and methods for evaluating claims. Chapter 1 introduces you to the nature of nutrition controversy. The next seven chapters discuss the nutrients and energy, with each chapter followed by such related issues as sweeteners, fiber, coronary heart disease, and weight control. The book concludes with a chapter on the U.S. diet and covers the topics of additives, alternative eating patterns, and cancer.

Written for college students and with the assumption that the reader has had little science background, the book is also useful for high school health education classes, continuing education classes, in-service courses, and community nutrition or health classes. The style is informal so that you can use the book not just as a text but as a guide to examining your own eating habits based on the information presented.

Patricia J. Long
Barbara Shannon

Nutrition Controversy: Whom to Believe?

1

Dick Cavett is a TV talker who is...nervous about diet promoters. Cavett's attitude may have been shaped partly by a tragic and depressing experience that happened to him....He taped an interview with Jerome Rodale, whose 'Rodale Press publishes *Prevention* magazine and a steady stream of books arguing with established medical views....He was promoting his publications about "organic foods," which he thought were better for people than foods grown with commercial fertilizers. During the Cavett interview, the 72-year-old Rodale bragged that he would live to be 100 because of his healthful eating habits. Cavett completed the interview and briefly turned his attention to somebody else. When he looked back, Rodale was dead in his chair.(1)

If Rodale had managed to fulfill his boast, many people would have jumped to devour both his books and his organically grown foods. Since he died at age 72, we can scoff at his theories. But what if he was right?

Since the beginning of recorded history, in an effort to prevent and cure illness, people have tried all kinds of rituals and concoctions—some reasonable, some odd, and some downright dangerous. Food and spices were often used as medicines. Take, for instance, the problem of sexual impotence. The early Romans ate truffles to cure the problem; and Italians of a later century insisted upon tomatoes; as late as the 1700s, others swore by pistachio nuts and the foot and snout of the hippopotamus. If these remedies failed, pigeons and turtle doves were recommended to lessen the heartbreak.(2)

In the sixteenth century, many people, including doctors, believed that fruits and vegetables had both healing and destructive properties. If someone indulged in a Jerusalem artichoke, with its shrunken, contorted roots, it would be no surprise if the person became grossly deformed with leprosy.(3) This theory lasted well into the 1800s: The pale, delicate women of Victorian times were often prescribed port wine in order to put a glow in their cheeks. (If the wine put color in their cheeks, it was for reasons other than its red color.)

In recent history, the nineteenth century would get the prize as the classic age of quackery. It was the heyday of the patent medicine craze, and faddists promoted such "health foods" as sodas, graham crackers, Grape-Nuts, postum, laxatives, and peanut butter.(4) The founding of the modern cereal industry in the United States is a tale of health sanatoriums, religious revivalism, and grab-bag remedies. Today we still have food fads, but the ingredients have changed. Granola replaced Grape-Nuts, and soda became junk food. Peanut butter is still holding its own, provided no preservatives appear on the label.

There is nothing wrong with preferring or promoting special foods, whether they are organically grown or fabricated in a factory. Quackery becomes a factor only when promoters make false claims about the benefits of consuming such products and charge prices well beyond the foods' value.

FOOD FADDISM AND QUACKERY

Where do these ideas come from? Do they have any merit? Mann(5) has identified five ways for food fads and quackery to get started: (1) through philosophical-religious beliefs, (2) hucksterism, (3) medical abandonment, (4) the influence of badly informed or adventurous scientists, and (5) fear of the orthodox food industry.

A number of groups such as those who follow the Zen macrobiotic diet, the New Vrindaban International Society for Krishna Consciousness, and the members of the Ehrets Mucusless Diet Healing System, have unusual eating practices for philosophical or religious reasons. Some of these groups refuse to eat animal products; others eliminate all food groups but one. Some of these diets may be nutritious and provide a religious bond among members, but they are not the best or the only way for everyone to eat.

In contrast to this emphasis on the spiritual, hucksterism is the blatant attempt to mislead the public for money. One thing you can be sure of: If half of humanity is searching for health and longevity, the other half is trying to sell it to them. Just look at all the diets advertised in newspapers and magazines, complete with physician sponsorship and money-back guarantees.

The third source, abandonment of the medical establishment, can come from a belief that doctors are conspiring to keep cures off the market so their businesses will thrive. This is best seen in the accusations aimed at the American Cancer Society by proponents of laetrile. Other persons who look outside the medical establishment are the terminally ill. In his book *Death Be Not Proud*, John Gunther tells the story of his 16-year-old son's battle with brain cancer. He recalls the family's search for bizarre cures such as calves' liver, vegetable juices, and health foods once the neurosurgeons diagnosed the son's condition as hopeless.(6)

This move away from traditional medical treatment can be seen in the holistic approach to health. Also known as wholistic, humanistic, alternative, new age or consciousness medicine, the approach emphasizes treating the whole person by focusing on life style and environmental factors. Holistic therapies include acupuncture, chiropractic, nutrition, herbal medicine, biofeedback, Rolfing, *shiatsu*, and psychic healing.(7) Although medical personnel have too long ignored a preventive approach to disease, the holistic movement is so new that there are few adequate standards to distinguish the capable practitioners from the incompetent, and the sound therapies from the ridiculous or dangerous.(8)

One of the most disturbing sources of misinformation is the badly informed scientist. Doctors and Ph.D.s have developed some of the most potentially dangerous diets, many of which have been widely publicized. Dr. Carlton Frederick's *Low Carbohydrate Diet* and Dr. Atkins' *Diet Revolution* are two examples.(9,10) Adelle Davis, who earned a master's degree in nutrition, wrote a number of best-selling nutrition books, all of them filled with misquotes, personal interpretations of data, and speculative conclusions.(9) A lawsuit has been brought against her estate and her publishers following the death of an infant who was treated by his parents according to information in one of her books.(11) One of her famous quotes, "I have yet to know a single adult to develop cancer who has habitually drunk a quart of milk daily," was proved wrong when she herself, an avid milk-drinker, died of cancer at the age of 70.(2)

Fear of the orthodox food industry is Mann's final category. Few people would hold that all our current methods of processing and distributing food are without problems. There are, however, many processed products, from frozen orange juice to pasteurized milk, that are nutritious. Those who refuse to use processed products may be putting too much faith in the alternatives.

Food faddism and quackery are not the same, though we have treated them together here. Faddism includes eating practices outside the norm, some of which, though unusual, are not harmful. Quackery implies a false and sometimes dangerous claim being made for such practices.

GUIDELINES FOR EVALUATING CLAIMS

Three areas to scrutinize when you read a statement or claim are these: promoter's intent, the flow of logic, and the research base (Table 1–1).

Promoter's Intent

Is the promoter biased? First look at the author's or announcer's approach. What is the purpose? To sell you a product (food or supplement)? To sell you an idea (book)? If you are being sold a product, does the promoter focus more on the package than the contents? Is there an unrealistic aura given to the product, such as a seductive woman sipping a diet soda?

Is the promoter trying to convince you you are unhealthy? Are you being asked to diagnose yourself? Is it suggested you avoid talking to a doctor or

TABLE 1–1   **Evaluating Nutrition Claims**

1. *Promoter's Intent*
   Sell product
   Sell idea
2. *Flow of Logic*
   Multiple-subject
     and multiple-object sentence
   Masking opinion as fact
   Use of qualifiers
   Generalizations
   Arrangement of sentences
     and words

Connotations of words
Inaccurate synonyms and half-truths
Dangling or unstated comparisons
Spurious comparisons
Deceptive omissions
Uniqueness
Unbalanced view

3. *Research Base*
   Anecdotal record
   Single-blind studies
   Double-blind studies

dietitian? Does the promoter imply that everyone's diet is poor and needs correction? Does the promotion use intimidating tactics? "If you love your child, you'll feed him product X."

Another indicator of possible bias is the type of publication in which an article is found. If the article appears in a sensational magazine sandwiched between a headline screaming about sex scandals on Capitol Hill and one prophesying a miracle cure for cancer, there is a good chance the nutrition information may not be reliable. If the information is in a scholarly journal, where all research articles are reviewed before publication, there is a greater likelihood the data are well supported.

Flow of Logic

Besides approach, examine the flow of logic. One common practice is to dispute the laws of nature. Does the promoter promise to cure diseases for which science has yet to find a cure (cancer, arthritis)? Are quick, dramatic results promised ("Eat all you want and lose weight" or "Twenty pounds in 10 days")? Because of this miracle cure, does the promoter claim to be a victim of persecution by the Food and Drug Administration and the established medical profession? Double check the claims; see what others' opinions are.

Certain grammatical patterns can also lead the reader or consumer to make incorrect assumptions.(12) For instance, an author may use a multiple-subject and multiple-object sentence: "Sugar, fat, cholesterol, and salt cause diabetes, cancer, hypertension and heart disease." As a reader, you have to decide which disease correlates with which nutrition component. Do all factors cause all the diseases? Does one factor cause all? Do all factors cause one disease?

Another tactic is to mask opinion as fact. "It is thought," "It is believed," and "It appears" are valid ways of presenting information as long as the reader is aware that opinions are not always facts. When you see phrases like these, ask yourself these questions: "Whose opinion is this?" "On what scientific information is it based?"

Authors can present information in a factual way, but buried in the text are words and phrases such as "may," "probably," "perhaps," "assuming," and "seems to." This use of qualifiers turns facts into possibilities. The use of generalizations like "Nine out of ten doctors believe" should lead you to ask: "Who are these doctors?" "How do you know this is what they believe?"

Certain arrangements of sentences and words can cause the reader to make a mental connection that is not necessarily valid. For example: "High intakes of saturated fats contribute to heart attacks. This product is low in saturated fat." Placing these sentences together makes it easy to conclude that the product prevents heart attacks, a conclusion that is not justified. Word connotations can make a product appear better than it actually is. Cream of Rice is claimed to "give 'em fast energy." Nutrament is the "body building energy food." Yogurt is described as the "new fruit and energy snack." The advertiser of each of these products chose the word "energy" to describe the benefits of consuming the product. What goes unstated is that a food can provide energy without providing many nutrients, so the amount of energy does not indicate the nutrient value or lack of it in the food. Other pairs of words with similar meanings but different connotations include "synthetic" versus "formulated," "cheap" versus "economical," and "coarse" versus "textured." Writers choose particular words to influence the reader's opinion.

Often nonscientists, by using inaccurate synonyms for scientific terms, change the meaning conveyed to the public. The meanings of the following terms are quite different:

SCIENTIFIC TERMS	INACCURATE SYNONYMS
hypothesis	fact
implications	results
suggests	proves
correlates	causes

Nonscientists often publish theories and call them facts; or refer to research proof when the findings are only highly suggestive. Pseudoscientific reports tend to be written simply, concisely, and convincingly. By contrast, scientific reports are often worded so carefully that they come across as ambiguous.(13) Read critically to see if assumptions are supported by sound data. Remember that medical assertions, unlike legal ones, are considered false until proved true.(3)

Promoters often use dangling or unstated comparisons, like "cholesterol intake is higher in the American diet." After reading this example, you are forced to ask: Cholesterol intake in America is higher than what? Than what we need? Than what other cultures consume? Than the amount of fat we eat? Another advertisement using an unstated comparison is the one for "light beer." What is this beer lighter than? The ad is often misinterpreted to mean you can drink large amounts without worrying about gaining weight.(14)

One of the most difficult techniques to recognize is the spurious comparison. For instance: "Fresh whole milk...an important food for children. With proteins, vitamins, minerals, but not much iron....And you need iron to help build healthy red blood. It would take 35, 8-ounce glasses of milk every day...to give you all the iron you get in one serving of enriched Cream of Wheat Cereal." This ad compares the nutritive value of a product to a food recognized as a poor source of a given nutrient. It is not surprising that Cream of Wheat has more iron than milk, since milk contains very little iron.(15)

Other techniques also affect the flow of logic. An example of one of these, deceptive omission, is the early commercial for the iron supplement Geritol that claimed a daily Geritol pill would relieve tiredness. A court order later forced the advertisers to admit that not all fatigue is caused by iron deficiency.(16)

Some ads use the technique of claiming uniqueness for a product when in fact it is of standard composition. Here is an example: "Our vegetable oil contains absolutely no cholesterol." What the reader may not know is that cholesterol is an animal product and is not found in any vegetable oil. Consider the advertising for brand X bread which claims it contains important vitamins and minerals needed for growth when, in fact, most processed breads are enriched with these nutrients.(16) Some writers present an unbalanced view by appearing to present both sides of an issue but weighting the evidence in one direction.

All these techniques indicate possible bias or inaccurate claims. Some promotional tactics are more obvious than others. One of the most difficult areas to evaluate is the research base, the data offered as supporting evidence.

Research Base

To review claims critically, you must examine certain aspects of the research. First, does the promoter cite an authority or leave the reader to guess who conducted the research? If an authority is cited, note the credentials. Is the researcher referred to only as "a leading nutritionist" or "a noted scientist"? Does the writer give the names of individuals who can later be contacted for verification of statements?

Check the degrees following the person's name. The M.D., D.O., D.Sc., M.S., M.A., R.D., and M.P.H. usually indicate the individual has a certain level of training in a particular field. But reputable science writers who do not have these degrees also produce well-written articles; remember that an M.D. is not a nutritionist, and that a nutritionist does not always know every aspect of the field. Doctoral degrees in nutrition can even be purchased through at least one health food organization.

In examining the research presented, look at the data. How recent are they? Can the original article even be found? Was the research conducted on animals or humans, and is this point made clear? Look closely at how the research was designed or set up. People are inclined to believe testimonials and unverified claims: "Before I took product X I could hardly walk. After just one week of eating it, I was able to jump out of my wheelchair and go dancing." Rigorous, scientific research sounds dull by comparison. Even so, the nature of the research design is what determines the validity of claims.

Researchers use three general types of data-collection techniques: the anecdotal record, single-blind studies, and double-blind studies.

The Anecdotal Records.   Anecdotal records are brief accounts of incidents in which individuals claim to have experienced "clear cases of cure" from various remedies. Testimonials from well-known personalities are especially popular. You should not confuse such observations with research that attempts to control all intervening factors except the one that is being tested.

For example, let us assume you develop cold symptoms and decide to try treating yourself with vitamin C. After taking 4 grams of the vitamin daily for two days, you note that you feel better and that the symptoms have not lasted as long as those of previous colds. You conclude that vitamin C is effective in combatting the common cold. This is anecdotal. You have no way of knowing whether the shorter duration of the symptoms was a result of the vitamin C or a less vigorous strain of the virus than those which caused your previous colds. Also, it is known that if you expect a response to occur, you are likely to experience that response, at least to some extent. This is called the placebo effect. Thus, in our example, you may have felt better because you expected to and not because of the vitamin.

Single-Blind Studies.   These studies involve two groups of subjects, a control and an experimental group. Researchers compare the two groups to assess the effect of a test substance. For example, if they are interested in assessing the effectiveness of vitamin C in reducing cold symptoms, they will give the vitamin to the experimental group and give the control group a placebo, a pill identical in appearance and taste to the vitamin but with no vitamin activity. The critical factor is that the subjects are unaware of which substance they are receiving. Researchers can then observe and record the cold symptoms experienced by the two groups over a period of time.

The problem with this type of design is that the researcher is aware of which group is taking the vitamin C and which the placebo. No matter how objective the researcher may be, there is always a tendency to view symptoms of the vitamin C group as different from those of the placebo group, depending on the expected effect. Therefore, such data may be unintentionally biased by the researcher.

Double-Blind Studies.   To avoid this bias, double-blind studies are designed so that neither the subject nor the researcher is aware of which individuals are receiving the placebo and which the vitamin C. Another person, completely unassociated with the study, randomly selects subjects to participate in the placebo or experimental group and codes the identities. This code is sealed and not broken until all the data have been collected and analyzed. The

TABLE 1–2 **Individuals and Organizations: Local Contacts for Nutrition Information**

City, county, or state public health department: Nutritionist*

Local hospital: Dietitian*

Local college or university: Food and Nutrition Science department: Dietetics program: Public Health/Nutrition department: Home Economics department

Landgrant university and county: Cooperative Extension Service

Local or state department of education: Nutrition Education and Training Program: Home Economics department

Community resources: Home Economists with supermarkets and utility companies: Nutrition Consultants*: Dietetic Consultants*

---

*Nutrition professionals who have a degree in nutrition, food science, or public health/nutrition or who are licensed by the American Dietetic Association as registered Dietitians (R.D.) are qualified to offer sound food and nutrition information.

Source: Jane A. Rubey, *Nutrition for Everybody* (Oakland, CA: Society for Nutrition Education, 1981), p. 21.

double-blind study is the best type of design, since it eliminates the placebo effect and at the same time avoids unintentional researcher bias.

Although it may be difficult to evaluate all the nutrition claims you will encounter in the future, there are individuals and organizations which can provide you with sound information (Table 1–2).

REFERENCES

1. M. Gunther, "The Worst Diet Advice," *TV Guide*, January 11, 1975, pp. 3–6.

2. R. Deutsch, *The New Nuts among the Berries* (Palo Alto, Calif.: Bull Publishing, 1977).

3. R. Gay, "Fear of Food," *American Scholar* 45(1976):437. Reprinted from THE AMERICAN SCHOLAR, Volume 45, Number 3, Summer, 1976. Copyright © 1976 by the United Chapters of Phi Beta Kappa. By permission of the publishers.

4. W.T. Jarvis, "Food Quackery Is Dangerous Business," *Nutrition News*, February–March, 1980.

5. G.V.V. Mann, "Food Quality: Is There Reason for Doubt?" *Panhandle Magazine* 6(1972):18–22.

6. H. Bruch, "The Allure of Food Cults and Nutrition Quackery," *Nutrition Reviews* 32(1974):62–66.

7. J.P. Callan, "Holistic Health or Holistic Hoax?" *Journal of the American Medical Association* 241(1979):1156.

8. G. Yahn, "The Impact of Holistic Medicine, Medical Groups, and Health Concepts," *Journal of the American Medical Association* 242(1979):2202–05.

9. E.H. Rynearson, "Americans Love Hogwash," *Nutrition Reviews* 32(1974):1–14.

10. American Medical Association, Council on Foods and Nutrition, "A Critique of Low-Carbohydrate, Ketogenic Weight Reduction Regimens: A Review of Dr. Atkins' Diet Revolution," *Journal of the American Medical Association* 224(1973):10.

11. L.A. Barness, "Who Gives Nutritional Advice: Who Follows It?" *Pediatrics* 65(1980):1045.

12. K. McNutt and D. McNutt, *Nutrition and Food Choices* (Chicago: Science Research Associates, 1978).

13. R.J. Wolff, "Who Eats for Health?" *American Journal of Clinical Nutrition* 26(1973):438–45.

14. *Proposed Trade Regulation Rule: Food Advertising. Report of the Presiding Officer, United States of America, before the Federal Trade Commission,* February 21, 1978. Public Record No. 215–40.

15. L. Schwartzberg, C. George, and M.C. Philipps, "Issues in Food Advertising—The Nutrition Educator's Viewpoint," *Journal of Nutrition Education* 9(1977):60–63.

16. K.B. Rotzoll, J.E. Haefner, and C.H. Sandage, *Advertising in Contemporary Society* (Columbus, Ohio: GRID, Inc., 1976).

The Nutrients
2

We lived for days on nothing but food and water.

W.C. FIELDS (describing a town that ran out of whiskey)

WHAT ARE NUTRIENTS?

Humans do not need specific foods for survival; rather, they need the components of food, called nutrients. The earliest organisms, somewhat like present-day bacteria, were able to create all the compounds necessary for survival. As these organisms evolved into more complex biological systems, they developed specialized cells, tissues, and organs. In terms of energy, it became inefficient for them to make all the necessary nutrients from scratch; instead, they lost the ability to synthesize many compounds abundant in the environment and became dependent on outside sources.

A human is one of the most highly organized and complex systems. Although the body can synthesize many vital compounds, others must be obtained from the diet. Dependable supplies of raw materials are needed for building tissues, and to provide energy for growth, maintenance, and work, as well as regulators for different biochemical reactions. Nutrients are the chemical components in food that perform these functions.

Essential nutrients (of which there are at least 45, possibly 50) are those humans must get from the diet. Either the body cannot synthesize them at all, or it cannot do so in sufficient amounts to support health. Each species has its own needs for particular nutrients. Most animals and plants, for instance, can make vitamin C. A few species, including humans, monkeys, guinea pigs, and the Indian fruit bat, must rely on food for this nutrient. Certain microorganisms are

| TABLE 2–1   Essential Nutrients |

Carbohydrates

Glucose*

Fats

Linoleic acid

Proteins

Amino acids:	Leucine	Valine
	Isoleucine	Threonine
	Lysine	Tryptophan
	Methionine	Histidine (for infants only)
	Phenylalanine	

Nonessential nitrogen

Vitamins

Fat-soluble:

A
D
E
K†

Water-soluble:

	Thiamin (B-1)	Pyridoxine (B-6)
	Riboflavin (B-2)	Cobalamin (B-12)
	Niacin	Pantothenic acid
	Biotin†	Ascorbic acid (C)
	Folacin	

Minerals

	Calcium	Copper
	Phosphorus	Cobalt
	Sodium	Molybdenum
	Potassium	Iodine
	Sulfur	Chromium
	Chlorine	Fluorine
	Magnesium	Vanadium
	Iron	Tin
	Selenium	Nickel
	Zinc	Silicon
	Manganese	

Water

*Can be synthesized by body but not in sufficient amounts.
†Can be synthesized by bacteria in the human digestive tract.

the only ones that can synthesize vitamin B-12. Table 2–1 shows the nutrients essential to humans based on current knowledge.

These nutrients are grouped into six general classes: carbohydrates, fats, proteins, vitamins, minerals, and water (see Table 2–2). Any substance that contains the element carbon is said to be organic. Except for water and minerals, all the classes contain the elements carbon, oxygen, and hydrogen. Protein also contains nitrogen. The arrangement of these elements determines the structure

TABLE 2–2 **The Classes of Nutrients and Their Component Elements**

Carbohydrates	Fats	Proteins*	Vitamins†	Water	Minerals
Carbon Hydrogen Oxygen	Carbon Hydrogen Oxygen	Carbon Hydrogen Oxygen Nitrogen	Carbon Hydrogen Oxygen	Hydrogen Oxygen	Each mineral is a distinct element (iron, zinc, calcium), not a combination of elements

*Some amino acids contain sulfur.
†Some vitamins contain sulfur, nitrogen, and cobalt.

of each nutrient. This arrangement, whether single threads, coils, branches, or loops, also influences the nutrient's characteristics.

Essential nutrients in each of the six classes play critical roles in overall health. Those needed in relatively large amounts (grams) are the macronutrients: carbohydrates, fats, proteins, and water. Nutrients required in smaller quantities (milligrams and micrograms) are called micronutrients and include the vitamins and minerals.

The differences in requirements between the macronutrients and the micronutrients are phenomenal. For adults, the recommended daily intake of protein is about 50 grams, while that of the trace mineral chromium is 200 micrograms. The protein recommendation is thus 25,000 times as large as that for chromium. Despite these vast differences micronutrients are just as important to health as macronutrients; long-term deficiencies of either will lead to severe abnormalities and, in many cases, death.

Energy and nutrients are not the same but sometimes they are erroneously thought of as the same. Several of the nutrients provide energy to fuel body functions but the nutrient must be broken down and the energy released before this can occur. In nutrition, energy is measured in units called kilocalories (kcals). Calories is the term more commonly used, but kilocalories is technically correct.

Each nutrient is dependent on the others for its functioning. For instance, in order for the body to break down carbohydrates into useful energy, it needs the vitamins thiamin, niacin, and riboflavin. Without certain amino acids available at the same time, none can be used to build new tissues. And without adequate protein, the intestine eventually loses its ability to absorb many of the other nutrients. Here we will examine the functions of each nutrient class separately, for each has its own idiosyncracies and behaviors. But keep in mind that none functions independently of the others. A summary of the nutrient classes and their main functions is presented in Table 2–3.

Carbohydrates

Carbohydrates are the body's main source of energy. Once broken down, they fuel both the mechanical work of movement (yawning, smiling, dancing) and the chemical work of biological reactions (changing amino acids to muscle protein).

TABLE 2–3 **The Nutrient Classes and Their Functions**

Nutrient Class	Functions
Carbohydrates	Energy (primary source)
Fats	Energy (concentrated) Supply essential fatty acids Carry fat-soluble vitamins
Proteins	Raw material for body tissues and compounds (enzymes, hormones, antibodies) Energy (secondary source)
Vitamins	Regulate body processes
Minerals	Regulate body processes Part of body tissues and compounds
Water	Hydration Aqueous environment for cells Regulates body temperature

Depending on level of physical activity, an individual may not need all the energy provided by the carbohydrate in the diet. A limited amount can be stored in the form of glycogen in the liver and in muscle. Since glycogen contains a lot of water, it is too bulky to be stored in any great quantity. During periods of food shortage glycogen can be converted to energy, but the supply is exhausted within 24 hours. If the individual eats more carbohydrate than needed for energy or glycogen storage, the excess is converted into fat.

Fat (Lipids)

Fats are also a major source of energy for the body, but they provide it in a more compressed form. Because of its chemical structure, fat can break down to release more than twice the energy per gram than carbohydrate. (This is why you should avoid a high fat diet when you want to lose weight.) Because they concentrate energy, fats are more efficient and compact storage units than carbohydrates. If the body stored an equivalent energy reserve of carbohydrate as glycogen, the person would gain about 130 pounds. This would be like backpacking with a grocery sack of beef, peas, carrots, and potatoes, rather than carrying a 6-ounce package of dehydrated beef stew.

Fats also supply essential fatty acids, the smaller units that make up most common fats. Essential fatty acids are precursors of hormonelike substances called prostaglandins, which are involved in controlling blood pressure and stimulating muscle contractions. Fats are also the vehicles for fat-soluble vitamins (A,D,E,K); these vitamins are carried within the fatty portions of food. In addition, fats are part of body tissues. They form a sheath around nerves and, when combined with protein, form many cell subunits, such as the cell membrane.

Protein

The primary function of protein is to provide the raw materials for building body tissues, antibodies, enzymes, and many of the hormones. Providing energy is not protein's main function, as it is with carbohydrates and fats.

Almost half the dry weight of the animal cell is protein. When bound to fat (a combination called a lipoprotein), proteins form many cellular structures (Figure 2–1). Proteins are composed of smaller units called amino acids. The kinds and arrangements of amino acids determine the protein's function—whether it will be part of the fingerlike projections lining the intestine, a milk-digesting enzyme, or an antibody destined to attack foreign substances.

Proteins are not stored in the sense that there are idle pockets floating around waiting to be put to work. All proteins in the body are actively engaged in maintaining the structure and function of tissue. If a person consumes more protein than required, it will be converted into carbohydrates and fats and shunted into the overall energy pool of the body. Proteins, however, are inefficiently converted into energy because the body cannot break down the nitrogen-containing portion. Instead, the nitrogen is converted into waste products, mainly urea and ammonia, to be excreted in urine. The maximum amount of usable energy contained in fats and carbohydrates is about 38 to 40 percent; the energy available from proteins is somewhat less—32 to 34 percent. The energy that is not usable or converted into waste is given off as heat.

The rationale for many high-protein reducing diets is that the inefficiency in converting proteins to energy results in a greater amount of energy

FIG. 2–1

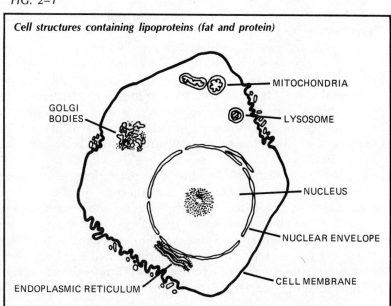

Cell structures containing lipoproteins (fat and protein)

GOLGI BODIES

MITOCHONDRIA

LYSOSOME

NUCLEUS

NUCLEAR ENVELOPE

CELL MEMBRANE

ENDOPLASMIC RETICULUM

wasted or "lost." Some people claim this is why proteins are "difficult to digest." In fact, they are just less efficiently converted into usable energy, making them very expensive sources of fuel. The body is fully equipped to digest protein and does not have difficulty doing so. Furthermore, the reduced efficiency does not help in losing weight. When carbohydrates are in short supply, as in carbohydrate-restricted diets, proteins are diverted from their primary function of providing raw materials for tissues to one of supplying energy. This can result in tissue breakdown and muscle wasting, and people on these diets often experience hair loss and sagging muscles.

Because they can be broken down to supply energy, carbohydrates, fats, and protein are called the fuel nutrients. This function, however, is usually reserved for carbohydrates and fats with proteins spared for tissue synthesis.

Vitamins and Minerals

All chemical reactions in the body require enzymes. An enzyme is a substance that can shorten the time of a reaction from weeks or months to seconds. (It would be difficult to survive if every time you consumed a meal it took three months before your cells came in contact with the nutrients.) Each enzyme is responsible for a specific reaction. In the following reaction:

$$A + B \xrightarrow[\text{enzyme X}]{} C + D$$

enzyme X speeds up the process of combining substrates A and B to form products C and D. The enzyme is not part of the reacting substances and will emerge from the reaction in the same form as it entered, whereas A and B will be transformed into C and D.

The enzyme is composed of protein but may require the addition of a vitamin and/or mineral to serve as a cofactor, or helper, before it can function properly. Vitamins and minerals, acting as cofactors, help biochemical reactions in several ways: They can keep the enzyme in its active form, or they can bind the enzyme to the reacting substances, a vital step before the reaction can proceed. As cofactors, they participate indirectly in the reaction. But like the enzyme, they are not part of the substrates or products and will not be changed by the reaction.

Neither vitamins nor minerals supply energy. But if they are deficient in the diet, the body will not have the cofactors necessary to convert carbohydrates, fats, and proteins into energy. On the other hand, popping vitamin and mineral pills will do nothing for the energy level if the fuel nutrients are not available for the breakdown process. Minerals have another function in addition to serving as cofactors: They can be incorporated into body tissues and become part of many important body compounds. Thus 99 percent of the body's calcium is in bones and teeth; 60 to 70 percent of the iron is in hemoglobin, the oxygen-carrying molecule that gives blood its red color; and iodine is an essential part of the thyroid gland. Minerals can also be part of other nutrients. Vitamin B-12 contains cobalt, and the vitamins thiamin and biotin both have sulfur in their chemical formulas. The ability of minerals to become components of tissues sets them apart from vitamins, which act mainly as cofactors.

Water

Water, often forgotten as a nutrient, comprises about 60 percent of the body by weight for men and 54 percent for women. The difference results from varying amounts of muscle and fat tissue. Men usually have greater muscle mass (high in water content) and less body fat (low in water content) than women.

Water has a number of functions in the body: It is necessary for general hydration, since it is part of the blood and lymph that transport nutrients to the cells and carry the waste products to the kidneys, lungs, and skin for excretion. Blood is about 80 percent water, urine about 97 percent. Water also comprises the intracellular fluid (fluid within the cells) and the extracellular fluid (fluid outside the cells), acts as a lubricant, and provides the body tissue with a medium well-suited for chemical processes. In addition, without water you would be hard pressed to keep your body temperature within a survivable range, because evaporation from the skin is the primary means for ridding the body of heat.

DIGESTION

Before nutrients can perform their functions, they must be released from food and absorbed into the blood for distribution to body cells. The process of breaking down food and releasing nutrients in a form suitable for absorption is called digestion.

The digestive tract (or gastrointestinal tract) is like a tube passing through the body. Food enters through the upper opening, the mouth, passes down the esophagus to the stomach, moves from the stomach through the small intestine, continues through the large intestine, with the final unabsorbed residue exiting through the anus. As it proceeds through the digestive tract, food is churned, mixed, and chemically broken down so nutrients can be released.

When you put food in your mouth, the mechanical action of chewing begins the breakdown. As it is broken into smaller particles, the food mixes with saliva, yielding a consistency that can be swallowed. In the stomach another type of mechanical action, peristalsis, occurs. The muscles in the stomach wall contract, kneading and churning the food. Peristalsis mixes the food with stomach secretions, forming chyme. It also moves the chyme through the stomach into the small intestine where peristalsis, along with another type of mechanical action, rhythmic segmentation, mix the chyme with intestinal secretions and propel it slowly through the small intestine.

The major chemical reactions that occur during digestion involve hydrolysis (hydro means "water" and lysis means "to split"). During this process a molecule is split and two or more new ones are formed. At the same time water molecules are also split and used in forming the new molecules. For most of the hydrolytic reactions of digestion to occur, enzymes are needed. The secretions of the digestive tract contain specific enzymes necessary for breaking apart carbohydrates, fats, and proteins. Saliva, secreted into the mouth and the juices secreted into the stomach, contain digestive enzymes. When the chyme enters the small intestine, the body sends messages to the gall bladder to release a substance called bile, which is necessary for fat digestion and absorption. It also notifies the pancreas to secrete enzymes to help break down any large molecules that are still present.

Most of the end products of digestion are absorbed in the small intestine. Extending from its walls are numerous small fingerlike projections called villi. Even smaller projections called microvilli cover the villi. The overall effect is to provide an enormous surface area within the small intestine for the absorption of nutrients (Figure 2–2).

The undigested residue of food passes into the large intestine (or colon), where the absorption of water and the action of microorganisms reduce it to feces. Contraction of the strong muscles in the wall of the large intestine expel the feces out of the body through the anus (Figure 2–3). Digestion and absorption of specific nutrients will be discussed in each nutrient chapter.

FACTORS AFFECTING NUTRIENT REQUIREMENTS

Body composition stays relatively constant over time, so your body is basically the same as it was a year ago (granted, you may have lost 50 pounds and be an exception). Your physical structure still contains protein, fat, and iron; yet these molecules are different from the ones you had last year. Picture a relay race where each participant runs a given distance and then hands off a baton to the next teammate. Although the team continues to compete as a group, the runners change. Cells, like these teams, continually replace their individual parts with new materials. To do this, they require constant nourishment.

Also, each type of cell has its own life span. Cells that must adjust to constantly changing circumstances tend to have short life spans. The cells lining the stomach and intestines, for instance, which must constantly adapt to different food intakes, die and are replaced every three days. Because of the constant turnover of nutrients within cells and the need for replacement of worn-out cells, humans must routinely eat. But the body can store nutrients and energy, so we can rely on meals instead of eating every minute of the day.

Certain nutrients are needed in larger amounts than others. Besides these differences, certain persons, depending on sex and genetic makeup, have

FIG. 2–2

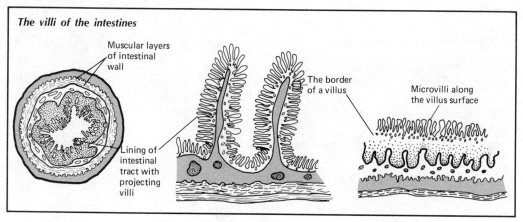

The villi of the intestines

Muscular layers of intestinal wall

Lining of intestinal tract with projecting villi

The border of a villus

Microvilli along the villus surface

a higher requirement for specific nutrients than others. Although humans need the same nutrients throughout life, the amounts change according to age, body size, physiological state, physical activity, state of health, and environment.

Infants and children demand a greater amount of nutrients and energy per unit of body weight than adults because of their rapid growth. Since muscle tissue requires more energy to function than fat, men generally have higher energy needs than women. Women, however, have higher iron needs due to

FIG. 2–3

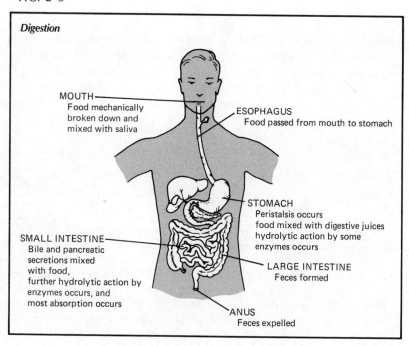

Digestion

MOUTH
Food mechanically broken down and mixed with saliva

ESOPHAGUS
Food passed from mouth to stomach

STOMACH
Peristalsis occurs
food mixed with digestive juices
hydrolytic action by some enzymes occurs

SMALL INTESTINE
Bile and pancreatic secretions mixed with food, further hydrolytic action by enzymes occurs, and most absorption occurs

LARGE INTESTINE
Feces formed

ANUS
Feces expelled

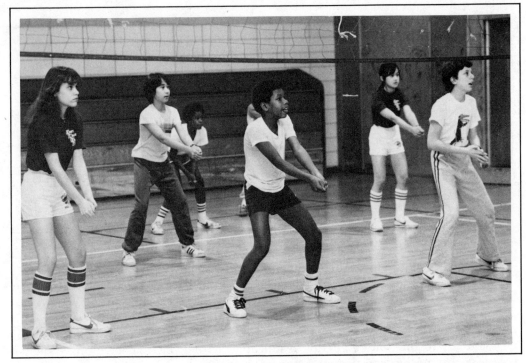

Children require greater amounts of nutrients than adults in order to meet the demands of both growth and physical activity.

the amount lost in the blood during menstruation. Pregnancy and lactation raise women's energy needs, as well as their needs for protein and most vitamins and minerals. Poor health increases the need for nutrients; during convalescence, the need is equivalent to that of a growth period. Finally, genetic makeup affects ability to use nutrients. Some people's bodies are more efficient than those of others. So no matter how many factors are held constant (age, sex, body size), no two persons require the same amount of each nutrient.

SUMMARY

Humans require food to live. More precisely, they require nutrients, the chemical components of food. The essential nutrients are those needed in the diet. Six classes of nutrients exist: carbohydrates, fats, protein, water, vitamins, and minerals. The first four are macronutrients because they are needed in relatively large amounts (grams); the last two are micronutrients because they are required in only microgram or milligram amounts. Foods differ in the kinds and amounts of nutrients they contain, although most foods supply representatives from a number of nutrient classes.

With the exception of water and minerals, each of the nutrient classes contains carbon, hydrogen, and oxygen. In addition, proteins contain nitrogen. The arrangement of these elements determines the structure and function of each nutrient. Carbohydrates and fats provide energy to the body; proteins mainly furnish the raw materials for tissue synthesis; vitamins and minerals regulate biochemical reactions; minerals also become part of body compounds; and water hydrates as well as provides a suitable environment for the cells.

Digestion is the process that breaks down food and releases the nutrients in a form that can be absorbed into the blood. The digestive tract includes the mouth, esophagus, stomach, small intestine, and large intestine.

Although the functions of each nutrient determine in part the quantity needed by the body, other factors, including age, sex, physiological state, illness, and genetic makeup also affect each individual's nutritional needs.

Issue

Nutrient Requirements

Michael Barnett is an aggressive, competitive prelaw student who tackles 20 credits each semester, works part time as a bartender (usually returning home at 3 in the morning), and is pushing hard to attain a position in the student government. At one point during his junior year he tired easily, his skin became sallow, and he got increasingly short-tempered. Instead of reducing his workload, Michael decided he suffered from malnutrition. Not knowing much about nutrition, he bought a book that not only explained the subject, but offered to evaluate the reader's nutritional status.

The instructions directed Michael to fill out a 52-item questionnaire that asked for height, weight, and medical history; dietary, smoking, and drinking habits; and level of work-related stress. He was to complete the questionnaire and send it along with $50 to the address given. His answers would be fed into a computer. A detailed analysis of his nutritional status and dietary deficiencies would then be sent to him.

Michael sent in the form and five weeks later found out he was deficient in B-vitamins and iron. After purchasing these supplements, he was greatly relieved to think his problems were now over.

If Michael had known how nutrient requirements are determined, he would probably have saved his $50 for a spring vacation. He would realize that no one can determine precise requirements by a questionnaire. To do so assumes that everyone has the same physiological needs. (Think of the people you know who bounce out of bed after three hours of sleep versus those who can't speak without a minimum of eight.) The only way you can come close to knowing your particular needs is to undergo expensive physical and biochemical testing that requires samples of blood, urine, and sometimes hair.

The so-called experts who evaluated Michael's diet probably calculated his nutrient intake by using a table of food composition and comparing that to the RDA for Michael's age-sex group. This approach is fine if all Michael wanted was a gross evaluation of his diet. It could not be the basis for diagnosing him as deficient in vitamins and iron.

Assume, however, that Michael decided to consult a doctor whose clinical and biochemical tests showed Michael to have marginal levels of iron and some B-vitamins. Are vitamin and mineral pills the best way to correct the problem? With only a few exceptions, nutrient requirements are easily met with a varied diet of ordinary foods. This is the safest and by far the most enjoyable way to meet nutrient needs. A poor diet supplemented with a vitamin-mineral pill can still fail to provide adequate amounts of nutrients, since supplements do not contain every nutrient (for further discussion of supplements, see Chapter 7). Assuming Michael did not have other intervening medical problems, he would be wise to take a few nutrition lessons rather than a vitamin-mineral pill.

DETERMINING REQUIREMENTS: THE RDA

Although there are no formulas to calculate exact requirements, there are ways to evaluate a diet based on a group of recommendations called the Recommended Daily Allowances (RDA). In the United States the Food and Nutrition Board (FNB) of the National Research Council, National Academy of Sciences, has the task of establishing nutrient requirements for the population. The board, composed of nutrition experts from universities, medical centers, and government, reviews data from nutrition research, conducted worldwide, prior to each revision. Members seek advice and counsel from nutritionists not involved in the revision process. The procedure takes three to four years, after which the board derives a standard called the RDA.

A *requirement* is the amount of a nutrient that must be consumed daily to avoid a deficiency. An *allowance* (like the RDA) provides a generous surplus to allow for differences in individual requirements so that practically everyone's needs are covered. The first RDA was developed in 1941; the most current revision was published in February 1980.(1)

The first step in setting the RDA is to estimate the average requirement for each nutrient to be included. Few data exist on certain nutrients like chromium and selenium, so they are not included in the RDA.

In addition, many factors (age, sex, body size) influence nutrient requirements. Two 20-year-old male roommates with the same weight and exercise patterns have different nutrient needs because their genetic backgrounds are different. A group of 20-year-old males, though, has closer requirements than a group of males and females ranging in age from 5 to 50 years. So it is possible to predict the average requirements for a group of people with similar characteristics.

The FNB uses data from different sources to estimate an amount of each nutrient which, in its best judgment, represents the average requirements of a particular age-sex group. After determining this amount, it decides how much individuals vary from the average and increases the average by an amount that covers the needs of practically all (97 to 98 percent) of the subjects studied. This becomes the recommended daily allowance for that nutrient for that particular age-sex group (Figure 2–4).

The allowances are set high enough to cover wide variations in individual requirements and differences in the way people digest and absorb nutrients. The levels prevent deficiency symptoms and provide adequate blood and tissue levels of the nutrients. They are not intended as optimal levels for every person. The board stresses two points about the RDA. First, they cover the requirements of practically all healthy people, but not those who are ill or have

FIG. 2–4

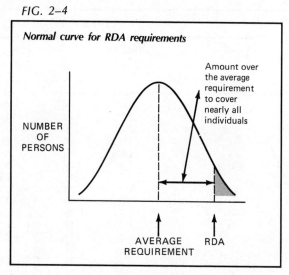

Source: Report by Comptroller General, CED-78-169, November 30, 1978.

special needs, such as the premature baby. Second, RDA should be met by eating a wide variety of foods and not by a pill, tonic, or single food fortified with nutrients. Since not all nutrients have RDA, a pill or fortified food that meets the allowances is still likely to be missing some essential nutrients. Meeting the RDA through pills and fortified foods may mean that fiber intake is

TABLE 2–4 **Recommended Daily Dietary Allowances, (Revised 1980)[a]**

	Age	Weight		Height		Protein	Fat-Soluble Vitamins		
							Vita-min A	Vita-min D	Vita-min E
	(years)	(kg)	(lb)	(cm)	(in)	(g)	(μg RE)[b]	(μg)[c]	(μg α-TE)[d]
Infants	0.0–0.5	6	13	60	24	kg × 2.2	420	10	3
	0.5–1.0	9	20	71	28	kg × 2.0	400	10	4
Children	1–3	13	29	90	35	23	400	10	5
	4–6	20	44	112	44	30	500	10	6
	7–10	28	62	132	52	34	700	10	7
Males	11–14	45	99	157	62	45	1000	10	8
	15–18	66	145	176	69	56	1000	10	10
	19–22	70	154	177	70	56	1000	7.5	10
	23–50	70	154	178	70	56	1000	5	10
	51+	70	154	178	70	56	1000	5	10
Females	11–14	46	101	157	62	46	800	10	8
	15–18	55	120	163	64	46	800	10	8
	19–22	55	120	163	64	44	800	7.5	8
	23–50	55	120	163	64	44	800	5	8
	51+	55	120	163	64	44	800	5	8
Pregnant						+30	+200	+5	+2
Lactating						+20	+400	+5	+3

	Water-Soluble Vitamins						
	Vita-min C (mg)	Thia-min (mg)	Ribo-flavin (mg)	Niacin (mg NE)[e]	Vita-min B-6 (mg)	Fola-cin (μg)	Vitamin B-12 (μg)
Infants	35	0.3	0.4	6	0.3	30	0.5
	35	0.5	0.6	8	0.6	45	1.5
Children	45	0.7	0.8	9	0.9	100	2.0
	45	0.9	1.0	11	1.3	200	2.5
	45	1.2	1.4	16	1.6	300	3.0
Males	50	1.4	1.6	18	1.8	400	3.0
	60	1.4	1.7	18	2.0	400	3.0
	60	1.5	1.7	19	2.2	400	3.0
	60	1.4	1.6	18	2.2	400	3.0
	60	1.2	1.4	16	2.2	400	3.0
Females	50	1.1	1.3	15	1.8	400	3.0
	60	1.1	1.3	14	2.0	400	3.0
	60	1.1	1.3	14	2.0	400	3.0
	60	1.0	1.2	13	2.0	400	3.0
	60	1.0	1.2	13	2.0	400	3.0
Pregnant	+20	+0.4	+0.3	+2	+0.6	+400	+1.0
Lactating	+40	+0.5	+0.5	+5	+0.5	+100	+1.0

TABLE 2–4   *Continued*

	Minerals					
	Cal-cium (mg)	Phos-phorus (mg)	Mag-nesium (mg)	Iron (mg)	Zinc (mg)	Iodine (µg)
Infants	360	240	50	10	3	40
	540	360	70	15	5	50
Children	800	800	150	15	10	70
	800	800	200	10	10	90
	800	800	250	10	10	120
Males	1200	1200	350	18	15	150
	1200	1200	400	18	15	150
	800	800	350	10	15	150
	800	800	350	10	15	150
Females	800	800	350	10	15	150
	1200	1200	300	18	15	150
	1200	1200	300	18	15	150
	800	800	300	18	15	150
	800	800	300	18	15	150
	800	800	300	10	15	150
Pregnant	+400	+400	+150	f	+5	+25
Lactating	+400	+400	+150	f	+10	+50

[a] The allowances are intended to provide for individual variations among most normal persons as they live in the United States under usual environmental stresses. Diets should be based on a variety of common foods in order to provide other nutrients for which human requirements have been less well defined.

[b] Retinol equivalents, 1 retinol equivalent = 1 µg retinol or 6 µg β carotene. Calculation of vitamin A activity of diets as retinol equivalents.

[c] As cholecalciferol 10 µg cholecalciferol = 400 IU of vitamin D.

[d] α-tocopherol equivalents. 1 mg *d*-α tocopherol = 1 α-TE, and calculation of vitamin E activity of the diet as α-tocopherol equivalents.

[e] 1 NE (niacin equivalent) is equal to 1 mg of niacin or 60 mg of dietary tryptophan.

[f] The increased requirement during pregnancy cannot be met by the iron content of habitual American diets nor by the existing iron stores of many women; therefore the use of 30–60 mg of supplemental iron is recommended. Iron needs during lactation are not substantially different from those of nonpregnant women, but continued supplementation of the mother for 2–3 months after parturition is advisable in order to replenish stores depleted by pregnancy.

Source: Recommended Dietary Allowances, Revised 1980, Food and Nutrition Board, National Academy of Sciences, National Research Council, Washington D.C..

too low. Fiber, though not a nutrient, helps regulate the movement of food through the intestinal tract and is part of good nutrition.

The 1980 Revision of the RDA

The latest revision of the RDA is shown in Table 2–4. Notice it does not list energy (kcalories) and several of the essential nutrients. In the case of energy, it is not wise to recommend an intake exceeding the requirements of most people, because many would then become obese. Instead, the board sets the energy recommendation at a level that meets the average needs of individuals in each age-sex group (Table 2–5). Since these values represent

Category	Age (years)	Weight (kg)	Weight (lb)	Height (cm)	Height (in.)	Energy Needs (with range) (kcal)[b]	
Infants	0.0–0.5	6	13	60	24	kg × 115	(95–145)
	0.5–1.0	9	20	71	28	kg × 105	(80–135)
Children	1–3	13	29	90	35	1300	(900–1800)
	4–6	20	44	112	44	1700	(1300–2300)
	7–10	28	62	132	52	2400	(1650–3300)
Males	11–14	45	99	157	62	2700	(2000–3700)
	15–18	66	145	176	69	2800	(2100–3900)
	19–22	70	154	177	70	2900	(2500–3300)
	23–50	70	154	178	70	2700	(2300–3100)
	51–75	70	154	178	70	2400	(2000–2800)
	76+	70	154	178	70	2050	(1650–2450)
Females	11–14	46	101	157	62	2200	(1500–3000)
	15–18	55	120	163	64	2100	(1200–3000)
	19–22	55	120	163	64	2100	(1700–2500)
	23–50	55	120	163	64	2000	(1600–2400)
	51–75	55	120	163	64	1800	(1400–2200)
	76+	55	120	163	64	1600	(1200–2000)
Pregnancy						+300	
Lactation						+500	

[a]The data in this table have been assembled from observed median heights and weights of children, together with desirable weights for adults for the mean heights of men (70 in.) and women (64 in.) between the ages of 18 and 34 years as surveyed in the U.S. population (HEW/NCHS data).

  The energy allowances for the young adults are for men and women doing light work. The allowances for the two older age groups represent mean energy needs over these age spans, allowing for a 2-percent decrease in basal (resting) metabolic rate per decade and a reduction in activity of 200 kcal/day for men and women between 51 and 75 years, 500 kcal for men over 75 years, and 400 kcal for women over 75 years. The customary range of daily energy output is shown in parentheses for adults.

  Energy allowances for children through age 18 are based on median energy intakes of children of these ages followed in longitudinal growth studies. The values in parentheses are 10th and 90th percentiles of energy intake, to indicate the range of energy consumption among children of these ages.

[b]Kcal stands for kilocalorie, a unit of measurement for energy. Calorie is the term more commonly used but kilocalorie is technically correct.

Source: Recommended Dietary Allowances, Revised 1980, Food and Nutrition Board, National Academy of Sciences, National Research Council, Washington, D.C.

average needs and are too high or low for many people, they should only be used as guides for *groups.* Individuals must gauge their own energy intake to meet their own needs. Energy intakes of children should be sufficient to allow for the weight gain required for growth but not for excessive fat accumulation. Adults should maintain ideal weight.

    The FNB currently has enough data to make recommendations for only 17 nutrients. The 1980 revision, however, includes a list of "estimated safe and adequate intakes" for 3 additional vitamins and 9 additional minerals. These appear as ranges of intakes (Table 2–6) because too little data exist for setting one level. When more data become available, the board will establish the RDA for these vitamins and minerals.

    How to Use the RDA. You should not use the RDA for precisely judging the adequacy of an individual diet. You can compare your nutrient intake to the RDA, but be sensible when interpreting the results. An intake less

TABLE 2-6   Estimated Safe and Adequate Daily Dietary Intakes of Selected Vitamins and Minerals

Vitamins

	Age (years)	Vitamin K (µg)	Biotin (µg)	Pantothenic Acid (mg)
Infants	0–0.5	12	35	2
	0.5–1	10–20	50	3
Children	1–3	15–30	65	3
and	4–6	20–40	85	3–4
Adolescents	7–10	30–60	120	4–5
	11+	50–100	100–200	4–7
Adults		70–140	100–200	4–7

Trace Elements*

	Age (years)	Copper (mg)	Manganese (mg)	Fluoride (mg)	Chromium (mg)	Selenium (mg)	Molybdenum (mg)
Infants	0–0.5	0.5–0.7	0.5–0.7	0.1–0.5	0.01–0.04	0.01–0.04	0.03–0.06
	0.5–1	0.7–1.0	0.7–1.0	0.2–1.0	0.02–0.06	0.02–0.06	0.04–0.08
Children	1–3	1.0–1.5	1.0–1.5	0.5–1.5	0.02–0.08	0.02–0.08	0.05–0.1
and	4–6	1.5–2.0	1.5–2.0	1.0–2.5	0.03–0.12	0.03–0.12	0.06–0.15
Adolescents	7–10	2.0–2.5	2.0–3.0	1.5–2.5	0.05–0.2	0.05–0.2	0.10–0.3
	11+	2.0–3.0	2.5–5.0	1.5–2.5	0.05–0.2	0.05–0.2	0.15–0.5
Adults		2.0–3.0	2.5–5.0	1.5–4.0	0.05–0.2	0.05–0.2	0.15–0.5

Electrolytes

	Age (years)	Sodium (mg)	Potassium (mg)	Chloride (mg)
Infants	0–0.5	115–350	350–925	275–700
	0.5–1	250–750	425–1275	400–1200
Children	1–3	325–975	550–1650	500–1500
and	4–6	450–1350	775–2325	700–2100
Adolescents	7–10	600–1800	1000–3000	925–2775
	11+	900–2700	1525–4575	1400–4200
Adults		1100–3300	1875–5625	1700–5100

*Since the toxic levels for many trace elements may be only several times usual intakes, the upper levels for the trace elements given in this table should not be habitually exceeded.

Source: Recommended Dietary Allowances, Revised 1980, Food and Nutrition Board, National Academy of Sciences, National Research Council, Washington, D.C.

than the RDA does not mean your diet is deficient, since it is unlikely that you are one of the few people with nutrient requirements as high as the RDA level. In fact, a percentage of the RDA, 66 to 77 percent, is a better standard against which to compare your intake. For instance, if you are a 17-year-old female, your RDA for calcium is 1200 milligrams. If your diet provides at least 75 percent of this, or 900 milligrams, you are probably getting enough. On the other hand, if your intake meets or exceeds the RDA, you can be almost 100 percent certain it is adequate. Be careful if you are ingesting nutrients in amounts that greatly exceed the RDA, because you could be doing yourself harm (see Chapter 7).

GUIDELINES FOR PLANNING FOOD INTAKE

Although the RDA serve as an essential tool for nutritionists and other professionals, most people find them too awkward to use in planning meals and evaluating diets. Your alternative is to look at food, not nutrients. By balancing and varying food choices, you can meet the RDA without counting nutrients. There are several guides designed to help individuals plan meals. The best known is the Essentials of an Adequate Diet.

Essentials of an Adequate Diet

Developed in the 1950s by the USDA,(3) this guide is commonly called the *Basic Four Food Groups* or just the *Basic Four* because it places food with similar nutrient composition into four groups: meat and meat substitutes, milk and milk products, fruits and vegetables, and breads and cereals (Table 2–7). These groups were originally intended to provide 10 nutrients: protein; carbohydrates; fat; the vitamins niacin, thiamin, riboflavin, A, and C; and the minerals iron and calcium. These 10 are called "leader" nutrients because supposedly if an individual eats the right foods to obtain them, the remaining nutrients automatically "follow."

Though the Basic Four system is easier to use than the RDA, it still has problems. In fact, many critics say it is so simple it is misleading. Obtaining the "leader" nutrients, they argue, does not guarantee that the person will obtain adequate intakes of other nutrients. Food processors and refiners remove many nutrients and do not add all of them back. Whole wheat flour, for instance, has much higher amounts of the trace mineral chromium than does white flour. Although processors add back to the white flour some of the vitamins and minerals removed from the whole grain, chromium is not one of them.

Foods in the same group have different nutritive value, so a person could consistently make poor food choices from any one group. There is also a problem with some fabricated foods that do not fit into any of the groups because the foods they physically resemble contain different nutrients than those added to the fabricated product. For example, breakfast bars resembling cake or candy often contain vitamins not ordinarily found in cake or candy. Combinations like pizza or enchiladas have a hard time finding a home in any of the four groups since they are assembled from foods belonging to each group.

If you follow an alternative eating pattern such as vegetarianism, you may not be able to use this guide. Although the meat group includes beans, peas, and nuts, the strict vegetarian who eats no animal products has to find

TABLE 2–7 The Basic Four Food Groups

Food Group and Sources	Main Nutrients Contributed	Recommendations for Adults
Meat group: Meat, poultry, fish, eggs, shellfish, legumes (dry peas and beans, peanuts), nuts, soybeans	Niacin, iron, thiamin, protein	Two or more 3-ounce servings daily
Milk group: Whole, low-fat, evaporated, and chocolate milk, buttermilk, nonfat dry milk, cottage cheese, ice cream, yogurt, cheeses	Protein, calcium, riboflavin, vitamin D (if fortified), vitamins A and D (in lowfat skim or nonfat milks)	Two or more servings milk (cup) or cheese (1 ounce) daily
Vegetables-fruits group: All fruits and vegetables, canned, frozen, fresh, dried; all citrus fruits, potatoes	Vitamins A, C, thiamin, riboflavin, niacin, and fiber, iron, calcium, some protein	Four or more half-cup servings daily; dark green leafy vegetables or orange-colored vegetable every other day; citrus fruit or other source rich in vitamin C daily
Bread and cereal group: All whole grain or enriched, fortified breads and cereals, macaroni, white or whole grain flour, spaghetti, noodles, tortillas, grits	Iron, thiamin, niacin, protein	Four or more servings daily

other sources of calcium, protein, and riboflavin to substitute for the milk group. (Chapter 5 provides special food groups for vegetarians.)

The Basic Four does not safeguard against excessive intakes, since even a diet grossly high in fat, sugar, salt, and energy can meet the requirements of the guide. Recently the USDA added a fifth group(4) to the Basic Four, a group that includes fats, sweets, and alcohol (Figure 2–5). It is called the Five Food Groups or the *Daily Food Guide.* What these foods have in common are kcalories with few nutrients. An individual should consume foods from this group only after meeting nutrient needs from the other groups, and providing the person still needs more energy.

The Exchange System

Another method of grouping foods is called the *exchange system.* Originally designed for diabetics, who have to exercise strict control over carbohydrate intake, the exchange system groups foods in lists according to carbohydrate content. Diabetics can exchange one food for another when planning their diets as long as they do not exceed their carbohydrate limit. The newest revision of these exchange lists organizes foods according to carbohy-

FIG. 2–5

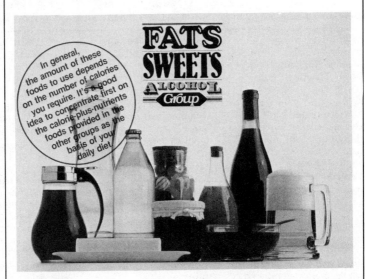

Daily food guide

FATS SWEETS ALCOHOL Group

In general, the amount of these foods to use depends on the number of calories you require. It's a good idea to concentrate first on the calorie-plus-nutrients foods provided in the other groups as the basis of your daily diet.

What's a Serving?

Includes foods like butter, margarine, mayonnaise and other salad dressings, and other fats and oils; candy, sugar, jams, jellies, sirups, sweet toppings, and other sweets; soft drinks and other highly sugared beverages; and alcoholic beverages such as wine, beer, and liquor. Also included are refined but unenriched breads, pastries, and flour products. Some of these foods are used as ingredients in prepared foods or are added to other foods at the table. Others are just "extras."

No serving sizes are defined because a basic number of servings is not suggested for this group.

What's in It for You?

These products, with some exceptions such as vegetable oils, provide mainly calories. Vegetable oils generally supply vitamin E and essential fatty acids.

Fats and oils have more than twice the calories, ounce for ounce, as protein, starches, or sugars, but keep hunger pangs away longer.

Pure alcohol has almost twice the calories per ounce as protein, starches, or sugars. However, few alcoholic beverages are 100 percent alcohol. Generally, the higher the alcohol content, the higher the calories, ounce for ounce.

Unenriched, refined bakery products are included here because, like other foods and beverages in this group, they usually provide relatively low levels of vitamins, minerals, and protein compared with calories.

drate, protein, fat, and energy content.(4) Appendix D provides more complete listings of the exchanges.

Individuals on weight control diets can use these lists by exchanging food on the basis of energy content. Dieters are allowed a certain number of exchanges from each group but can choose the types of foods within each exchange that they enjoy eating. (Sample diets and meal plans for reducing diets are given in Chapter 6.) Exchange lists are valuable for individuals on special diets where one or two factors must be monitored closely, but they are more complex and time-consuming than the Daily Food Guide.

Both the Daily Food Guide and the exchange system explain the amounts of different types of food an individual should eat, but they neglect to say which foods within each group or exchange are better than others. For instance, a slice of whole wheat bread and five ginger snaps are both considered one bread exchange, but are they nutritionally equivalent? Should some foods (or nutrients) be eaten only in moderate amounts or avoided altogether?

In the United States, certain health problems, such as obesity and heart disease, have been linked to overconsumption of nutrients. Many health professionals feel the public needs a guide to help avoid excessive consumption of suspect nutrients like salt and fat. They believe that the incidence of many chronic degenerative diseases could be reduced if the population changed its eating habits. Other groups believe the evidence for the diet-disease link is shaky. They point out that much of the data for this link are taken from epidemiological or population studies. Such studies are useful for predicting disease rates in populations, but not in individuals. If the population of the United States, for instance, consumes a high-fat diet and also has a high rate of heart disease, it does not mean that you, as an individual, will get heart disease if you eat a lot of fats. This group also argues that the chronic degenerative diseases are caused by many factors, not just diet, so changing the diet will not necessarily reduce the incidence of the diseases. Dietary recommendations, then, may create false hopes.

A number of dietary recommendations have been released that show these different attitudes toward the problem of diet and disease. Many of the controversies concerning the impact of diet on disease are discussed in the remaining chapters.

Dietary Goals for the United States. One of the first documents to give specific diet recommendations aimed at reducing the incidence of chronic degenerative disease was the *Dietary Goals for the United States,* prepared by the staff of the Select Committee on Nutrition and Human Needs of the U.S. Senate and published in February 1977. The committee print was later revised and issued as a second edition in December 1977.(5) The revised Dietary Goals are shown in Table 2–8.

TABLE 2–8 **The Dietary Goals**

1. To avoid overweight, consume only as much energy (kcalories) as is expended; if overweight, decrease energy intake and increase energy expenditure.
2. Increase the consumption of complex carbohydrates and "naturally occurring" sugars from about 28 percent of energy intake to about 48 percent of energy intake.
3. Reduce the consumption of refined and processed sugars by about 45 percent to account for about 10 percent of total energy intake.
4. Reduce overall fat consumption from approximately 40 percent to about 30 percent of energy intake.
5. Reduce saturated fat consumption to account for about 10 percent of total energy intake; and balance that with polyunsaturated and monounsaturated fat, which should account for about 10 percent of energy intake each.
6. Reduce cholesterol consumption to about 300 milligrams a day.
7. Limit the intake of sodium by reducing the intake of salt to about 5 grams a day.

Source: Dietary Goals for the United States. 2nd Ed., U.S. Senate Select Committee on Nutrition and Human Needs. (Washington, D.C.: U.S. Government Printing Office, 1977).

TABLE 2–9   **Dietary Guidelines for Americans**

1. *Eat a variety of foods*
   Include selections from:
      Fruits.
      Vegetables.
      Whole grain and enriched breads, cereals, and grain products.
      Milk, cheese, and yogurt.
      Meats, poultry, fish, eggs.
      Legumes (dry peas and beans).

2. *Maintain ideal weight*
   To improve eating habits:
      Eat slowly.
      Prepare smaller portions.
      Avoid "seconds."
   To lose weight:
      Increase physical activity.
      Eat less fat and fatty foods.
      Eat less sugar and sweets.
      Avoid too much alcohol.

3. *Avoid too much fat, saturated fat, and cholesterol*
      Choose lean meat, fish, poultry, dry beans and peas as your protein sources.
      Moderate your use of eggs and organ meats (such as liver).
      Limit your intake of butter, cream, hydrogenated margarines, shortenings, and
         coconut oil, and foods made from such products.

4. *Eat foods with adequate starch and fiber*
      Substitute starches for fat and sugar.
      Select foods which are good sources of fiber and starch, such as whole grain breads
         and cereals, fruits and vegetables, beans, peas, and nuts.

5. *Avoid too much sugar*
      Use less of all sugars, including white sugar, brown sugar, raw sugar, honey and
         syrups.
      Eat less of foods containing these sugars, such as candy, soft drinks, ice cream, cake,
         cookies.
      Select fresh fruits or fruits canned without sugar or light syrup rather than heavy
         syrup.
      Read food labels for clues on sugar content: if the names sucrose, glucose, dextrose,
         lactose, fructose, or syrup appear first, then there is a large amount of sugar.
      Remember, how often you eat sugar is as important as how much sugar you eat.

6. *Avoid too much sodium*
      Learn to enjoy the unsalted flavors of foods.
      Cook with only small amounts of added salt.
      Add little or no salt to food at the table.
      Limit your intake of salty foods, such as potato chips, pretzels, salted nuts and pop-
         corn, condiments (soy sauce, steak sauce, garlic salt), cheese, pickled foods, cured
         meats.
      Read food labels carefully to determine the amounts of sodium in processed foods
         and snack items.

Source: Nutrition and Your Health: Dietary Guidelines for Americans, U.S. Department of Agriculture and U.S. Department of Health, Education & Welfare (Washington, D.C.: U.S. Government Printing Office, 1980).

Critics of the goals said they were premature; that nutritionists did not have enough data to justify such widespread changes in the American diet. Critics also believed that stating nutrient recommendations in terms of percentages and grams was too complex to be useful to consumers. For instance, the report recommends that you limit salt intake to 5 grams per day. But how do you know what 5 grams looks like? How do you know when fats have reached 30 percent of your energy intake?

Dietary Guidelines for Americans. The idea of setting specific recommendations like those of the Dietary Goals was picked up by two federal agencies. The USDA, along with the former U.S. Department of Health, Education, and Welfare (HEW), developed the brochure *Nutrition and Your Health—Dietary Guidelines for Americans,* which was published in 1980.(6) It offers practical advice on ways to choose and prepare nutritious meals by moderating intake of certain nutrients like fats, cholesterol, sugar, and sodium (Table 2–9). It contains general descriptions without percentages.

By using these guidelines with the Daily Food Guide you have more specific directions for diet planning than with either alone. The Daily Food Guide specifies numbers of servings you should eat from each group; the Guidelines point out which foods from each group to emphasize and which to eat in moderate to low amounts.

Toward Healthful Diets. About six months after USDA-HEW published the *Dietary Guidelines for Americans,* the Food and Nutrition Board of the National Research Council published its own dietary recommendations, entitled *Toward Healthful Diets.*(7) Notice that these are similar to the USDA-HEW guidelines in that the board emphasizes eating a variety of foods and adjusting energy intake and expenditure to maintain desirable weight (Table 2–10).

The FNB recommendations place less emphasis on avoiding excesses of such things as fat, sugar, and cholesterol. According to the board, the assumption that dietary change will reduce the occurrence of degenerative diseases such as cancer and heart disease is controversial. The board does not think current scientific evidence justifies recommending major dietary changes for the general population. Individuals with a family history of the degenerative diseases or other factors that place them at high risk of developing these diseases

---

TABLE 2–10 **Dietary Recommendations, *Toward Healthful Diets***

■ Select a nutritionally adequate diet from the foods available by consuming each day appropriate servings of dairy products, meats or legumes, vegetables and fruits, and cereal and breads.

■ Select as wide a variety of foods in each of the major food groups as is practical in order to ensure a high probability of consuming adequate quantities of all essential nutrients.

■ Adjust dietary energy intake and energy expenditure to maintain appropriate weight for height; if overweight, achieve appropriate weight reduction by decreasing total food and fat intake and by increasing physical activity.

■ If the requirement for energy is low (e.g., reducing diet), reduce consumption of foods such as alcohol, sugars, fats, and oils, which provide kcalories but few other essential nutrients.

■ Use salt in moderation; adequate but safe intakes are considered to range between 3 and 9 grams of sodium chloride daily.

Source: Toward Healthful Diets, Food and Nutrition Board (Washington, D.C.: National Research Council, National Academy of Sciences, 1980).

should follow the diet therapy recommended by their physicians. (See Chapter 4 for details on one of the most controversial diseases: atherosclerosis.)

If you follow the Dietary Guidelines, you may want to reduce your intake of sugar, fats, oils, and alcohol. If you follow the recommendations in *Toward Healthful Diets,* you may want to reduce your intake of these items only if you are overweight. Both guides suggest you watch intake of salt.

Judging Nutritional Value

Notice that the guides agree on a diet that is balanced, varied, and moderate. Now, how are you supposed to know when you look at your plate of fried chicken, corn bread, and beans whether it is balanced, varied, and moderate enough? How do you know if you should eat the chicken because it is a good protein source or skip it because it is high in fat since it was fried. How do you know if the cornmeal you used for the bread is enriched? It would help to have some way of judging the nutritional value of the food itself. There are two tools for just that purpose: the U.S. Recommended Daily Allowances and nutrient density.

U.S. Recommended Daily Allowances (U.S. RDA). During the 1960s, people, concerned about the worth of processed foods, demanded food labels to help them determine the nutrient value of the products they purchased. It was not an easy demand to meet. If a company simply printed on the label the amount of each nutrient in a product, most people would have no idea if that amount was low or high compared to other foods or compared to their needs. A standard was needed that would relate the amount of nutrients in a food to the amount recommended for human diets. Why not just print the nutrient amounts in terms of the RDA?

The problem was that the only label large enough to squeeze in the RDA for all age-sex groups would be those the size of a 25-pound bag of dog food. The solution was to develop a less detailed standard, and the job fell to the U.S. Food and Drug Administration (FDA), the federal agency charged with food labeling. After much research and pilot testing, the FDA came up with a nutrient standard specifically for use in labeling called the *U.S. Recommended Daily Allowance (U.S. RDA).*(8)

The FDA began with the RDA and whittled it down to form the U.S. RDA. Instead of an allowance for each age-sex group, there was only one allowance for each nutrient. Since the standard had to cover the needs of most people, the highest RDA (from the 1968 RDA table) for the various age-sex groups (except pregnant and lactating women) became the U.S. RDA. Calcium and phosphorus are exceptions. The U.S. RDA for each of these nutrients is the amount recommended for adult men rather than the much higher amount recommended for adolescent boys. Although there is no RDA for copper and for the vitamins biotin and pantothenic acid, the FDA estimated U.S. RDA levels for

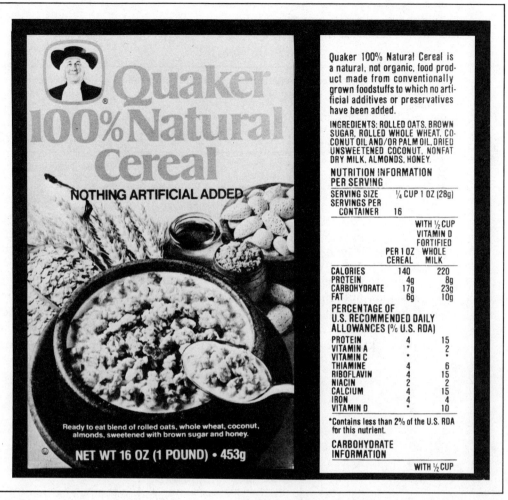

Quaker 100% Natural Cereal is a natural, not organic, food product made from conventionally grown foodstuffs to which no artificial additives or preservatives have been added.

INGREDIENTS: ROLLED OATS, BROWN SUGAR, ROLLED WHOLE WHEAT, COCONUT OIL AND/OR PALM OIL, DRIED UNSWEETENED COCONUT, NONFAT DRY MILK, ALMONDS, HONEY.

NUTRITION INFORMATION PER SERVING

SERVING SIZE ¼ CUP 1 OZ (28g)
SERVINGS PER CONTAINER 16

	PER 1 OZ CEREAL	WITH ½ CUP VITAMIN D FORTIFIED WHOLE MILK
CALORIES	140	220
PROTEIN	4g	8g
CARBOHYDRATE	17g	23g
FAT	6g	10g

PERCENTAGE OF U.S. RECOMMENDED DAILY ALLOWANCES (% U.S. RDA)

PROTEIN	4	15
VITAMIN A	*	2
VITAMIN C	*	*
THIAMINE	4	6
RIBOFLAVIN	4	15
NIACIN	2	2
CALCIUM	4	15
IRON	4	4
VITAMIN D	*	10

*Contains less than 2% of the U.S. RDA for this nutrient.

CARBOHYDRATE INFORMATION

WITH ½ CUP

NOTHING ARTIFICIAL ADDED.

Ready to eat blend of rolled oats, whole wheat, coconut, almonds, sweetened with brown sugar and honey.

NET WT 16 OZ (1 POUND) • 453g

Food labels provide both ingredient and nutrition information. The format is standardized and is only required if a claim is made about the product or if nutrients are added to the product as in fortification or enrichment.

all three. Table 2–11 compares several nutrients in terms of the U.S. RDA and the RDA ranges for the different age-sex categories.

One hundred percent of the U.S. RDA generously meets the RDA for most age-sex groups. For example, 10-year-olds need only 70 percent of the U.S. RDA for vitamin A to obtain their RDA, whereas a 25-year-old woman needs 100 percent to obtain the RDA for her group. The U.S. RDA is not meant to be a rigid prescription for individual nutrient needs.

If you look at food labels, you may notice that a specific format has been established.(8) The container must list the number of servings (by common portions) and specify the grams of carbohydrate, protein, and fat. It must also

TABLE 2–11 **U.S. RDA for Selected Nutrients**

Nutrient	U.S. RDA	Range of RDA
Protein	45 to 65 grams depending on quality of the protein	30 to 56 grams
Vitamin C	60 milligrams	40–60 milligrams
Calcium	1 gram	0.8–1.2 grams
Iron	18 milligrams	10–18 milligrams
Vitamin E	30 milligrams	6–10 milligrams
Zinc	15 milligrams	10–15 milligrams

Source: Adapted from B. Peterkin, J. Nichols and C. Cromwell, *Nutrition Labeling—Tools for Its Use.* Publ. A1B–382, U.S. Department of Agriculture, Washington, D.C., 1975; and from *Recommended Dietary Allowances, Revised 1980,* Food and Nutrition Board, National Academy of Sciences, National Research Council, Washington, D.C.

include the percentage (per serving or portion) of the U.S. RDA for protein, vitamin C, thiamin, niacin, riboflavin, calcium, and iron. If a serving of food contains less than 2 percent of the U.S. RDA, an asterisk (*) must appear next to that particular nutrient. An explanation appears at the bottom of the label. Manufacturers can list additional nutrients if they wish. Special labels for food low in saturated fats and cholesterol appear on certain products. A sample label is shown in Figure 2–6. A serving of this product would contain 2 ounces of dry

FIG. 2–6

Sample food label

LASAGNA
Nutrition Information

Serving size . . . . .2 ounces-dry
Servings per package 8
Calories. 210
Protein . . . . .7 grams
Carbohydrate . . . . .41 grams
Fat . . . . 1 gram

% U.S. RECOMMENDED
DAILY ALLOWANCE

Protein 10
Vitamin A. . . . .*
Vitamin C . . . .*
Thiamin. 35
Riboflavin 15
Niacin 15
Calcium. . . . .*
Iron. .10

*Contains less than 2% U.S. Recommended Daily Allowances of these nutrients.

lasagna. Less than 2 ounces would provide a smaller percentage of the nutrients, while a larger serving would increase these amounts. The label indicates that this product is high in carbohydrate, low in fat, and is a poor source of calcium and vitamins A and C. Manufacturers must label foods only if they make a special nutritional claim about the product such as "high in vitamin C" or when they add nutrients, as in the cases of enriched bread, fortified margarine, or breakfast cereals. In spite of its voluntary nature, many food companies have gone ahead and labeled all their products.

The purpose of labels is to help shoppers compare the nutritive value of foods. For example, you can figure out which baby food provides more nutrients per serving or which cereal has the most iron. Labeling can allow you to take a critical look at the foods you normally purchase. But nutritionists have several concerns about the use of the U.S. RDA on labels. Consumers can develop a false sense of security and believe that by eating a serving of a food that contains 100 percent of the U.S. RDA for 8 to 10 vitamins and minerals, they meet their nutrient needs. Some breakfast cereals, for example, are fortified so that one serving, with a cup of milk, provides 100 percent of the U.S. RDA for the vitamins and minerals listed. If you believe that the one serving takes care of all your nutrient needs for the day, you may eat poorly the rest of the day. But not all vitamins and minerals have a U.S. RDA value and will even appear on the label. Some labels list MDR instead of U.S. RDA. The MDR stands for the Minimum Daily Requirement of five vitamins and four minerals and are the amounts suggested for daily consumption to prevent signs of deficiency. They are obsolete and have been revised and replaced by the U.S. RDA. If you see any labels using the MDR, you know the product has been on the shelf for some time or the company has failed to update its nutrition labeling.

Nutrient Density.   With the concern about excesses in the diets of Americans, particularly excess energy, nutritionists felt the public should be able to evaluate food by comparing the levels of nutrients in the food to its energy content. They came up with the concept of nutrient density. Foods that have high nutrient density provide, along with energy, a large percentage of the human requirement for several nutrients. Foods with low nutrient density provide little other than energy.

The index of nutrient quality (INQ) is a mathematical expression of nutrient density.(9) The INQ for each nutrient in a food is calculated by dividing the percentage of the nutrient requirement supplied by a food by the percentage of the energy requirement supplied by that same food. For example, assume you eat a portion of food X that supplies 30 milligrams of vitamin C and 200 kcalories. Assume also that you need 60 milligrams of vitamin C and 2000 kcalories of energy per day. You calculate the INQ of the food as follows:

$$\frac{\text{vitamin C in food} \div \text{vitamin C needed daily}}{\text{kcalories in food} \div \text{kcalories needed daily}} = \frac{30 \div 60}{200 \div 2000} = \frac{0.5}{0.1} = 5.0$$

If the INQ for a nutrient in a food is 1, the amount of the food that supplies daily energy needs also meets daily nutrient needs. The vitamin C INQ of food X is 5.0, indicating that the food meets vitamin C needs well before it meets energy needs. If the food contained several other nutrients with an INQ of 1 or more, it would qualify as being nutrient dense.

ALCOHOL CONSUMPTION

Alcohol (more accurately called ethanol) is both a nutrient and a drug. Throughout time, people have considered alcohol a food, a medicine, and a sign of hospitality. The Romans believed it was a necessary part of the diet; they gave it freely to the poor, mixed it with herbs for the sick, and made sure every soldier received his allotment.(10)

Alcohol is produced by the action of yeast on the carbohydrates in starting materials such as grains, fruit, and molasses. Yeast is unable to grow in the presence of large amounts of alcohol, so the "hard" liquors (whiskey, vodka, gin, and rum) must undergo a special distillation process. The alcohol is drained from the original fermenting material and concentrated. This process removes any traces of the nutrients, although some amounts remain in beer and wine.(11) To figure out how much alcohol is in distilled spirits, divide the "proof" number on the label by half (100 proof whiskey is about 50 percent alcohol, so 2 ounces of the whiskey contains about 1 ounce of alcohol.) Table 2–12 gives the composition of some alcoholic beverages. One drink or 12 milliliters of alcohol, is equivalent to a 1-ounce jigger of 80 proof spirits, a 3.5-ounce glass of table wine, a 12-ounce glass of light beer, or a 10-ounce glass of ordinary American beer.(12)

As a food, alcohol provides kcalories (7 kcalories per gram) and limited amounts of vitamins and minerals. Less than one-fourth of ingested alcohol is absorbed from the diet directly by the stomach. The remaining alcohol passes into the body through the small intestine, just like any food, except that it moves through much faster.(10) Alcohol is metabolized in the liver, but is limited in its ability to detoxify it. The average person can break down about 0.1 gram of alcohol for each kilogram (2.2 pounds) of weight per hour. This means that if you weigh 60 kilograms (132 pounds), you can handle one glass of sherry or half a glass of California red wine in a given hour. If you wanted to detoxify the alcohol in a 12-ounce glass of beer in one hour, you would have to weigh about 293 pounds.(11) When you exceed your capacity to break down alcohol (easily enough done), the alcohol builds up in the tissues and blood, causing intoxication. Until you metabolize it, the alcohol continues to affect the nerve centers of the brain. You cannot store the kcalories from alcohol; the body uses them immediately, before those from food. Yet the conversion of alcohol kcalories to body fat is not efficient because the detoxification process in the liver

TABLE 2–12 **Composition of Some Alcoholic Beverages**

Beverage and Usual Serving	Kcalories	Alcohol (g)	Carbohydrate (g)
Ale (12 oz)	225	22	16
Beer (12 oz)	165	15	15
Gin (1 jigger)	126	18	—
Whiskey (1 jigger)	112	16	—
Vodka (1 jigger)	135	19	—
Daiquiri (1½ jiggers rum)	180	22	5
Manhattan (1½ jiggers whiskey)	200	28	1
Martini (1½ jiggers gin)	220	31	1
Dry champagne (champagne glass, 135 g)	105	13	3
Sweet champagne (135 g)	160	13	17
California red wine (claret glass, 120 g)	100	12	4
California white wine (120 g)	95	11	4
Port (sherry glass, 30 g)	50	5	4
Sherry (30 g)	45	5	2

Source: C. Robinson, *Normal and Therapeutic Nutrition*, 14th ed. (New York: 1972), p. 698. Figures are averages.

is very inefficient and wastes a lot of energy.(13) About 60 million Americans indulge in alcohol, with about 6 to 10 million drinking to excess. Because such sizable numbers use this drug, it is important to look at the effects of alcohol on nutrition and health.

Effects on Nutrition. Although it has been suggested that some people are more prone to alcoholism because they have an unusually high requirement for B vitamins or are deficient in certain hormones, there is little supporting evidence for this. And although poor nutrition does not cause alcoholism, alcohol certainly affects nutritional status. Alcohol displaces the protein-, vitamin-, and mineral-containing foods in the diet; interferes with the digestion and absorption of nutrients; requires vitamins, minerals, and protein to be detoxified; and increases loss of nutrients through the kidneys.

Alcoholics take in many of their kcalories from alcohol instead of from nutritious foods. For instance, 2 ounces of 86 proof liquor contains about 1500 kcalories, roughly one-half to two-thirds of the normal daily requirement. The alcoholic may lose a lot of weight from eating irregularly, abstaining from food during drinking sprees, and from associated factors like depression, heavy cigarette smoking, intoxication, liver disease, and nausea.(13) In addition to the decreased intake of nutrients, alcoholics poorly absorb and metabolize a number of nutrients, including thiamin, niacin, B-12, folacin, calcium, magnesium, sugars, and proteins. To compound the problem, the metabolism of alcohol in the liver requires protein, vitamins, and minerals, none of which are provided in sufficient quantities by the alcohol itself.

Nutritional anemias are common in alcoholics because chronic alcohol ingestion damages the cells involved with blood formation. Alcoholics also need more of the nutrients required for healthy blood: folacin, B-6, and B-12. Alcoholics may show deficiencies of thiamin and niacin. In moderate amounts alcohol acts as a diuretic, causing increased elimination of water from the body. When a large amount of water is flushed out through the kidneys, other nutrients (water-soluble vitamins, sodium, potassium, chloride, magnesium) follow.(11)

Ironically, certain alcoholics may suffer from obesity and overdoses of vitamins and minerals. The obesity results when the alcoholic is frequently exposed to social occasions that provide food and drink (although the kcalories from alcohol are "wasted," they do add up). In order to compensate for poor eating habits, many people with drinking problems become heavy users of vitamin preparations. Overdoses of vitamin A and niacin are most common. Individuals who are genetically disposed to absorb iron with great efficiency can get iron overdoses if they drink too much wine.(13)

Effects on Health. Alcoholism is probably the most common nutrition-associated health problem in the U.S. adult population. The damage is most often to the liver, the central nervous system, the blood, and the gastrointestinal tract.

Fat accumulates in the liver from both poor nutrition and from the toxic effects of the alcohol itself. (Alcohol can damage the liver even if the person eats a good diet.) Further liver damage can lead to alcoholic hepatitis and irreversible cirrhosis. Alcohol is a depressant that exerts its most obvious effects on the central nervous system. In the gastrointestinal tract, alcohol prevents proper digestion and absorption. It also interferes with the activity of cells that form the constituents of blood. Alcohol can damage the lining of the mouth, throat, stomach, and intestine, increasing the risk of cancer, especially in those who smoke.(11)

One of the most devastating effects of alcohol, though suspected for years, has just recently come to public attention. Fetal alcohol syndrome (FAS) is estimated to affect one out of every 2000 children born in the United States each year. Children suffering from this syndrome show slow growth before and after birth, small heads, facial irregularities such as narrow eye slits and sunken nasal bridges, defective hearts and other organs, malformed arms and legs, genital abnormalities, and mental retardation. Behavioral problems like hyperactivity, extreme nervousness, and poor attention span may also exist.(14) Since it passes easily through membranes, alcohol consumed by a pregnant woman flows from her blood through the placenta to the fetus. The blood of the fetus has the same concentration of alcohol as the mother's. If the mother is drunk, so is the baby. The fetus is worse off because it is much smaller than the mother and its liver is not fully developed. Unable to detoxify the alcohol, the fetus is forced to "hold" it until the concentration in the mother decreases.(14)

There are still many questions to be answered concerning fetal alcohol syndrome. Are there certain points in time during pregnancy when the most damage will occur? Do all kinds of alcohol have the same effects? What if the mother smokes at the same time? Despite the lack of answers, researchers do know that there is a definite risk in drinking 3 ounces or more of alcohol per day (6 drinks or more). Even drinking 1 to 3 ounces of alcohol per day (2 to 6 drinks) may be unsafe. Mothers who drink this much have a higher rate of stillbirths, and their babies weigh less. The best advice to the pregnant woman is to avoid alcohol completely. Short of that, she would be wise to have no more than 2 drinks per day. Women who are attempting to become pregnant should be cautious about their alcohol intakes, since damage can be done during the first month of pregnancy, a time when many women are not yet aware of their condition and the fetus is especially vulnerable.

For all its potential damaging side effects, alcohol does present a good side. It can help relax people and improve appetite. In patients, it can induce sleep and create a better state of mind for recovery.(10) There is some basis to suggest that moderate drinking may reduce the risk of heart disease and lower cholesterol levels (see Chapter 4). It may also help to lower blood pressure in hypertensive individuals. The key to consumption is moderation, for heavy drinkers are at higher risk of liver cirrhosis, cancer, and stroke.(12)

Effects on Drugs. Machinery in the liver designed to detoxify alcohol is also the center for the detoxification of certain drugs. A very curious situation results. The detoxification center in chronic alcoholics becomes so efficient at its job that the alcoholic can handle higher levels of drugs than the nonalcoholic. If, however, alcoholics take drugs and liquor at the same time, the drugs are broken down very slowly.

Moderate drinkers are advised to avoid alcohol when taking any type of drug. Alcohol does not mix well with antibiotics, anticoagulants, antidiabetic drugs (including insulin), antihistamines, high blood pressure drugs, MAO inhibitors, and sedatives.

SUGGESTIONS FOR SAFE USE
1. Moderate your intake of alcohol. A glass of wine with dinner or 2 to 3 drinks during an evening is moderate.
2. Eat food along with alcohol so that the food will slow down the rate of absorption of alcohol into the bloodstream.
3. Avoid alcohol during pregnancy, especially during the first three months.
4. Do not take alcohol while taking drugs, since alcohol can increase the potency of the drug or destroy its effectiveness.
5. Try to encourage moderation in friends and family. Have nonalcoholic alternatives available for social occasions (apple juice, club soda with lemon or lime slices, tomato juice, tea, coffee, sparkling cider).(11).

REFERENCES

1. Food and Nutrition Board, *Recommended Dietary Allowances*, 9th ed. (Washington, D.C.: National Research Council, National Academy of Sciences, 1980).

2. A.A. Hertzler and H.L. Anderson, "Food Guides in the United States," *Journal of the American Dietetic Association* 64(1974):19–28.

3. U.S. Department of Agriculture, *Food*. Home and Garden Bulletin No. 228, Washington, D.C., 1980.

4. American Diabetes Association and American Dietetic Association, *Exchange Lists for Meal Planning* (New York and Chicago, 1976).

5. U.S. Senate, Select Committee on Nutrition and Human Needs, *Dietary Goals for the United States*, 2nd ed. (Washington, D.C.: U.S. Government Printing Office, 1977).

6. U.S. Department of Agriculture and U.S. Department of Health, Education & Welfare, *Nutrition and Your Health: Dietary Guidelines for Americans* (Washington, D.C.: U.S. Government Printing Office, 1980).

7. Food and Nutrition Board, *Toward Healthful Diets* (Washington, D.C.: National Research Council, National Academy of Sciences, 1980).

8. B. Peterkin, J. Nichols, and C. Cromwell, *Nutrition Labeling—Tools for Its Use*. Publ. AIB-382, U.S. Department of Agriculture, Washington, D.C., 1975.

9. R.G. Hansen, "An Index of Food Quality," *Nutrition Reviews* 31 (1973):1–7.

10. "To Your Health," *The Professional Nutritionist*, Winter 1977, pp. 11–13.

11. "The Sober Facts about Alcohol," *Environmental Nutrition* (July–August 1979):1–5.

12. W.J. Darby, "The Benefits of Drink," *Human Nature*, November 1978, pp. 31–37.

13. D.A. Roe, "Nutritional Concerns in the Alcoholic" *Journal of the American Dietetic Association* 78 (1981):17–21.

14. F.P. Witti, "Alcohol and Birth Defects," *FDA Consumer*, May 1978, pp. 20–22.

Carbohydrates
3

Dieters cringe at the mere mention of them, yet athletes stuff them in until their stomachs bulge. What is it about carbohydrates that makes them cursed and loved at the same time? Maybe it is that they are nearly impossible to avoid.

Today in the United States, about 50 percent of dietary energy is from carbohydrate, including the starches from cereals and grains as well as sugars from fruits and sweetened products. The American diet, typical of most contemporary Western diets, includes an increasing proportion of carbohydrate kcalories from sugary foods rather than starchy ones. Although both starches and sugars are carbohydrates, their food sources are different. Starches are generally consumed as vegetables, breads, and cereals that, on the whole, provide other nutrients (protein, vitamins, minerals, water), whereas most of the sugar is refined and consumed in products providing few other nutrients. Starches and sugars also have different compositions and structures.

All carbohydrates are composed of three elements: carbon, hydrogen, and oxygen. There are always two hydrogens to every oxygen, a pattern also found in water. The hydrogens and oxygens are attached like appendages to a carbon backbone or chain, with the number of carbons in the chain varying from as few as three to more than a thousand.

CLASSES OF CARBOHYDRATES

Based on size, carbohydrates fall into three categories: monosaccharides, disaccharides, and polysaccharides. The mono- and disaccharides are simple carbohydrates, or *sugars;* the polysaccharides are complex carbohydrates, or *starches*. The prefixes *mono-*, *di-*, and *poly-* refer to the number of sugar units forming the particular carbohydrate. Monosaccharides contain only a single unit of sugar, disaccharides contain two units, and polysaccharides contain multiple units.

Monosaccharides

The single monosaccharide units are usually chains of six carbons, the three most common sugars in this class being glucose, fructose, and galactose (Figure 3–1). Each of these sugars is different because their hydrogens and oxygens are arranged differently around the carbon skeleton. These slight variations in arrangement give each sugar distinctive properties, such as sweetening power.

Glucose is sometimes called blood sugar because it is the major sugar found in the general circulation of the body. All carbohydrates are ultimately broken down or converted to glucose in the intestines or liver before being used by the cells. Another name for glucose is *dextrose,* a term often seen on food labels. *Fructose,* the sweetest of the sugars, is found with glucose in fruits, vegetables, and honey. *Galactose* does not exist in nature as a single sugar, but is part of other larger carbohydrates.

Disaccharides

Attaching two monosaccharides together forms the second class of carbohydrates, the disaccharides. Sucrose, lactose, and maltose are the most common sugars in this group.

Sucrose is a combination of the monosaccharides glucose and fructose. More widely known as the sweetener refined from cane sugar and sugar beets, it takes the form of molasses, brown sugar, and both white powdered and granulated (table) sugar. The major food sources of sucrose are sweetened foods (pastries, sodas, ready-to-eat cereals), although there are many less obvious sources, such as ketchup and peanut butter. Sucrose is naturally present in sorghum, pineapple, and carrot roots.

Lactose is a combination of glucose and galactose. Since it is present only in milk, it is called milk sugar. Of all the sugars, it is the least sweet. Lactose increases absorption of calcium, and promotes the growth of beneficial bacteria in the intestines.

Two glucose units together give *maltose*. Outside of malt and germinating grains, it does not exist freely in nature. Rather, certain agents like dry heat and enzymes break down longer chains of glucose to form the two-unit maltose. This is the reason bread tastes sweeter after toasting; maltose has been created upon browning of the bread. Enzymes used in the brewing process segment off maltose units from long glucose chains in barley and wheat, which then serve as

FIG. 3–1

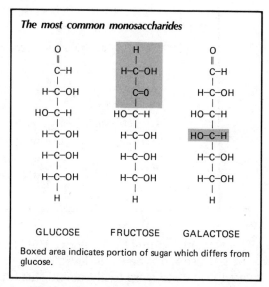

The most common monosaccharides

| GLUCOSE | FRUCTOSE | GALACTOSE |

Boxed area indicates portion of sugar which differs from glucose.

flavorings for beer and whiskey. It is the removal of maltose units from beer that produces "light" beer.

Because of differences in composition, each sugar has its own sweetening power. Fructose is more than half again sweeter than sucrose. Not long ago food scientists concluded that if you used fructose instead of sucrose, you could get the same sweetness for about 30 percent fewer kcalories. When they tried substituting fructose for sucrose, though, they found that in many cases its sweetening power was much less than predicted.(1,2)

Polysaccharides

Polysaccharides, the final class of carbohydrates, are formed from repeating linkages of glucose, some adding up to 10,000 units. The glucose chains assume a variety of configurations, depending on whether they are straight or branched (Figure 3–2). The three principle polysaccharides are starch, glycogen, and cellulose.

Starch is the storage form of carbohydrate in plants, and is found in wheat, rice, and corn, in tubers (potatoes, yams, and cassava), and in peas, beans, as well as other plants. The enzymes in the human digestive tract do not break down starches efficiently unless the starches are cooked. The long glucose chains in raw starch are packed together in a way that makes them inaccessible to digestive enzymes. Cooking causes the chains to spread out so enzymes can break them down into their separate glucose units so they can be absorbed from the intestines. Thus, some starch in food is lost if you eat foods raw.

FIG. 3–2

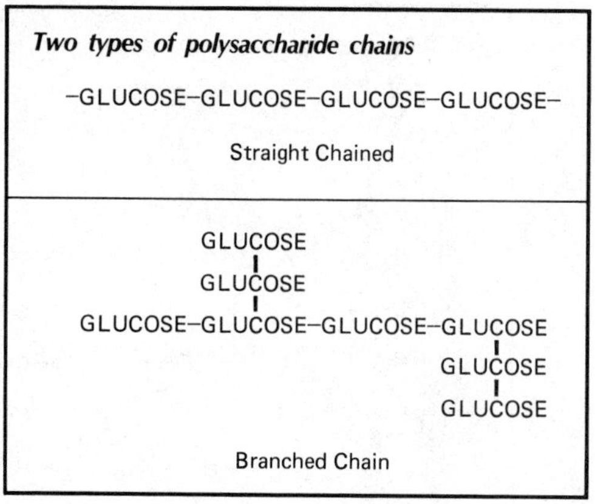

```
┌─────────────────────────────────────────────────┐
│  Two types of polysaccharide chains              │
│                                                   │
│   -GLUCOSE-GLUCOSE-GLUCOSE-GLUCOSE-              │
│                                                   │
│                 Straight Chained                 │
├─────────────────────────────────────────────────┤
│                                                   │
│                  GLUCOSE                          │
│                     |                             │
│                  GLUCOSE                          │
│                     |                             │
│   GLUCOSE-GLUCOSE-GLUCOSE-GLUCOSE                │
│                              |                    │
│                           GLUCOSE                 │
│                              |                    │
│                           GLUCOSE                 │
│                                                   │
│                 Branched Chain                   │
└─────────────────────────────────────────────────┘
```

Glycogen is manufactured by the body. The bloodstream can hold only a certain level of glucose, so when this level has been reached, the liver and muscles convert the extra glucose to glycogen. This stabilizes the sugar level in the blood. Glycogen is the storage form of carbohydrate in animals. Sometimes called animal starch, it acts as an energy store in animals much as starches do in plants. This storage is a more rapidly accessible, though less extensive, energy reserve than fat. It is available for energy during active muscular work.

Cellulose gives plants rigidity in a way similar to the calcium skeleton in humans. Like starch and glycogen, cellulose is composed of glucose units, but the way in which they are linked makes cellulose resistant to human digestive enzymes. Cellulose, along with other indigestible matter from plants, is also known as dietary fiber.

DIGESTION OF CARBOHYDRATES

An enzyme in saliva called ptyalin or α-amylase begins the breakdown of starches into smaller units. If a cracker is chewed and held in the mouth for a few minutes it tastes sweet, a result of the sweeter maltose units being formed. Few people chew their food long enough, however, to have much digestion take place in the mouth. Food mixed with saliva is carried to the stomach, where the ptyalin from the saliva continues to act on the starches for a short time. The major site of carbohydrate digestion and absorption is the small intestine. An enzyme from the pancreas, also called α-amylase, works to continue the breakdown of starches to form shorter chains of glucose.

On the surface of the cells lining the intestinal tract are enzymes that break down the short glucose chains into single glucose units. There are also specific enzymes on the surface of the cells that break down maltose, lactose, and sucrose to their component monosaccharides. These enzymes are, respectively, *maltase, lactase,* and *sucrase*. Some people have difficulty digesting lactose and cannot consume large amounts of milk without becoming ill. This condition, known as lactose intolerance, results from too little of the enzyme lactase. Without enough of the enzyme, lactose remains in the intestinal tract for a long time, fostering the growth of bacteria and leading to abdominal bloating, flatulence, and watery diarrhea. Lactose intolerance affects at least 30 million people in this country. Its prevalence varies among different population groups, affecting 70 to 75 percent of blacks, 70 percent of the adult Jewish population, almost all Orientals, and 5 to 10 percent of whites. Most of these people can tolerate small quantities of milk and many can eat cured cheese and yogurt because much of the lactose is broken down in the fermentation process. Lactase can be purchased under the trade name Lact-Aid® and added to dairy products to predigest the milk sugar.

The end products of carbohydrate digestion are monosaccharides. These are mainly glucose, but there is also some fructose from sucrose digestion and galactose from lactose digestion. These monosaccharides pass through the intestinal wall, enter the bloodstream, and are transported to the liver. Most of the fructose and galactose are converted to glucose in the liver and released to the blood. They circulate to other tissues, where the glucose is used for energy or converted to glycogen or fat and stored (Figure 3–3).

The body digests and absorbs sugars rapidly. If you have not eaten in a few hours, you feel hungry because your blood sugar level is low. A soda or candy, composed mostly of sugar, gives a quick lift, because the sugar rushes into the bloodstream. The sugar influx causes the body to release insulin, a hormone required for the cells to use glucose. This rapid rise in insulin can overcompensate for the amount of glucose available and cause blood sugar level to drop to a point lower than the precandy level. The individual ends up feeling tired and dizzy. Complex carbohydrates, on the other hand, take a longer time to be broken down into simple sugars and enter the bloodstream gradually. A more sensible snack would be some combination of protein, fat, and carbohydrate, such as cheese and fruit or peanut butter and crackers. The fat and protein take a longer time to digest, so the person feels full for a longer period of time.

FIG. 3–3

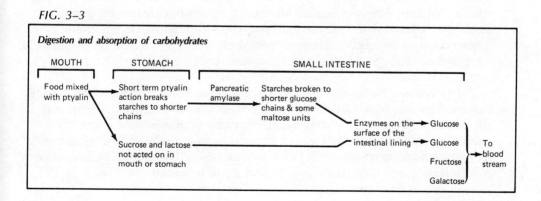

Digestion and absorption of carbohydrates

They are also released gradually into the bloodstream, so the body does not experience wide fluctuations in blood sugar level.

The body has several controls to keep the level of blood glucose constant. This is important, since the brain relies almost exclusively on glucose for its functioning. When a surge of glucose enters after a meal or snack, the cells (under the influence of insulin) take up the excess from the blood and store it as liver glycogen, muscle glycogen, or fat in the fat cells.

Glycogen is a highly-branched carbohydrate with glucose units hanging from the ends of the branches. Enzymes can quickly break off these ends when the body needs energy. The glycogen in the liver (a storage only large enough to last about 12 hours) is released into the bloodstream for use by body tissue; the glycogen in the muscles is used by the muscles themselves. If the glucose circulating in the blood and the glycogen stores are all full, any remaining glucose is converted into fat and stored in fat cells. There are few limits on the amount of fat the body can store.

If the blood glucose level falls too low, two hormones, epinephrine (also known as adrenalin) and glucagon, cause the glucose from the liver glycogen to be released into the bloodstream, thus raising the level of blood glucose. If the body needs more glucose than is stored in the liver, it can synthesize more from certain amino acids. Glucagon starts this process.

FUNCTIONS OF CARBOHYDRATES

Once absorbed into the bloodstream carbohydrates can function in a number of capacities, the major one being provision of energy but other important functions are also discussed below.

Provide Energy.   Carbohydrates are the cheapest and most readily accessible form of energy. Most tissues can use proteins, carbohydrates, or fats for energy, but some tissue, like that of the brain, lungs, and nerves, needs glucose. Proteins can be converted into glucose to meet this need, but fats cannot. Proteins, however, are not stored in the body but are actively engaged in tissue synthesis and maintenance. Using them for energy diverts them from other necessary functions. Thus, carbohydrates "spare" protein by providing the glucose. (See the discussion of low-carbohydrate diets in Chapter 6.)

Maintain Water and Sodium Levels in the Body.   Researchers do not fully understand how carbohydrates maintain normal balances of both water and sodium. There is no dietary requirement for carbohydrates, but without a minimum amount in the diet (about 40 to 60 grams), the body sets in motion a series of adaptations similar to those for starvation. Symptoms include water and sodium loss, along with fatigue and protein breakdown.

Part of Body Tissues.   Carbohydrates, combined with proteins or fats, serve as components of many body tissues. They also form many essential compounds like heparin, a factor that prevents blood clotting.

Stimulate Growth of Intestinal Bacteria.   Carbohydrates provide energy to many bacteria that inhabit the intestinal tract. Although some of these bacteria may not be welcome (such as those that cause abdominal pain and diarrhea), others synthesize important vitamins like biotin.

Aid in Absorption of Other Nutrients.   Certain sugars enhance the absorption of nutrients from the digestive tract. Glucose has a positive effect on the absorption of sodium, while lactose helps calcium absorption.

Provide Fiber or Bulk.   Cellulose, because it is resistant to human digestive enzymes, moves quickly through the digestive tract. It helps to keep the intestinal muscles in tone and to regulate the movement of food through the intestines.

Add Flavor, Color, Texture.   If carbohydrates were eliminated from the diet, there would be few food choices left. Almost all that would remain would be meat, fish, poultry, and eggs.

FOOD SOURCES OF CARBOHYDRATES

Plant Sources

The major food sources of carbohydrates are plants, but different types of plants provide varying amounts of sugars and starches. Most of the sugars consumed in affluent societies take the form of white table sugar, brown sugar, honey, maple syrup, and corn syrup, a substance widely used in the food industry. These sweeteners consist mostly of sucrose; exceptions are honey and corn syrup, composed in large part of separate glucose and fructose units.

Fruits and berries contain more sugar than vegetables, which are high in starch. The amount of sugar found in fruits varies with the water content. Fresh fruits can be 6 to 20 percent sugar, compared to 70 percent for dried fruit. The sugar content of canned fruit depends on whether or not a sweetener has been added. A sugar is a sugar regardless of the source. Table sugar, however, contains only minimal amounts of other nutrients, while fruits offer vitamins, minerals, fiber, and water in addition to the sugar. Nutritionally, they are better sources of sugars. Keep in mind, though, that by eating fruits you are consuming kcalories in the form of sugar, so unlimited consumption is not recommended.

Vegetables can be from 3 to 35 percent carbohydrate, the carbohydrate taking the form of sugars, starch, and cellulose. Grains are the seeds of a variety of grasses and the main source of starch for most of the world. The most common are rice, wheat, rye, corn, oats, barley, and millet. Due to their low moisture content, nuts are concentrated sources of both fats and proteins. They contain about 10 to 27 percent carbohydrate, with 1 to 2 percent as fiber.

Animal Sources

Milk and milk products containing lactose are the primary animal sources of carbohydrate. The only other animal source is shellfish, with about 5 percent by weight being carbohydrate. Meats contain little carbohydrate because once rigor mortis sets in after the animal's death, the glycogen in the muscle converts to another compound called lactic acid. The animal exhausts all its own glycogen at slaughtering time.

FIBER

Fiber is usually mentioned with carbohydrates because most food fibers are carbohydrates or carbohydratelike substances. Fiber is largely indigestible, so it is not a true nutrient (nutrients must be absorbed). Until recently, nutritionists have ignored fiber. Now, however, it is known to play a vital role in the digestive tract and has become a source of controversy because of the exaggerated claims that have been made for it. (See the discussion later in this chapter.)

SUMMARY

Carbohydrates are composed of three elements: carbon, hydrogen, and oxygen. Based on size, carbohydrates can be classified as monosaccharides (one sugar unit), disaccharides (two sugar units) or polysaccharides (multiple sugar units). The sugars include the monosaccharides (glucose, fructose, and galactose) and the disaccharides (sucrose, lactose, and maltose). Polysaccharides are the complex carbohydrates (starches, cellulose, glycogen).

All carbohydrates are broken down into glucose for circulation in the bloodstream. Once in the bloodstream, carbohydrates are used by the body for many functions, the primary one being as a source of energy. If too much glucose is available in the blood, the body converts it into a short-term energy store, glycogen, or a long-term store, fat.

Dietary sources of carbohydrates are mainly plants: sugars, fruits, vegetables, nuts, and grains. A small contribution comes from dairy products.

Fiber, a carbohydratelike substance, is resistant to human digestive enzymes and aids in maintaining the tone of intestinal muscles.

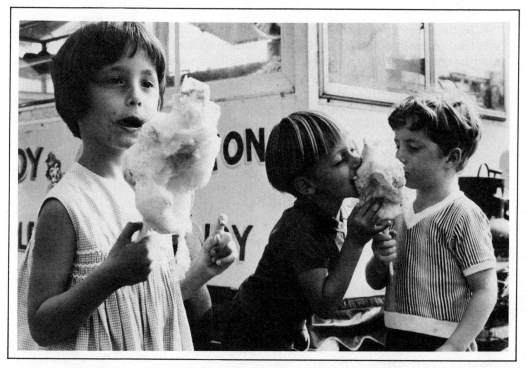

Are people really born with a sweet tooth, or is the desire for sweets learned in childhood?

Issue

Sweeteners—Health Hazard?

"Good common sense tells you that the earth is flat and that the natural sugar in raisins is better for you than the added sugar in chocolate candy bars. Existing scientific data doesn't back up either of those views."

Carol Tucker Foreman
USDA Assistant Secretary, 1979

When a drop of bitter solution is placed on a newborn's tongue, the baby's face puckers up into an expression of displeasure. But when the drop is from a sweetened solution, the baby's face lights up with surprise and joy. Though it is still not known whether babies really like sweets (or whether humans have an innate desire for sugar), they certainly react as if they do. Children also readily accept candies and other sweet foods, though there is no evidence to support the belief that eating sugar during infancy and childhood leads to a "sweet tooth" later in life.(3) On the contrary, the overall taste sensation of sweetness appears to lessen as people get older. The preference for sweet mixed drinks shifts to more bitter, "straight" drinks with age, a result not only of changing social expectations, but of changing taste sensations.(4)

Over the centuries humans have tried to satisfy their desire for sweets in different ways. Dates, figs, and honey were popular in prehistoric times. In ancient Greece sugar was called a "kind of honey made from reeds." From the eleventh to the fifteenth centuries, sugar was used to hide the nasty tastes of medicines; but because it was extremely expensive and scarce, only the nobility could afford it.(5) It has only been fairly recently that refined white sugar has become widely available. Now, when almost anyone can afford to purchase it, sugar is being proclaimed a health hazard and a poison.

Some people fear that the consumption of sugar is the cause for many current health problems, such as obesity and heart disease. Some have even suggested that sugar be banned from sale in this country. One observer wryly noted that this "might result in such ludicrous situations as candy bar smuggling and Mafia gumballs."(6)

TYPES OF SWEETENERS

What is the evidence behind these accusations? Do we need sugar in the diet? Are there limits on how much the body can handle before the level becomes dangerous to health? Are Americans becoming "sugar addicts"? What about switching from sugar to artificial sweeteners? Is this just increasing the risk of cancer and other disorders?

There are many types of sweeteners. Some are used mainly in the home, others by industry. Although many are different forms of sucrose, several sweeteners have been developed specifically for those who wish to cut back on sucrose intake. In general, sweeteners are classified into two groups: those that provide energy (nutritive) and those that do not (nonnutritive).

Nutritive Sweeteners

Nutritive sweeteners are simply those that provide kcalories. Sugars, syrups, molasses, sugar alcohols, and honey fall into this category, and all provide the same number of kcalories gram for gram.(7) The most common sweetener is sucrose or *table sugar*.

With the possible exception of blackstrap molasses, none of these sweeteners provide significant amounts of nutrients other than simple carbohydrates (Table 3–1). There are a few other nutritive sweeteners, but they are not often used, either because they have only recently become available or because they carry questionable health risks.

One method of reducing the number of kcalories obtained from sweetening is to find a substance so sweet that a small amount gives the desired effect. Many people's hopes were raised when a synthetic sweetener made from a combination of two amino acids was found to be 200 times sweeter than sugar. The substance, called *aspartame,* was approved in 1981 for use in dry products such as cereals, chewing gum, and powdered beverages. Aspartame has limited uses, though, since it loses its sweetness in bottled beverages after 6 to 8 weeks of shelf life and breaks apart in baked goods when exposed to high temperatures.

Proponents of the sweetener fructose claim that because it is sweeter than sucrose, smaller amounts can be used in recipes to achieve the desired taste with fewer kcalories.(7) The fact is that fructose is sweeter than regular sugar only in dilute solutions, and its sweetening power in food varies, as mentioned earlier. Fructose has been billed as a "natural" sweetener because it is present in many fruits. In reality, the new manufacturing process for fructose begins with starch which is broken into individual glucose units, many of which are then converted through enzyme action to fructose. This fructose is actually more highly processed than sucrose, and more expensive. It is available in bulk and in packets through health food stores.

Another way to obtain the sweetness of sugar without the quick rise in blood sugar is to use a sugar that is not well absorbed during digestion. Three of these are available: sorbitol, mannitol, and xylitol, all types of sugar alcohols. They occur naturally in fruits but are also commercially produced. Xylitol is present in berries, yellow plums, and mushrooms and is produced from birch tree chips. Although it has a sweetness equal to sucrose, it is about 14 times more expensive. In Scandinavia, it is used in sugarless gum and candy. In the United States it is only permitted in chewing gum and may be banned soon altogether by the Food and Drug Administration because of possible health risks.(8) Sorbitol and mannitol are about half as sweet as sucrose. Because these sugars are not well absorbed, they are used in dietetic products like gum, candy, and wafers. If consumed in abnormally large amounts (about 25 sticks of gum daily), they can cause severe diarrhea.

Nonnutritive Sweeteners

Diabetics and dieters frequently use nonnutritive sweeteners because these sweeteners have no kcalories. For many years the only nonnutritive sweetener approved by the FDA was *saccharin.* It is an artificial sweetener derived from coal tar that has a sweetening power about 300 times that of sucrose. Previously it was used in combination with *cyclamates,* whose sweeten-

TABLE 3–1 Food Values of Nutritive Sweeteners

	Recommended Daily Dietary Requirements Male 154 lb 5'9" 22–35 yr	Female 128 lb 5'4" 22–35 yr	White Granulated Sugar	Powdered Sugar	Dark Brown Sugar	Light Molasses	Medium Molasses	Blackstrap Molasses	Strained Honey	Corn Syrup	Maple Syrup
1 tablespoon Weight (grams)			12	11	14	20	20	20	21	20	20
Kcalories	2800	2000	46	42	52	50	46	43	64	57	50
Carbohydrate (gm)			11.9	10.9	13.4	13	12	11	16.4	14.8	12.8
Fat (gm)	65	55									
Protein (gm)									0.1		
Sodium (mg)					3.4	3	6	20	1	17	3
Calcium (mg)	800	800	tr.		11	33	60	137	4	6	33
Phosphorus (mg)	800	800			5	9	14	17	3	3	3
Potassium (approx.)(mg)	1000	1000			32	200	213	600	11	tr.	26
Magnesium (mg)	350	300				9	16	52	0.6		
Iron (mg)	10	18			0.4	0.8	1.4	3	0.2	0.8	0.6
Thiamin (mcg)	1400	1000				14		56	2	tr.	
Niacin (mg)	18	13				tr.		0.4	tr.		
Vitamin A (IU)	5000	5000									
Riboflavin (mcg)	1700	1500				12		50	14	2	
Ascorbic acid (mg)	60	55							1		
Vitamin D (IU)		55									0.1

Source: Questions Most Frequently Asked About Sugar, The Sugar Association, Inc., 1511 Kay Street NW, Washington, D.C. Calculated from *Food Values of Portions Commonly Used,* 11th Ed. Bowes & Church; and *Composition of Foods,* Agricultural Handbook No. 8, United States Department of Agriculture, 1963.

ing power was discovered in 1944. In the mid-1950s manufacturers found that by mixing 10 parts cyclamate to 1 part saccharin they could obtain a product 55 times as sweet as sugar without the bitter aftertaste of saccharin alone. In 1969, cyclamates were banned as carcinogens when studies showed they caused bladder tumors in rats.(9)

SUGAR CONSUMPTION IN THE UNITED STATES

It is often stated that the amount of sugar Americans consume is increasing to staggering levels. When we examine the data, though, it appears that the average consumption of sucrose in the United States has not changed in the past 50 years. Because it is difficult to measure accurately how much an individual consumes, the best indicator for average intake is USDA consumption figures. According to these figures, the bulk of sweeteners consumed in this country are refined sugar and corn syrup (Figure 3–4).

From 1960 to 1974, the amount of refined sugar consumed in the United States remained steady, about 100 pounds per person per year; in 1978, this amount declined to about 93 pounds. This decline in sugar consumption is offset by an increase in the use of corn sweeteners, from 19 pounds in 1970 to almost 34 pounds in 1978. This rise is a result of growing industrial use of sweeteners, especially in the soft drink industry. The consumption of complex carbohydrates, especially cereals and flour, has declined. Thus, even though the consumption of refined sugar has not increased, the fact that consumption of

FIG. 3–4

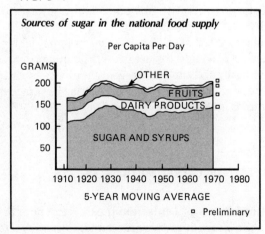

Source: L. Page and B. Friend, "Level of use of sugars in the United States," in H.L. Sipple and K.W. McNutt, eds., *Sugars in Nutrition* (New York: Academic Press, 1974), p. 97.

total complex carbohydrates has decreased and the use of corn syrup has risen means that a higher proportion of kcalories is coming from sweeteners.(11) At present, Americans are consuming about 24 percent of their total kcalories as sugar, of which 3 percent is from fruits and vegetables, 3 percent from dairy products, and the balance from added sugar.(10)

One of the most noticeable changes has been not in the amount of sugar consumed, but in who is adding it to food. Increasingly, industry is the prime user of sweeteners. Sixty-five percent of refined sugar is used by the food and beverage industries, whereas only 24 percent is used in food prepared at home.

Uses of Sugar

Despite the similarities among different types of sweeteners, white sugar gets most criticism. How many people want to ban honey? Is there any use for sugar in the diet, or is it merely a luxury that has become more of a hazard than a blessing?

Sugar is called the ultimate empty kcalorie food. It does not provide any nutrients, just carbohydrate kcalories. The kcalories in sugar, however, are not inferior to other kcalories. And, proponents argue, sugar is rarely eaten alone. Since it makes other foods taste good, it can enhance the consumption of bitter or sour foods people otherwise might not eat.

Some nutritionists feel that the growing child may have difficulty obtaining adequate kcalories without moderate intake of sucrose, unless fats are increased.(12) Increasing the amount of starchy foods can add so much fiber to the diet that children feel full before they have consumed enough kcalories for their energy needs. For some people, such as children with advanced kidney disease, it is important that protein be spared as much as possible. Nutritionists have found that these children will eat popsicles and hard candy, which provide enough kcalories so that their bodies will not have to break down protein for energy.(13)

Sugar is used as a preservative in jams, jellies, syrups, and candies. It ties up the water needed for the growth of microorganisms that may spoil food. Sugar provides a medium for the growth of yeasts and fermenting agents in the manufacture of pickles, bread, and alcoholic beverages. (Sugar is used up in the process, and is not present in the final product.)(7)

DISEASE AND SWEETENER CONSUMPTION

Sugar is often named as a culprit in the development of obesity, diabetes, certain diseases of the heart, and hypoglycemia. Other sweeteners, such as saccharin, are linked to cancer. Is our national sweet tooth really leading us to early graves?

If we examine the evidence, we will find that many of these accusations are unfounded.

Obesity

It is claimed that eating a nutritionally adequate diet rich in sugar may supply all the needed nutrients but lead to overconsumption of kcalories and obesity. If obesity did occur, then certainly too many kcalories were consumed. But it is difficult to distinguish between the effects of sugar intake on weight gain and the effects of kcalories from all other foods. This claim assumes that the obese consume sugar in greater amounts than people of normal weight. Research studies show just the opposite: Fat people consume less sugar than do lean people.(14) In societies with high-fat diets, sugar consumption is not related to obesity.(14) In short, obesity is not caused by eating sugar, but by an imbalance in kcalorie intake and energy expenditure. Many nutritionists now agree with the Nutrition Council of the Netherlands in its conclusion that eating sugar does not play a primary role in causing obesity or shortening life.(15) For people who want to lose weight, nutritive sweeteners, fats, and alcohol are usually restricted because foods rich in sugar, fat, or alcohol are often poor in other nutrients.

A small number of people are unable to control their intake of kcalories if they have too much carbohydrate in the diet. With increased starches and sugars, these people lose control of their appetite and go on carbohydrate binges. The number of these "carboholics," however, is quite low.(16)

Claims that fructose helps suppress hunger are not proved. Since its sweetening power when mixed with many foods is not as high as claimed, it has to be used in amounts similar to sucrose. The kcalorie level of most fructose-sweetened foods is only slightly lower than that of those sweetened with regular sugar.

Diseases of the Heart and Blood Vessels

A number of claims supposedly link sugar consumption and cardiovascular disease or disease of the heart and blood vessels. (When only the heart is involved, it is generally called coronary heart disease or CHD.) Studies of a link between sugar consumption and elevated blood lipids have produced mixed results. In some population studies, high sugar intakes were associated with both high levels of fats in the blood and increased deaths from heart disease. These same populations, however, also had an increased rate of obesity that was more closely related to fatty deposits in arteries than to the rate of sugar consumption. In many of the countries where these studies were conducted, consumption of fats is also high. If complex carbohydrates in the diet are replaced by fats, then fats become the issue, not sugars. Carbohydrates, even in the form of simple sugars, may be good if they help reduce fat consumption. Animal experiments in which results suggested a link between sugar consumption and heart disease were based on consumption of amounts of sugar abnormally high when extrapolated to the human population of the United States.(17)

Diabetes

Diabetes is an inherited disease in which the ability of glucose to enter body cells is impaired. Insulin, a hormone secreted by the pancreas, is required for glucose entry, and diabetics lack the hormone, or their cells are not sensitive enough to its action to allow normal entry of glucose.

Diabetes takes two forms: Type I (also referred to as early onset or juvenile onset) and Type II (late onset or adult onset). Type I, which usually occurs during childhood or early adulthood, is caused by a lack of insulin due to a malfunction in the pancreas. Type II, generally appearing in middle age or thereafter, occurs in individuals who have insulin but are not sufficiently sensitive to it. In fact, insulin levels in the blood of Type II diabetics are often higher than normal. Regardless of whether the diabetes is early or late onset, glucose cannot enter body cells or enters at a rate slower than normal. Glucose appears in high levels in the blood and is often excreted in the urine if the condition is not treated. Insulin also influences the use of body fat. High levels of the hormone depress the breakdown of stored fat. Thus the body fat of Type II diabetics often is not as readily withdrawn and used for energy as that of nondiabetics.

The cause of the pancreatic malfunction or insulin insensitivity of cells is not known, but people who are predisposed by heredity to diabetes are more likely to develop the condition if they are overfat. The U.S. National Diabetes Commission states that the chance of becoming diabetic more than doubles for every 20 percent of excess weight;(18) and excess weight, of course, results from overconsumption of kcalories regardless of food source.

Whether the level of sugar in the diet plays a role in the development of diabetes is not known. One experiment with laboratory animals showed that rats fed sucrose developed diabetes, while those fed starch did not.(19) The effect of complex carbohydrates versus sugar on the prevention of diabetes has not been established in humans. Some studies reveal that those who developed the disease had a lower sugar intake than nondiabetic controls.(14) In population groups that have moved to a Westernized diet high in sugar, fat, and kcalories, the incidence of diabetes has increased, but so too has the incidence of obesity. Epidemiological data show that the risk of diabetes occurs less often in some populations where carbohydrate and sugar consumption are high, and more often where fat consumption and total kcalories are high.(14)

The treatment of diabetes involves control of total kcalories to attain ideal body weight.(20) This means the kcalorie restriction of all foods, but especially fat, sugars, and alcohol. There was a time when diabetics were prescribed diets high in fat and low in carbohydrates of all types, but nutritionists now know that it is more desirable to allow moderate amounts of complex carbohydrates and reduce the level of fat. Such diets lend themselves better to weight control programs than do diets high in fat.

Hypoglycemia

True hypoglycemia occurs in only a few rare individuals and is caused by the pancreas consistently releasing too much insulin. The result is low blood sugar levels and feelings of faintness, hunger, and anxiety. In order to control the insulin response, these persons must eat a diet high in protein, with no sugars.

Every one of us experiences a mild form of hypoglycemia throughout the day when we go without food for a few hours. We begin to feel hungry and weak, and we may start to get a headache. The best advice is to eat something, particularly a well-balanced meal instead of a high-sugar snack. Although sugar and starches are not the cause of hypoglycemia, they are usually reduced to control the problem.(21)

Vitamin and Mineral Depletion

In order to use the energy in food, the body requires vitamins and minerals. Since sugar provides no nutrients, some people argue that the body has to use up vitamins and minerals already in storage or from other foods to break down the sugar. It is true that the need for thiamin (a B-vitamin) is increased with increased carbohydrates, complex as well as simple. But researchers do not know whether this is of practical significance when diets contain amounts of thiamin in the range of the RDA. Despite the current consumption of sugar, there is no thiamin deficiency in the United States. In fact, most sugars are eaten with other foods or as part of other foods that contain the nutrients needed to use sugar.

Dental Caries

Caries, or cavities, have occurred in populations that have never used sugar or processed foods.(22) Peoples of ancient civilizations had caries, though fewer than modern people.(23) Caries is an infectious disease, but aspects of the diet do play a role. Three factors are required for the development of caries: bacteria, fermentable carbohydrate, and a susceptible tooth.

Many factors influence whether a person will develop cavities, and many are more important than the amount of sugar consumed. The length of time the teeth are exposed to the fermentable carbohydrate is crucial. Thus fruits such as figs and gooey candies will stay in contact with the teeth for a longer period of time than less sticky sweets. Frequency of sugar eating has a greater effect than the total amount of sugar consumed. Another important factor is whether most sugary foods are eaten during a meal or as between-meal snacks. Sweet foods eaten during a meal are accompanied by liquids that help cleanse the mouth area. In addition, people are more likely to brush their teeth after a meal than after a snack.

The physical properties of a food influence its effect on tooth decay. Liquid foods promote cavities less than solid foods that adhere to the tooth surface. Some foods contain protective factors. The sucrose in chocolate appears to be counterbalanced by other ingredients in the candy, though it is not yet certain whether the fats, proteins, or even the extract of cocoa powder is responsible.(24)

General state of health and dentition determine susceptibility to cavities, as can dental hygiene habits. Fluoride can reduce tooth susceptibility to cavities (fluoride is discussed in more detail in Chapter 9). Regular and thorough brushing and flossing to remove plaque are necessary to good oral hygiene and can protect against caries.

Cancer

The only sweetener linked to cancer that is currently available on the market is saccharin. Cyclamates, shown to be carcinogens (cancer-causing agents), were banned in 1969. Upon learning of a possible ban on saccharin in 1977, consumers responded by hoarding the substance. This response was triggered by the fact that the $2 billion saccharin industry provides the only nonnutritive sweetener on the market today. Diabetics who must control sugar intake and dieters, worried about kcalories, have come out in force in favor of leaving saccharin on the market.

Saccharin was initially found to be carcinogenic in a Canadian animal study in which rats given saccharin in their feed showed an increased occurrence of bladder cancer. A later Canadian study on humans found that men who consumed saccharin suffered from a higher rate of bladder cancer than those who used sugar.(25) No other laboratory studies to date, however, have duplicated and confirmed these results.

In late 1979 the National Cancer Institute (NCI) and the FDA released the preliminary results of a $1.5 million epidemiological study that included interviews with more than 3000 bladder cancer patients and almost 6000 people from the general population who did not have cancer.(26) The data failed to show a major association between bladder cancer and the use of artificial sweeteners. The study did indicate that certain groups may have an increased risk of bladder cancer: users who smoke cigarettes, pregnant women, and diet soda drinkers or anyone with a heavy saccharin intake. "Heavy" use was defined as two or more 8-ounce diet drinks daily or six or more servings of sugar substitutes. (One packet of sweetener contains 30 milligrams of saccharin, compared to the 80 milligrams in an 8-ounce diet soda.) Risk is also greater for men who smoke two or more packs of cigarettes per day and for women who smoke one or more packs per day.

The relationship of cigarette smoking and saccharin to cancer is a curious one. Saccharin is a weak carcinogen that can enhance the activity of other cancer-causing agents like cigarettes. (A weak carcinogen does not produce a weak form of cancer, but rather affects fewer people than a strong carcinogen.) If you use only a packet or two of saccharin a day or have a diet drink every other day, your risk of bladder cancer is minimal. The risk increases, however, if you are a heavy smoker. The report released by the NCI and FDA recommended that saccharin not be consumed by pregnant women or women of childbearing age, nondiabetic children and youths, and heavy smokers, while excessive use by anyone should be avoided.

One of the primary users of saccharin is the dieter, yet saccharin's use is of doubtful significance in weight loss. There are other low kcalorie foods and drinks that do not carry the added risk of cancer (see Chapter 6).

HOW MUCH SUGAR SHOULD YOU CONSUME?

Banning sucrose is unnecessary and probably impossible. The main consideration when deciding how much sugar, or any of the sweeteners, an individual should consume is the overall quality of the diet. If enough nutritious foods are eaten throughout the day but the need for kcalories is still not met, then sweet foods, in moderation, are acceptable. Obviously, active individuals will have a high energy requirement and be in a better position to eat desserts and sweet snacks with few undesirable effects. The form of the sweetener (sucrose, honey, maple syrup) is not of primary importance.

There are a number of ways to increase the nutrient content of sweetened foods, especially of snack foods for children. Yogurt can be mixed with fresh or frozen fruit, or fruit juices can be frozen in popsicle containers. Instead of baking sugar cookies, you can make what some cooks fondly call "kitchen sink" cookies. These contain such combinations as oatmeal, raisins, cheddar cheese, apple chunks, nuts, and seeds. Or you can make a zucchini-nut bread or a carrot cake.

Sugar, however, as well as some other nutritive sweeteners, does contribute to the development of dental caries. For those who would prefer not to incorporate sweets into the diet for this or any other reason, there are some

TABLE 3–2 Substitutes for Sweetened Foods

Food Group	Eat More of These	Eat Less of These*
Dairy	Milk, cheese cubes, plain yogurt, cottage cheese, some dips and spreads (see label)	Chocolate milk, ice cream, shakes, pudding, cocoa, commercially prepared yogurt, sherbet
Fruits and vegetables	All fresh fruits and vegetables and their unsweetened juices, water-packed fruits or vegetables	Dried fruits, fruits packed in syrups, sweetened canned fruit and vegetable juices, powdered drinks, jams, jellies, preserves, dips with added sugar, vegetables with sugared glazes or added sugar
Bread and cereals	Popcorn, soda crackers, toast, pretzels, pizza	Cookies, pies, cakes, mints, caramels, doughnuts
Meat and fish	Nuts, eggs, peanut butter, some bean dips, leftover meats and fish	Meats with sugared glazes or added sugar, candy-coated nuts
Other	Olives, dill or sour pickles, club soda with lemon or lime	Gum, candy, Jello, syrups, frosting, soups and sauces with sugar added, caramels, toffee, coffee and tea with sugar

*When possible, sugar-rich foods should be limited to mealtime consumption.

Source: Adapted from Diet and Dental Health, American Dental Association, 1980.

delicious substitutes that do not contain added sugar or sweeteners (Table 3–2). You can get the effect of sweetness without using sweeteners by using sweet spices and herbs, such as cinnamon, nutmeg, coriander, cardamon, basil, ginger, or mace. You can caramelize the sugar naturally present in fruits and vegetables by broiling grapefruit, bananas, or tomatoes. Shredded coconut also makes fruits taste sweet.

TABLE 3–3 Percentage of Hidden Sugar in Selected Foods

Cremora nondairy creamer	56.9%	Ritz crackers	11.8%
Coffee-mate nondairy creamer	65.4	Wish Bone Italian Dressing	7.3
Skippy creamy peanut butter	9.2	Wish Bone French Dressing	23.0
Delmonte whole kernel corn	10.7	Wish Bone Russian Dressing	30.2
Libby's peaches, halves	17.9	Jell-O	82.6
Dannon blueberry low-fat yogurt	13.7	Hershey's milk chocolate	51.4
Wyler's beef flavor boullion	14.8	Heinz tomato ketchup	28.9
Hamburger Helper	23.0	Shake'n Bake, crispy style	14.7
Ragu spaghetti sauce	6.2	Shake'n Bake, barbeque style	50.9
Cool Whip	21.0		

Source: Consumer Reports, March 1978.

Be careful to read labels when you shop if you hope to reduce sugar consumption. An ingredient label that reads:

INGREDIENTS: granola (rolled oats, *brown sugar*, coconut oil, raisins, *honey*, sesame seeds, salt, soy lecithin, natural flavor), *sugar, malto dextrin, dextrose*, ground raisins, coconut oil, nonfat milk, *corn syrup*, salt, whey, egg white, soy lecithin, natural flavor.

indicates that the product contains sugar from at least six sources. Some products not usually thought of as sweet many contain "hidden" sugar (Table 3–3). Many products are available with or without sugar (peanut butter, hot dogs, lunch meat, cereals, fruit juices), so it is important to read labels.

A product billed as "natural" or as a "health" food does not necessarily have a reduced sugar content. A comparison of the sugar levels in ready-to-eat cereals versus their "natural" granola counterparts is presented in Table 3–4.

In short, it is possible to cut back on sugar intake, but remember that sugar can be enjoyed in moderation with little hazard to health, especially with good dental hygiene.

TABLE 3–4 **Sugar Content of 62 Ready-to-Eat Cereals**

Product	Total Sugar[†]	Sucrose
Sugar Smacks (K)	56.0%	43.0%
Apple Jacks (K)	54.6	54.0
Froot Loops (K)	48.0	48.0
Sugar Corn Pops (K)	46.0	39.0
Super Sugar Crisp (GF)	46.0	36.0
Crazy Cow, chocolate (GM)	45.6	42.0
Corny Snaps (K)	45.5	45.0
Frosted Rice Krinkles (GF)	44.0	43.3
Frankenberry (GM)	43.7	38.0
Cookie Crisp, vanilla (R-P)	43.5	43.0
Cap'n Crunch, crunch berries (QO)	43.3	42.0
Cocoa Krispies (K)	43.0	41.0
Cocoa Pebbles (GF)	42.6	42.0
Fruity Pebbles (GF)	42.5	42.0
Lucky Charms (GM)	42.2	36.0
Cookie Crisp, chocolate (R-P)	41.0	40.0
Sugar Frosted Flakes of Corn (K)	41.0	39.0
Quisp (QO)	40.7	40.0
Crazy Cow, strawberry (GM)	40.1	38.0
Cookie Crisp, oatmeal (R-P)	40.1	39.0
Cap'n Crunch (QO)	40.0	40.0
Count Chocula (GM)	39.5	35.0
Alpha Bits (GF)	38.0	38.0
Honey Comb (GF)	37.2	37.0
Frosted Rice (K)	37.0	35.0
Trix (GM)	35.9	33.0
Cocoa Puffs (GM)	33.3	32.0

TABLE 3–4 Continued		
Product	Total Sugar[†]	Sucrose
Cap'n Crunch, peanut butter (QO)	32.2	31.0
Country Morning (K)*	31.0	18.0
Raisin Bran (GF)	30.4	15.0
Golden Grahams (GM)	30.0	27.0
Craklin' Bran (K)	29.0	27.0
Raisin Bran (K)	29.0	11.0
C.W. Post, Raisin (GF)*	29.0	11.0
Nature Valley Granola, Fruit and Nut (GM)*	29.0	20.0
C.W. Post (GF)*	28.7	20.0
Quaker 100% Natural, Raisin and Date (QO)*	28.0	15.0
Vita Crunch—Almond (OM)*	28.0	25.0
Vita Crunch—Raisin (OM)*	27.0	23.0
Heartland—Raisin (P)*	26.0	18.0
Frosted Mini Wheats (K)	26.0	26.0
Nature Valley Granola, Cinnamon and Raisin (GM)*	25.0	18.0
Quaker 100% Natural, Apple and Cinnamon (QO)*	25.0	18.0
Vita Crunch—Regular (OM)*	24.0	23.0
Familia (BF)*	23.0	17.0
Heartland, Coconut (P)*	22.0	19.0
Quaker 100% Natural, Brown Sugar & Honey (QO)*	22.0	18.0
Country Crisp (GF)	22.0	18.0
Life, cinnamon (QO)	21.0	21.0
100% Bran (N)	21.0	19.0
All Bran (K)	19.0	16.0
Fortified Oat Flakes (GF)	18.5	18.0
Life (QO)	16.0	16.0
Team (N)	14.1	12.0
Grape Nuts Flakes (GF)	13.3	7.0
40% Bran (GF)	13.0	10.0
Buckwheat (GM)	12.2	10.0
Product 19 (K)	9.9	8.1
Concentrate (K)	9.3	9.0
Total (GM)	8.3	7.0
Wheaties (GM)	8.2	7.0
Rice Krispies (K)	7.8	7.0
Grape Nuts (GF)	7.0	—
Special K (K)	5.4	5.0
Corn Flakes (K)	5.3	3.0
Post Toasties (GF)	5.0	3.0
Kix (GM)	4.8	4.0
Rice Chex (R-P)	4.4	4.0
Corn Chex (R-P)	4.0	4.0
Wheat Chex (R-P)	3.5	2.0
Cheerios (GM)	3.0	3.0
Shredded Wheat (N)	0.6	0.6
Puffed Wheat (QO)	0.5	0.5
Puffed Rice (QO)	0.1	0.1

*Granola-type cereal.
[†]Total sugar = sucrose, glucose, fructose, maltose, lactose.

Notes: (1) Sugar content is percent of dry weight of the product. (2) Letters in parens following product name indicate manufacturers: General Foods (GF), General Mills (GM), Kellogg (K), Nabisco (N), Quaker Oats (QO), Ralston-Purina (R-P), Bio-Familia (BF), Organic Milling (OM), Pet (P).

Source: Research News, USDA, June 1979.

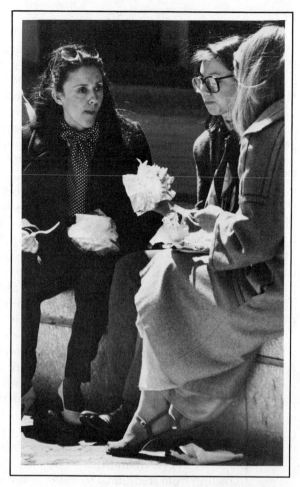

The traditional American diet is changing. City workers, for example, tend to frequent quick-service restaurants at lunchtime.

Issue

Can Fiber Prevent "Diseases of Civilization"?

There was a time, not long ago, when you couldn't buy a box of prunes in a supermarket without everyone in the checkout line snickering. Now shopping carts are filled with Bran Buds, Kellogg's All Bran Flakes, and Nabisco's 100% Bran, and no one even cracks a smile. The demand for fiber-rich foods has increased so much that one bakery began marketing loaves of bread with added sawdust.

Part of the reason for this change in attitude toward foods billed as "keeping you regular" is due to the work of a British physician named Denis Burkitt. Dr. Burkitt has amassed a great deal of evidence supporting his claim that, because of diet, Western societies have higher rates than developing countries of many chronic degenerative diseases. Other researchers, after examining Burkitt's evidence, still have doubts.

As populations become modernized, disease patterns change dramatically: they move from one predominantly of infection to one of degenerative disease. Colon cancer, diverticular disease, and heart disease are rare in developing countries, yet commonplace in Western nations. The transition from traditional to modern society is also accompanied by reduced physical activity and changes in diet. Although both factors are linked to heart disease, dietary changes in particular might be important in the development of other disorders.

One of the major dietary changes is a decrease in consumption of fiber-containing or bulk-forming foods. Fiber, or *roughage* as your grandparents called it, is the component in plant foods that is resistant to human digestive en- zymes. Fiber is not present in animal products, and refining, as well as certain types of processing, reduces the amount found in plant foods. Whole grain breads and cereals contain more fiber than refined ones, while fresh fruits contain more fiber than juices.

In the United States during the past seventy years, the change in food consumption patterns that has had the most significant effect on fiber intake is the decline in the consumption of cereal grains. USDA food consumption data show that, on a per capita basis, present consumption of wheat flour and flour products is only half that of 1910. Consumption of other cereals has declined even more. Until the turn of the century, the most popular flour was whole wheat. Today people use mostly white flour that contains very little fiber, though a shift back to whole grain is emerging. A 75 percent reduction in the fiber content of breads occurred after the shift to refined white flour. Fruit consumption has increased because more people are drinking fruit juice (low in fiber), but consumption of raw fruit (high in fiber) has declined. People are eating more vegetables except for white and sweet potatoes, which have suffered a decline. Both are high in fiber. It is estimated that the overall fiber intake from fruits and vegetables has declined by 20 percent and that from cereals by 50 percent during this century.(27) Considering all these factors, the decline in fiber intake since the beginning of this century could be as high as 83 percent.

Burkitt, aware of this decline in fiber consumption among Westernized societies, compared the dietary patterns and disease rates of people living in regions south of the Sahara to those of people living in modern societies.(28) From these comparisons he developed a theory that low-fiber diets are major factors in the development of "diseases of civilization." The problem with much of the evidence supporting Burkitt's theory is that it is drawn largely from population and historical studies. For instance, in countries where there has been a transition from rural to urban living, changes in fiber consumption were accompanied by changes in intakes of animal protein and fat, sucrose, and refined grains. The population data are based on only one major geographical area in Africa.

When you draw conclusions from historical studies of changing disease rates, you must take into consideration that old records of sickness and death are frequently inaccurate and that many diseases went unreported. It is difficult to compare the occurrence of heart disease today to the occurrence 100 years ago, when many deaths from heart disease were classified simply as death from "old age." Finally, the data available from experimental studies are far from conclusive.(29)

Despite the shortcomings of the research, Burkitt's work did raise the awareness of nutritionists and physicians to the importance of fiber and the fact that it is not useless bulk. Both groups had paid little attention to fiber previously. Since it is resistant to human digestive enzymes and cannot be considered a nutrient, fiber was generally believed to be of little consequence in human health and disease. Simply stated, no one had ever identified a fiber deficiency disease. Fiber is now known to play an important role in regulating the passage of food through the gastrointestinal tract and in exerting an influence on events that occur within the intestine, particularly the large intestine.

DIETARY FIBER

The fiber in food is actually a group of substances found in plants that cannot be broken down by human digestive enzymes. These substances, collectively called *dietary fiber*, make up the semi-rigid walls that surround plant cells. Within the boundaries of the cell wall are flexible membranes, comparable to those surrounding animal cells. Plant fibers differ in composition because of genetics, the age and stage of growth of the plant, and changes produced by different processing techniques.(29)

The different types of dietary fiber include:

- certain gums and mucilages
- pectins
- hemicellulose
- cellulose
- lignin

Each is either a carbohydrate or carbohydratelike substance, except lignin. Pectins are not stringy but soft and formless; it is pectin that causes jams and jellies to gel. Pectins differ from the other dietary fibers in that they dissolve during cooking and are often discarded with the cooking liquid. Cellulose and lignin give rigidity to cell walls. As plant cells age, the amount of lignin increases, giving a woodiness to older portions of the plant. Little lignin is obtained in the diet because the older wood portions of plants are usually not eaten.

Formerly the fiber in food was called crude fiber. Crude fiber is the residue left after a food sample is treated with hot acid and hot alkali. This treatment is much harsher than that of digestive enzymes, so values obtained by this method grossly underestimate the amount of dietary fiber. As shown in Table 3–5, crude fiber can represent as little as 8 percent of the dietary fiber in food. Most food composition tables still list the crude fiber content of food because the techniques for determining dietary fiber content are relatively new. Some food labels now list the dietary fiber content of the product.

Physical Properties of Fiber

Fiber is often called indigestible. Indigestible means it passes through the digestive system intact and is recovered in the feces. Many carbohydrate fibers, however, though resistant to digestive enzymes, are fermented by bacteria in the colon, or lower segment of the large intestine. In a sense, they disappear and are not found in the feces.(29) Other fibers are carried the length of the intestinal tract intact.

Fiber's resistance to human digestive enzymes gives it a number of unique physical properties which include:

- absorption of water (bulking effect)
- binding with toxic substances such as heavy metals and drugs
- binding with essential minerals such as calcium, phosphorus, magnesium, and iron

When you eat plants, your body digests the inner components of the cells, leaving the cell wall just an empty shell. The empty spaces fill with water as they

TABLE 3–5 Fiber Values for Various Foods*

Food	Hemicellulose, Cellulose, Lignin	Pectin	Dietary Fiber	Crude Fiber
Fruits and vegetables				
Apples (peeled)	12	17	29	9
Cabbage	14	5	19	8
Carrots	9	19	28	6
Lettuce	17	4	21	12
Oranges (peeled)	4	12	16	3
Potatoes (peeled)	5	7	12	1
Squash	15	3	18	6
Grains (whole kernel)				
Whole barley	27	tr	27	7
Whole corn	13	tr	13	3
Whole oats	31	tr	31	13
Whole wheat	14	tr	14	3
Corn bran	60	tr	60	14
Wheat bran	45	tr	45	11
Rice bran	24	tr	24	13

*Grams per 100 grams dry matter.

Source: G.A. Spiller and S.G. Sorenson, "Dietary Fiber and Human Intestinal Microflora." In *Dietary Fiber: Proceedings of the Miles Symposium* (Nova Scotia, 1976).

are carried through the intestine and excreted. As a result, fecal material formed from high-fiber foods is greater in volume and weight than that from foods low in fiber. This water-absorbing property of fiber is called the *bulking effect*. Not only are the feces greater in volume, but they are softer and move through the intestinal tract faster so they are excreted easily without straining.

Several of the components of fiber can bind with other substances as they pass through the gastrointestinal tract. When fiber binds to a substance, the substance cannot be absorbed and passes out of the body with the fiber in the feces. Fiber can bind both macronutrients and micronutrients. This property of fiber is a blessing and a detriment. Fiber helps pull out toxic metals like lead and drugs from the body, but also increases the loss of valuable minerals like calcium, phosphorus, magnesium, iron, and zinc. For instance, less iron is absorbed from whole wheat bread than white even though the whole wheat might have more iron.(30) (As you will see in Chapter 8, grains contain other substances that bind metals, hindering their absorption.)

Unless the binding effect of fiber is temporary or the body can adapt, certain people might find this a problem. Those with low iron or calcium intakes, such as the elderly or vegetarians, or those who have an increased need for these minerals, such as pregnant women, might not be able to absorb sufficient amounts to meet their needs. These people should be careful if they are using bran to treat constipation or diverticular disease.

Many microorganisms inhabit the large intestine of humans. Normally, the ones that predominate are harmless because they have achieved a symbiotic relationship with their human host over centuries of evolution. Under some circumstances, however, pathogenic (harmful) microorganisms take over, causing disease.

Microorganisms feed on the material that passes through the intestines. Fiber is particularly important because it passes through the stomach and small intestine virtually intact. In the large intestine, the microorganisms break down some of the fiber for nourishment. The amount and type of fiber in the diet affects the type and growth of intestinal microorganisms. The by-products of these microorganisms determine the environment within the intestine. For example, *Lactobacillus acidophilus* is one of the harmless bacteria that inhabit the human intestinal tract. It converts lactose (milk sugar) to lactic acid. When lactose is bound to fiber in the upper intestine, it is carried to the lower intestine intact, where lactobacilli grow on it and produce lactic acid, making the environment within the colon acidic. This type of environment is hostile to certain pathogenic microorganisms. Thus the host benefits.

FIBER AND DISEASE

Based largely on epidemiological (population) data, low-fiber diets have been associated with the incidence of a number of noninfectious diseases. Although many of these conditions are unrelated, they can be grouped into three categories: disorders of the digestive tract, circulatory diseases, and metabolic diseases.(31)

Disorders of the Digestive Tract

The more refined the diet, the slower the feces move through the intestines. So food residues, low in fiber, remain in the colon for several days. The daily stool specimen of a rural African weighs over 450 grams and has a transit time of less than a day, while the average American, whose diet is low in fiber, may have a stool weight of 115 grams and a transit time of two or more days. A bowel movement every three to four days, while "regular," may not be healthy. Some researchers believe this is the reason behind a number of gastrointestinal problems.

The muscles of the intestinal wall are arranged so that the intestine is segmented. As food is digested, the contraction of the muscle in the first segment pushes the material being digested into the second segment, and so on.

Feces excreted by individuals on low-fiber diets tend to be small, dense, and hard (less moisture), compared to the large, soft feces excreted by those who consume high-fiber diets. The colon muscles must contract more to expel them. The layer of muscles in the walls of the colon thicken, due to the increased work required to force low-fiber feces through the lower intestine and out of the body (Figure 3–5). When the thickened walls contract, there is less space within the segment, particularly where the contracting segment and the next one meet. Pressure builds up within the colon similar to the pressure buildup that occurs in an inflated balloon if you attempt to squeeze all the air to one end. If the pressure becomes too great, the balloon bursts. The colon does not burst, but protrusions or "blowouts" of the colon lining may push through the overlying muscle. These protrusions, or diverticula, are part of the overall conditions called diverticulosis. If feces become trapped in these pockets, the diverticula become inflamed and result in diverticulitis.

Low-fiber diets are now believed to play a major role in the onset of diverticulosis. In addition, several researchers have reported successful treatment of diverticulitis with bran, which is high in dietary fiber. Fibers with the greatest bulking effect are most effective in preventing and treating diverticulosis.

A low-fiber diet is suggested as a contributing factor in the development of *appendicitis*. The initial problem is believed to be a blockage of the opening of the appendix into the intestine by a hardened mass of fecal material or by a spasm of the muscle in the wall of the appendix. Both could result from firm feces such as those formed when the diet is low in fiber. The obstruction raises the pressure high enough to allow invasion by bacteria. This theory is not

FIG. 3–5

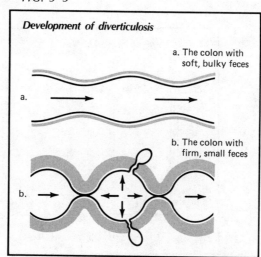

Development of diverticulosis

a. The colon with soft, bulky feces

a.

b. The colon with firm, small feces

b.

Source: From D.P. Burkitt, "Some Mechanical Effects of Fibre-Depleted Diets." In *Dietary Fiber: Proceedings of Miles Symposium* (Nova Scotia, 1976).

supported by statistics, which show the incidence of appendicitis in the United States decreasing by 40 percent from 1955 to 1975, while fiber intake during this period remained low.(31) It seems more likely that several other factors are involved.

The increases in pressure in the colon brought about by low fiber intakes might be linked to the development of hiatus hernia, varicose veins, deep vein thrombosis and hemorrhoids. In the case of hemorrhoids, the straining to excrete hard feces causes relaxation of the muscles surrounding the anus, the opening of the colon to the exterior. Once these muscles contract, they place pressure on the veins that drain the colon, preventing them from dilating. The veins are allowed to dilate only once the muscles relax. Repeated and prolonged straining allow the veins to dilate so much that hemorrhoids are formed (Figure 3–6).

Colon cancer is another disorder of the digestive tract that has been linked to low-fiber diets. Among adults who die of cancer, the death rate due to colon cancer is second only to that for lung cancer. The American male is six times more likely to develop cancer of the intestines than his counterpart in less developed nations.

It is far from clear what the relationship between fiber and colon cancer is. The rationale behind the association is that fiber might in some way protect the colon from excessive exposure to carcinogens in the diet or from intestinal microorganisms that produce carcinogens. A number of theories explain how this might work.

One speculation is that high intakes of fiber create an intestinal environment hostile to the growth of microorganisms which produce carcino-

FIG. 3–6

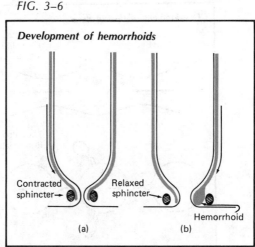

Development of hemorrhoids

Contracted sphincter→   Relaxed sphincter→   Hemorrhoid

(a)   (b)

Source: From D.P. Burkitt, "Some Mechanical Effects of Fibre-Depleted Diets." In Dietary Fiber: Proceedings of Miles Symposium (Nova Scotia, 1976).

gens. The second explanation for fiber's possible protective effects suggests that increased fiber causes food residues to move through the colon faster, reducing the time the tissue is exposed to any carcinogens in the feces. Another theory holds that a diet high in fiber is lower in substances used by microorganisms to make carcinogens. Finally, since fiber increases the water content of the feces, the concentration of any carcinogen would be diluted. Obviously, much more research is needed to determine whether fiber does offer any protection against colon cancer.

Heart Disease

The major cause of heart disease is atherosclerosis, a condition in which the coronary arteries (those that provide blood to the heart) become clogged with fatty deposits rich in cholesterol. As a result, the heart is not nourished well and weakens. Cholesterol is a waxy, fatlike substance found in the diet as well as made in the body. The cause of atherosclerosis is not known, but the disease occurs more frequently in people with high levels of cholesterol in their blood. There is substantial evidence that diets rich in animal fats and cholesterol raise the risk of developing atherosclerosis and ensuing heart disease (see Chapter 4).

Few records exist of heart disease in Westernized nations prior to the end of the nineteenth century, when roller-milling of grains replaced the earlier fiber-preserving process of stone grinding. As mentioned earlier, this could be the result of poorly kept records. It could also result from a reduction in the fiber content of diets. Data suggest that high intakes of fiber provide some protection against atherosclerosis. The first indication came when researchers, working with rabbits, observed that those fed a diet containing little or no fiber developed fatty deposits in their coronary arteries, whereas the rabbits fed diets containing large amounts of alfalfa (rich in fiber) had much smaller or no fatty deposits in their arteries. Further studies revealed that experimental animals fed high levels of fiber had low levels of cholesterol in their blood and carcasses.

The prevalence of heart disease in humans was investigated with 1,154 age-matched Irish brothers, half of whom lived in Ireland and half in Boston.(32) Only 29 percent of all deaths of the men in Ireland were from heart disease, compared to 42 percent of the deaths of the Americans. The brothers had similar blood cholesterol levels, even though the Irish diet is higher in total fat and animal fats. The brothers consumed similar amounts of sugar, protein, cholesterol, and alcohol, and had similar cigarette habits. Irish brothers ate more starch than the Americans. As a nation, the Irish consume more potatoes and cereal products than Americans, but Americans consume more vegetables and fruit.

Some researchers propose that the different incidence of heart disease in this study was due to the higher intake of fiber among the Irish. But how can fiber possibly lower the cholesterol levels in arteries? The answer involves the way cholesterol is eliminated from the body. The main route for getting rid of cholesterol is through bile secreted into the intestine. Bile is synthesized from cholesterol in the liver and stored in the gall bladder. It is secreted into the small intestine, where it helps digest fats. Once bile has finished its task in the intestine, most of it is reabsorbed and returned to the liver. Fiber can bind some of the constituents of bile (bile salts), forcing them to pass out of the body in the feces. With more fiber in the diet, more bile salts are excreted. Since fewer bile salts are returned to the liver, more have to be synthesized from available cholesterol (Figure 3–7). Also, fiber not only draws on the cholesterol from the liver, but binds some of the cholesterol from the diet, dragging it out with the feces. In this way, fiber plays both a direct and an indirect role in ridding the body of cholesterol.

Researchers do not know if fiber's ability to bind cholesterol and bile salts helps prevent or reverse atherosclerosis. They have conducted a few studies to determine the effect of increasing fiber intake on blood cholesterol of humans. Results indicate that some fibers are better able to reduce blood cholesterol than others.(33) Fibers in fruits (pectin) and cereals (hemicellulose) have this ability; bran does not. More research is needed to determine whether increasing consumption of fiber offers protection against heart disease and if so, which fiber sources are most effective.

FIG. 3–7

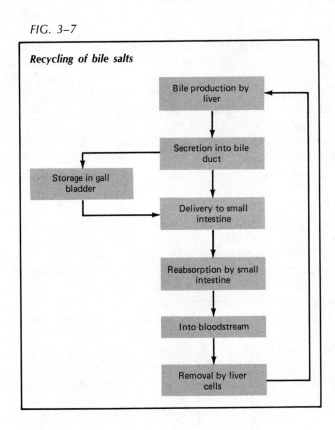

72   CARBOHYDRATES

Low-fiber diets are associated with higher rates of diabetes and obesity.(31) Some nutritionists propose that fiber, by binding the macronutrients and making them unabsorbable, decreases the kcalories available from food, a benefit to those on weight-control diets. A recent study,(34) however, showed that increasing fiber to 38 grams per day, about twice the amount usually consumed in Western societies, only increased the loss of energy in the feces by 40 to 80 kcalories per day. This amount of energy is equivalent to a piece of bread and will hardly be the deciding factor in the success of a reducing diet. High-fiber foods do provide some bonuses for weight watchers because they can replace high kcalorie foods. They also take longer to chew, helping to slow down food intake and to promote feelings of fullness. A graphic summary of the ways by which fiber is hypothesized to prevent disease is presented in Figure 3–8.

FIG. 3–8

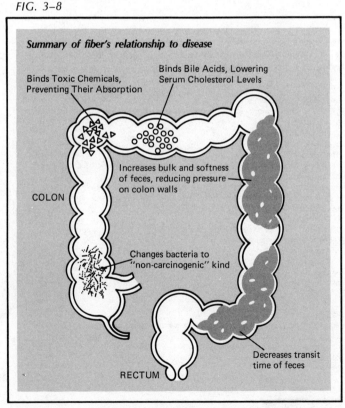

Source: R.D. Smith, "Checking Out the Fiber Fad," *The Sciences* (March/April 1976), p. 27.

All foods of plant origin contain fiber, but in varying amounts. Whole grain cereals are a major source of dietary fiber, but most fiber is lost in the milling process, when portions of the wheat are removed. The parts of a kernel of wheat and the nutrients contained in each are presented in Figure 3–9. Millers remove the germ of grain because it contains fat, which limits the amount of time the food can be kept before developing off flavors. White flour has also had the bran of the wheat removed, resulting in a lower fiber content than whole wheat flour.

The cell walls of foods differ in how easy they are to digest. Those of onions and bran are much more difficult to break down than those of other vegetables. In general, the cell walls of cereals are the hardest to digest, followed by those of vegetables and fruits. Some portions of foods high in fiber are discarded by the consumer. Pectin is present in most fruits and berries such as apples, citrus fruits, and those used in making jellies. In citrus fruits, most of the pectin is in the white inner rind and connective tissue, which is not ordinarily eaten and is not present in juice.

FIG. 3–9

A cross section of a kernel of wheat and the nutrients in each of the three parts—endosperm, bran, and germ

ENDOSPERM
    . . . about 83% of the kernel
Source of white flour. Of the nutrients in the whole kernel the endosperm contains about:
       70–75% of the protein
         43% of the pantothenic acid
         32% of the riboflavin   } B-complex
         12% of the niacin   vitamins
          6% of the pyridoxine
          3% of the thiamin
Enriched flour products contain added quantities of riboflavin, niacin and thiamin, plus iron, in amounts equal to or exceeding whole wheat—according to a formula established on the basis of popular need of those nutrients.
 BRAN. . . about 14½% of the kernel
Included in whole wheat flour. Of the nutrients in whole wheat, the bran, in addition to indigestible cellulose material contains about:
         86% of the niacin
         73% of the pyridoxine
         50% of the pantothenic acid
         42% of the riboflavin
         33% of the thiamin
         19% of the protein
 GERM. . . about 2½% of the kernel
The embryo or sprouting section of the seed, usually separated because it contains fat which limits the keeping quality of flours. Available separately as human food. Of the nutrients in whole wheat, the germ contains about:
         64% of the thiamin
         26% of the riboflavin
         21% of the pyridoxine
          8% of the protein
          7% of the pantothenic acid
          2% of the niacin

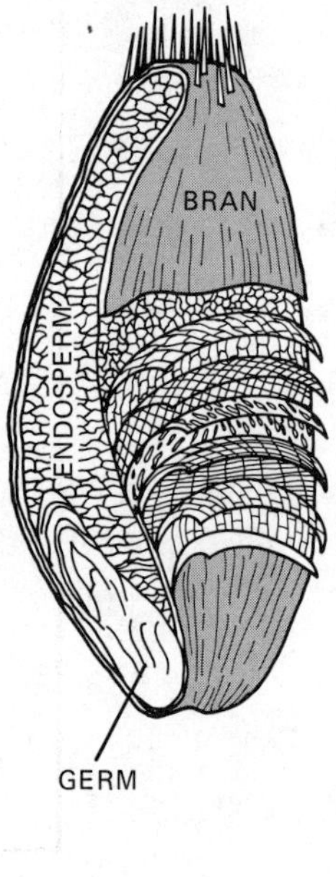

BRAN

ENDOSPERM

GERM

Source: Kansas Wheat Commission.

No recommended dietary allowance has been set for fiber mainly because there are no data indicating how much would be adequate or optimal. Rural black populations in Africa that eat large amounts of vegetable products obtain 50 grams or more of fiber per day. These groups seem to be free from some of the diseases suffered by Western, industrialized populations that consume about 20 grams of fiber per day.(35) Increasing intake to 30 to 60 grams might be both possible and "protective" for Western populations.(36)

The problem with this suggestion is that obtaining the right combinations of the different fibers could be as important as the total intake. Very little is known about the different types of fibers consumed by various groups and how they relate to the incidence of disease. For instance, the African tribes studied by Burkitt, who showed such a low incidence of the disorders mentioned here, derive most of their fiber from corn and legumes. Americans obtain most of their fiber from wheat, potatoes, fruits, and vegetables. Whether an increase in bran and whole grains in the American diet will lead to a reduction of disease rates remains to be seen.(37)

Since the different types of fiber have different effects, you should try to vary your sources. Whole grain cereals, rich in cellulose, should not be emphasized over fruits and vegetables, rich in pectin, or vice versa. If you increase consumption of whole grains, vegetables, and fruits at the expense of foods rich in fat and sugar, you will reduce the kcalorie value of your diet. Substituting beans, fruits, and vegetables for some of the meat and dairy products will also reduce intake of cholesterol. Remember, though, that simply substituting whole for milled grains will not affect how much cholesterol you consume, though it could affect how much you excrete because of fiber's binding effect on cholesterol.

For the time being, the best advice is to consume a wide variety of fiber-rich foods such as products made from coarsely ground whole grains and fruits and vegetables (keeping the edible skins and peels on but washing them before eating). It is not necessary to buy special high-fiber foods like bran in order to increase the amount of fiber in the diet. Changing to whole wheat or cracked wheat bread, selecting cereals high in fiber, and incorporating more fruits and vegetables in daily meals will automatically increase fiber intake. Certain fibers, such as bran and other bulk producers, should not be eaten dry because they can obstruct the esophagus.(38) Large amounts of bran can also temporarily increase flatulence (intestinal gas).

A number of processing and preparation practices affect the composition and quantity of fiber in food. Grinding fiber into fine particles reduces its effects on the gastrointestinal tract. There are some exceptions to this, such as *tofu* (bean curd). Overcooking foods can increase the proportion of fiber to other food components, since the other components might be lost. Certain cooking reactions cause amino acids and carbohydrates to condense into fiberlike chains, so that toasting a piece of white bread can actually increase its fiber content.(29)

You should be cautious when making dramatic increases in fiber intake, since little is known about the effects of excessive intakes—or, for that matter, how much constitutes an excess.

REFERENCES

1. R.M. Pangborn, "Relative Taste Intensities of Selected Sugars and Organic Acids," *Food Science* 28(1963):726.

2. A.V. Cardello, D. Hunt, and B. Mann, "Relative Sweetness of Fructose and Sucrose in Model Solutions, Lemon Beverages and White Cake," *Journal of Food Science* 44(1979):748–51.

3. J.J. Wurtman and R.J. Wurtman, "Sucrose Consumption Early in Life Fails to Modify the Appetite of Adult Rats for Sweet Foods," *Science* 205 (July 20, 1979):321–22.

4. H.R. Moskowitz, "The Psychology of Sweetness," In *Sugars in Nutrition,* edited by H.L. Sipple and K.W. McNutt. (New York: Academic Press, 1974), pp. 37–64.

5. W.R. Aykroyd, "Sugar in History." In *Sugars in Nutrition,* edited by H.L. Sipple and K.W. McNutt (New York: Academic Press, 1974), pp. 3–9.

6. S.A. Miller, "Sugar and Caries: Regulation of a Nonmortal Hazard," *Food Technology,* January 1980, pp. 77–80.

7. The Institute of Food Technologists, Expert Panel on Food Safety and Nutrition, "Sugars and Nutritive Sweeteners in Processed Foods, A Scientific Status Summary," *Food Technology,* May 1979, pp. 101–105.

8. "Confectionary Ingredients." From *Confectionary Facts,* National Confectioners Association, National Candy Wholesalers Association, and Retail Confectioners International, pp. 9–12.

9. S.R. Kruglicoff de Dennis, "Metabolic Effects of Saccharin Ingestion." In *First International Sugar Research Conference, The International Sugar Research Foundation,* March 1970, pp. 15–28.

10. "Sugar, How Sweet It Is—And Isn't," *FDA Consumer,* February 1980, pp. 21–23.

11. L. Page and B. Friend, "Level of Use of Sugars in the United States." In *Sugars in Nutrition,* edited by H.L. Sipple and K.W. McNutt (New York: Academic Press, 1974), pp. 93–107.

12. F.J. Stare, "Role of Sugar in Modern Nutrition." In "Sugar in the Diet of Man," edited by F.J. Stare, *World Review of Nutrition and Dietetics* 22 (1975):239–47.

13. E.M. Hamilton and E. Whitney, *Nutrition: Concepts and Controversies* (St. Paul, Minn.: West, 1979).

14. E.L. Bierman, "Carbohydrates, Sucrose, and Human Disease," *American Journal of Clinical Nutrition* 32 (1979): 2712–22.

15. K.M. West, *Epidemiology of Diabetes and Its Vascular Lesions* (New York: Elsevier, 1978), pp. 224–74.

16. T. S. Danowski, S. Nolan, and T. Stephan, "Obesity." In "Sugar in the Diet of Man," edited by F.J. Stare, *World Review of Nutrition and Dietetics* 22 (1975): 270–79.

17. F. Grande, "Sugar and Cardiovascular Disease." In "Sugar in the Diet of Man," edited by F.J. Stare, *World Review of Nutrition and Dietetics* 22 (1975): 248–69.

18. National Commission on Diabetics, *The Long-Range Plan to Combat Diabetes* (Washington, D.C.: USDHEW, DHEW Publ. No. 76–1018, Vol. 1, 1975).

19. A.M. Cohen, "High Sucrose Intake as a Factor in the Development of Diabetes and Its Vascular Complications." In *Sugar in Diet, Diabetes, and Heart Disease, Hearing before the Select Committee on Nutrition and Human Needs of the U.S. Senate,* 1973, pp. 167–198.

20. E.L. Bierman and R. Nelson, "Carbohydrate, Diabetes, and Blood Lipids." In "Sugar in the Diet of Man," edited by F.J. Stare, *World Review of Nutrition and Dietetics* 22 (1975): 280–87.

21. T. S. Danowski, S. Nolan, and T. Stephan, "Hypoglycemia." In "Sugar in the Diet of Man," edited by F.J. Stare, *World Review of Nutrition and Dietetics* 22 (1975): 288–303.

22. *Evaluation of the Health Aspects of Sucrose as a Food Ingredient,* Federation of American Societies for Experimental Biology. Prepared for the Food and Drug Administration, 1976.

23. S.B. Finn and R.B. Glass, "Sugar and Dental Decay." In "Sugar in the Diet of Man," edited by F.J. Stare, *World Review of Nutrition and Dietetics* 22 (1975): 304–26.

24. M. C. Alfano, "Nutrition, Sweeteners, and Dental Caries," *Food Technology,* January 1980, pp. 70–74.

25. G.R. Howe, J.D. Burch, and A.B. Miller, "Artificial Sweeteners and Human Bladder Cancer," *Lancet,* September 17, 1977, pp. 578–81.

26. *HEW News,* p. 79–40, December 20, 1979.

27. J. Scala, "Fiber: The Forgotten Nutrient," *Food Technology* 28 (1974):34–36.

28. D.P. Burkitt, "Economic Development—Not All Bonus," *Nutrition Today,* January–February 1976, pp. 6–13.

29. P.J. Van Soest, "What Is Fiber?" *The Professional Nutritionist,* fall 1978, pp. 7–10.

30. E.M. Widdowson and R.A. McCance, "Iron Exchanges of Adults on White and Brown Bread Diets," *Lancet* 1 (1942): 588.

31. "The Role of Fiber in the Diet," *Dairy Council Digest*, January–February 1975.

32. J. Brown et al., "Nutritional and Epidemiological Factors Related to Heart Disease," *World Review of Nutrition and Dietetics* 12 (1970): 1–42.

33. "Lower Cholesterol from High-Fiber Bread," *Agricultural Research* 27 (1978):11.

34. D.A.T. Southgate et al. "Metabolic Responses in Dietary Supplements of Bran," *Metabolism* 25 (1976): 1129–35.

35. S. Bingham, J.H. Cummings, and N.I. McNeil, "Intakes and Sources of Dietary Fiber in the British Population," *American Journal of Clinical Nutrition* 32 (1979): 1313–19.

36. A.I. Mendeloff, "Dietary Fiber and Human Health," *New England Journal of Medicine* 297 (1977): 811–14.

37. K. McNutt, "Perspective—Fiber," *Journal of Nutrition Education* 8 (1976): 150–52.

38. "Dietary Fiber? The Medical Profession Demurs," *Nutrition Today*, January–February 1976, p. 14.

Fats

4

A recent TV commercial featured a slice of "new improved" cheese strutting through a woman's patio, proudly announcing that it is low in fat. The woman naturally reacts with surprise—not because the cheese has arms and legs and is speaking, but because it has less fat and fewer kcalories than her regular brand. Another commercial shows a tub of margarine yapping about the hazards of consuming butter. The producers of both commercials, as well as those of numerous other ads, are taking advantage of the American consumer's concern over fats in the diet. Though there has been much publicity about fats and cholesterol in recent years, and much confusion, the subject is not as difficult to understand as it first appears.

THE STRUCTURE OF FATS

Fats and fatlike substances are classified under the general term lipids. They are defined as substances that are insoluble in water but soluble in fat solvents like ether, acetone, and chloroform. Most fat in the diet is in the form of triglycerides. A triglyceride is a compound composed of one glycerol molecule and three fatty acids (Figure 4–1).

Glycerol, a kind of alcohol, forms the backbone of the triglyceride. Extending from this backbone are three fatty acids, so that the entire configuration when drawn resembles a capital letter E. Triglycerides, like carbohydrates, are composed of carbon, hydrogen, and oxygen. Some substances derived from petroleum oil are not true fats—for example, lubricating oil and mineral oil. These substances contain carbon and hydrogen but no oxygen and can be harmful to humans because they interfere with the absorption of nutrients. Attached to the glycerol can be any combination of fatty acids, usually a mixture

FIG. 4-1

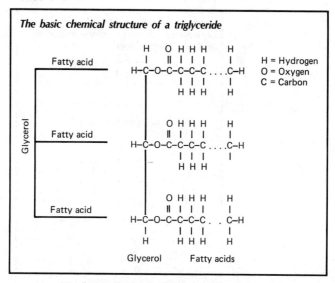

The basic chemical structure of a triglyceride

Glycerol

Fatty acid

Fatty acid

Fatty acid

H = Hydrogen
O = Oxygen
C = Carbon

Glycerol   Fatty acids

of two or three different types. The type and arrangement of the fatty acids identify a particular triglyceride. A triglyceride composed of fatty acids A, B, and C may be liquid at room temperature, whereas one composed of fatty acids A, A, and C may be solid.

Compared to carbohydrates and proteins, fats in nature have fewer oxygens to the number of carbons and hydrogens, so more occasions exist for adding oxygens when fats are broken down in the body, producing more usable energy per gram than either carbohydrates or protein (see Chapter 6).

Structurally, a fatty acid is a series of carbons strung out into chains varying both in length and in the way the carbons are connected or bonded together. The length ranges anywhere from short (2 to 6 carbons), to medium (8 to 12 carbons), to long (16 to 20 carbons). The carbons in the fatty acid chain bond in a number of ways. Based on the bonding arrangement, fatty acids fit into one of three groups: saturated, monounsaturated, and polyunsaturated. If you look at the carbons within the fatty acid chain, you see many hydrogens attached. If a fatty acid has all links in the carbon chain bound to hydrogen, it is called saturated (Figure 4-2). In a saturated fatty acid each carbon is attached to two hydrogens (the end carbon is an exception and is not considered within the chain). When two adjacent carbons are missing a hydrogen, they each share their free bond, forming a double bond. An unsaturated fatty acid will have one or more such double bonds in the carbon chain. If there is only one double bond, the fatty acid is monounsaturated; with more than one double bond, a polyunsaturated fatty acid (sometimes written PUFA) is formed (Figure 4-2). If one or more PUFA is attached to a triglyceride, the fat itself becomes polyunsaturated.

Many of the different physical properties of fats are determined by the degree of saturation of their fatty acids. Most saturated fats are solid at room

FIG. 4-2

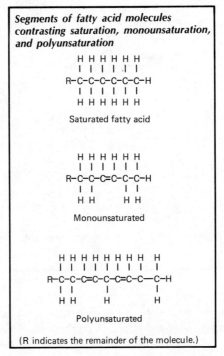

Segments of fatty acid molecules contrasting saturation, monounsaturation, and polyunsaturation

Saturated fatty acid

Monounsaturated

Polyunsaturated

(R indicates the remainder of the molecule.)

temperature, whereas polyunsaturated fats are usually liquid. The area between the double bonds of a polyunsaturated fat is weak and susceptible to destruction by oxidation. (This is why oils become rancid more rapidly than solid fats and why refrigerating an oil will retard this process.) Food manufacturers convert unsaturated oils into saturated fats in a process called hydrogenation. During this process, the chains of a polyunsaturated fat are bombarded with hydrogens, converting some or all of the double bonds, into single ones (Figure 4–3). Margarines and vegetable shortenings are products of hydrogenation. The more double bonds that are broken in this manner, the more saturated and more solid the fat becomes so that, in general, soft margarines are less hydrogenated than the stick margarines.

FIG. 4-3

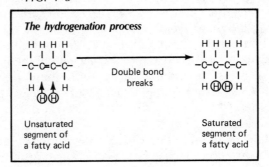

The hydrogenation process

Double bond breaks

Unsaturated segment of a fatty acid

Saturated segment of a fatty acid

Cholesterol

Cholesterol comes from fat but is chemically more complex than triglycerides. It can be considered a cross between an alcohol and a fat, although technically it is related to a family of compounds called sterols. Cholesterol is composed of scaly crystals that are sparkling white and soapy to the touch.

Lately diets high in cholesterol have taken the blame for being one of the primary factors involved in the development of heart disease (Table 4–1). The

TABLE 4–1 **Fatty Acid Composition of Selected Foods**

Food	Total Fat (%)	Fatty Acids%*		
		Saturated	Monounsaturated	Polyunsaturated
Salad and cooking oils				
Safflower	100	10	13	74
Sunflower	100	11	14	70
Corn	100	13	26	55
Cottonseed	100	23	17	54
Soybean	100	14	25	50
Sesame	100	14	38	42
Peanut	100	18	47	29
Olive	100	11	76	7
Coconut	100	80	5	1
Vegetable fats, shortening	100	23	23	6–23
Table spreads				
Margarine, first ingredient on label				
Safflower (liquid)—tub	80	11	18	48
Corn oil (liquid)—tub	80	14	26	38
Corn oil (liquid)—stick	80	15	33	29
Partially hardened or hydrogenated fat	80	17	44	14
Butter	81	46	27	2
Animal fats				
Poultry	100	30	40	20
Beef, lamb, pork	100	45	44	2–6
Fish, raw				
Salmon	9	2	2	4
Tuna	5	2	1	2
Mackerel	13	5	3	4
Herring, Pacific	13	4	2	3
Nuts				
Walnuts, English	64	4	10	40
Walnuts, black	60	4	21	28
Brazil	67	13	32	17
Peanuts or peanut butter	51	9	25	14
Pecan	65	4–6	33–48	9–24
Egg yolk	31	10	13	2
Avocado	16	3	7	2

*Total is not expected to equal "total fat."

Source: *Fats in Food and Diet*. Agriculture Information Bulletin No. 362. Washington, D.C.: U.S. Department of Agriculture, 1974.

case against cholesterol is often too simply stated. In fact, it serves a number of essential functions in the body. It is used to produce bile and several hormones including testosterone, the regulator of sexual development in males. Cholesterol is a precursor of vitamin D and a structural component of the brain and of the sheath or coating of nerves. As a component of cell membranes, it plays a large role in determining what substances pass through the cell wall. Present in the outer layer of skin, cholesterol helps prevent water from soaking through your hand when you place it in a pan of water and it slows water evaporation from the skin.(1)

Cholesterol is not only available from the diet; it is also synthesized by all tissues of the body. Less than half of the cholesterol in the blood comes from the diet, even when a high-cholesterol diet is consumed. Rich dietary sources include liver, eggs, and foods high in saturated fats (Table 4–2). Cholesterol is found only in animal products.

In certain people, cholesterol accumulates in tissues and blood vessels leading to the heart, resulting in heart disease. This has led researchers to suspect that high levels of cholesterol in the diet may increase the chances of cholesterol accumulation in the arteries. The problem is that some individuals have very low cholesterol intakes, yet they have high cholesterol levels in their blood. Others have high intakes, yet have low blood levels. In population groups, however, there is a strong correlation between high blood levels and intakes of cholesterol or saturated fats. It is because of this strong correlation that so much research has focused on the relationship of heart disease to cholesterol and dietary fat. (We will discuss many of the findings and unsolved questions in the section on atherosclerosis.)

TABLE 4–2 **High Cholesterol Foods**

Food	Portion	Cholesterol Content (in milligrams)
EGGS		
Chicken	1 large	250
Roe	4 oz.	400
ORGAN MEATS		
Brains	4 oz.	225
Heart	4 oz.	310
Kidney	4 oz.	910
Liver: beef, calf,		
pork, lamb	4 oz.	500
chicken	2 oz.	420
Sweetbread	4 oz.	525
SHELLFISH		
Clams	1 cup	110
Crabmeat (fresh)	1 cup	125
Lobster	1 cup	120
Oysters	1 cup	120
Shrimp	4 oz.	170

Source: Adapted from J. Mayer, *Fats, Diet and Your Heart* (New York: Newspaperbooks, 1976).

FAT DIGESTION

Fat digestion begins in the stomach, where churning action and chemicals separate the fat from other nutrients. Carbohydrates and proteins are digested first and leave the stomach more quickly than fats. This is why fats make you feel full longer; they are the last nutrients to leave the stomach and enter the intestine.

Unlike carbohydrates and proteins, fats, which are not soluble in water, tend to float on the surface—they behave like the oil in a vinegar and oil salad dressing that is left standing in a bottle. In order to be absorbed, fat must be broken down into tiny particles so that digestive enzymes will have a greater surface area on which to work. The substances that break up the fat are called bile salts. They are made in the liver, then stored in the gall bladder until needed. Once fat passes from the stomach into the small intestine, the gall bladder is stimulated to pour bile, containing bile salts, into the intestine. These salts not only break up the fat into tiny particles, but keep the particles separated. Lipase, a fat-splitting enzyme secreted by the pancreas, then attacks the fat particles. It removes the outer two fatty acids from triglycerides, leaving one center fatty acid attached to the glycerol. The result is free fatty acids and a fatty acid attached to a glycerol (called a monoglyceride). Occasionally only one of the outer fatty acids is removed, in which case one free fatty acid is formed and the glycerol is left with two fatty acids attached (a diglyceride). The end products of fat digestion are mainly free fatty acids and monoglycerides with a few diglycerides. Bile salts, after breaking up the fat, remain attached to it until they reach the intestinal wall near the site of absorption. Both the fat and the bile salts are absorbed through the wall, but the bile salts are recycled back to the liver.

Once past the intestinal wall, the length of the fatty acid chain determines what happens next. Short- and medium-chain fatty acids separated from their glycerol backbone enter the bloodstream and adhere to proteins, forming a substance called lipoprotein. Unlike free fatty acids, lipoproteins are soluble in blood. The glycerol, already water-soluble, also enters the bloodstream. Longer-chain fatty acids are unable to pass intact into the blood. Instead, they are packaged as minuscule droplets coated with a thin layer of protein. This package, a special type of lipoprotein called a chylomicron, is water-soluble and enters the lymphatic system, an alternate circulatory system. Later the chylomicrons will enter the bloodstream. The lipoprotein packages that carry the fat through the blood have been the subject of much debate. These fat-protein complexes are classified according to density. The two most controversial are high-density and low-density lipoproteins. (We will discuss them in more detail in the section on atherosclerosis.)

Once digested and absorbed, fats can go in one of three directions. They can be broken down and used as energy; they can combine with carbohydrates and proteins to form body components; or they can be stored in fat cells. In order to be stored in fat cells, the fatty acids circulating in the blood must be

FIG. 4–4

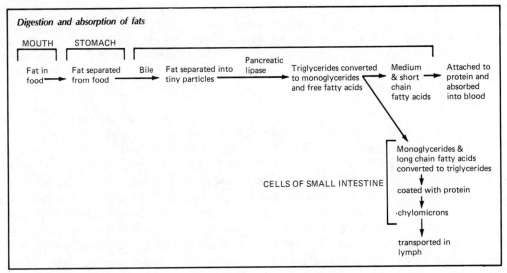

reattached to the glycerol molecule to re-form triglycerides. The triglyceride that is finally deposited in the adipose cell may have different fatty acids than the triglyceride that was ingested through food. Figure 4–4 outlines the process of fat digestion, absorption, and utilization.

FUNCTION OF FATS

In 1929 an experiment conducted on young rats revealed that a diet totally free of fat led to poor health and eventual death. The animals experienced such severe complications as delayed growth, difficulty in reproducing, decreased resistance to a number of stresses, scaly skin, hair loss, and death from kidney failure. Not only health, but survival itself depended on a dietary source of fat. Later research revealed that all these symptoms could be prevented by the addition of a polyunsaturated fat called linoleic acid to the diet.

Linoleic acid is an essential fatty acid; that is, it cannot be made by the body and must be obtained through food. Actually there exists a family of essential fatty acids. Along with linoleic acid which has two double bonds, there is linolenic acid with three and arachidonic with four. Arachidonic can be made in the body from linoleic acid when the need arises, so of these two fatty acids, linoleic is essential since it cannot be synthesized. Linolenic acid cannot be synthesized from linoleic acid and there are some functions that it performs which cannot be performed by linoleic acid. This certainly indicates that some small amount of linolenic acid must be provided by the diet and that technically it should also be considered essential. Researchers, however, are not sure whether linolenic acid deficiency symptoms have ever been exhibited so there is some disagreement about whether linolenic acid should be classified as a dietary essential.

Both linoleic and linolenic acids are polyunsaturated. The body can manufacture other fatty acids from them provided these two are available from the diet. Since the best sources of both these fatty acids are vegetable oils (corn, peanut, cottonseed, soybean, and safflower), you do not have to eat animal products in order to obtain them.

Despite the bad press they have received lately, fats do have some important functions in the body, as the researchers conducting the 1929 experiment discovered. The primary function of fat is to act as a long-term energy reserve. Because they have less water than glycogen (the storage form of carbohydrate), fats are a concentrated source of energy, an advantage for storage purposes. They can provide energy for all tissues except those of the brain, lungs, and nerves. In fact, the heart muscle relies exclusively on fats for energy. A few companies have capitalized on the fact that fat is a concentrated source of energy. One example is the product Energol, advertised as a special formulation providing strength, energy, and endurance. The "formulation," however, turns out to be simply three different vegetable oils.

Many body tissues such as the brain, muscle, bone marrow, and cell membranes, have portions composed of fats. In storage, fats provide a padding for body organs such as muscles and mammary glands. The subcutaneous fat (fat under the skin) acts as insulation against the environment. Certain vitamins (A, D, E, and K) are only soluble in fatty substances and are present in the fat portions of foods. They must also be incorporated into a tiny droplet containing fat before they can be absorbed from the intestine. The essential fatty acids are present along with other fats in the fatty portions of foods as well. Thus, the primary function of fat is to serve as an energy source or long-term energy reserve. Secondary functions include insulating and padding for body organs, carrying fat-soluble vitamins, providing essential fatty acids, serving as components of body tissue, and increasing the flavor and satiety value of food.

Fats are considered the bane of many a dieter. Because they provide more kcalories per gram than carbohydrates or proteins, their intake should be moderated on a weight-reduction program. Fats, however, are digested more slowly than either carbohydrates and proteins and tend to give a feeling of satiety for a longer period of time. In addition, fat makes food taste good, partly because the flavor components of food are dissolved in it. One of the many factors by which meats are graded is fat content. The more marbling (tiny streaks of fat in the lean) a steak has, the higher grade it receives because the marbling produces a tastier, more tender meat. Grading changes in recent years have allowed meats with less marbling to bear the higher grades. Some consumer groups, concerned about the high levels of fat in the American diet, are asking for further changes in the method of grading, since many people assume that a higher-grade meat is automatically better.

Although humans need fat in their diets, the amount necessary for good health is currently a subject of debate. Forty percent or more of the total kcalories in the American diet come from fat. Figure 4–5 shows the trend in fat consumption since the turn of the century as estimated by "disappearance data." Such data is calculated by subtracting from the quantity of food produced in the United States, the food exported and used for purposes other than feeding humans. The remainder is considered to have "disappeared" into civilian consumption. There were three periods during this century when fat levels increased (Figure 4–5):(1) in the 1920s, (2) in the late 1930s and 1940s, and (3) in the late 1960s and early 1970s. (2) From 1972 to 1975 there was a decrease in fat consumption. This trend has been confirmed by data from the most recent nationwide food consumption survey in which data about food intake were collected directly from individuals. This survey showed that average fat intakes decreased for all age groups between 1965 and 1977. For almost half of these groups the decrease was about 20 percent. (3) Nutritionists are still unclear as to why fat consumption has decreased since 1972, although public health campaigns aimed at lowering fat and total kcalorie intake may be a factor.

Ninety percent of the fats in the American diet come from three main sources: fats and oils; meats, poultry, and fish; and dairy products. Most of the fat consumed still comes from animal sources, although vegetable sources are providing an increasingly larger share (Figure 4–5). Salad and cooking oils have increased in popularity both for home use and within the fast food industry for frying potatoes, chicken, and fish. Use of margarine has exceeded that of butter since the mid-1950s. Consumption of both margarine and butter has declined,

FIG. 4–5

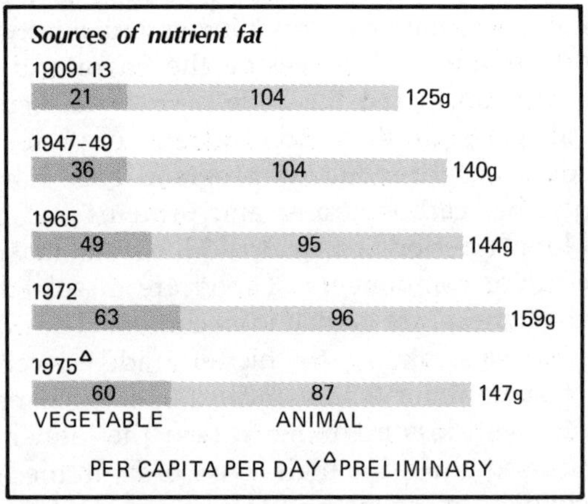

Sources of nutrient fat

1909–13
21 104 125g

1947–49
36 104 140g

1965
49 95 144g

1972
63 96 159g

1975△
60 87 147g
VEGETABLE ANIMAL

PER CAPITA PER DAY△PRELIMINARY

Source: C. Chandler and R. Marston, "Fat in the U.S. Diet," CFEI, USDA, May–August, 1979.

possibly due to the decrease in consumption of foods like bread and potatoes, with which they are often served. Shortening has replaced lard in many households.

In the meat, poultry, and fish group, beef consumption has increased, supplying a larger amount of fat to the diet. Pork consumption has dropped, but it is still the major fat supplier from the meat group due to its high fat content. It supplies almost one-half the total amount of fat from this group. Poultry, because it is low in fat, has increased very little as a supplier of fat to the diet. In the dairy group, whole milk and cream are providing a smaller share of fat, though they still contribute quite a lot; cheese consumption is increasing, and ice cream and frozen desserts are holding their own.(2) Overall, the proportion of kcalories from fat in the diet is much higher today than 70 years ago. This is due to the increased consumption of fats and to the decreased consumption of carbohydrate foods derived from grain products (Table 4–3). The shift toward a decrease in fat intake that has occurred since the early 1970s is due to decreases in home use of fats, oils, and milk products. Use of fatty pork products (such as bacon) and luncheon meats also decreased.(2)

Food Sources of Fats

Most foods contain some amount of fat unless it has been intentionally removed, as in skimmed milk products. The amount and type of fat, however, will vary. Animal products are higher in saturated fats, while polyunsaturated fats are present in greater amounts in vegetable products. The quantity of animal fat varies with each species, the highest content being in beef, pork, and lamb.

TABLE 4–3 Fat in the U.S. Diet from Animal and Vegetable Sources, Selected Years

	Animal Sources					Vegetable Sources				
Year	Meat, poultry, fish	Eggs	Dairy products ex. butter	Butter, lard, edible beef	Total* per capita	Other fats and oils	Dry beans, peas, nuts, soy products	Flour and cereal products	Other foods	Total* per capita
1909–13	46.4g	4.8g	18.6g	33.8g	103.5g	12.3g	2.4g	4.8g	1.8g	21.3g
1947–49	46.8	6.0	24.5	27.4	104.8	25.1	4.7	2.6	3.3	35.8
1965	48.4	5.1	21.2	20.4	95.1	38.2	5.5	2.1	3.2	49.0
1972	55.3	5.0	19.6	15.7	95.6	51.5	5.8	2.1	3.6	63.0
1975†	50.2	4.4	19.4	12.8	86.8	49.6	5.4	2.1	3.2	60.3

*Components may not add to total due to rounding.
†Preliminary.

Source: C. Chandler and R. Marston, "Fat in the U.S. Diet," CFEI, USDA, May–August, 1979.

Aside from differences in total fat content, the percentage of saturated fat in animal products varies. Recent research indicates that the proportion of saturated and polyunsaturated fat in animal products can be altered by varying the fat composition of the feed given the animal.

If you are interested in cutting down on kcalories, you should eliminate the foods that are richest in fats first. Instead of beef or pork, try substituting chicken, turkey, or fish. Switch to skim milk and part-skim dairy products and uncreamed cottage cheese; try using less margarine, butter, and oils. An advertisement from the Potato Board, while obviously focusing on the merits of the potato, illustrates the point (Figure 4–6).

FIG. 4–6

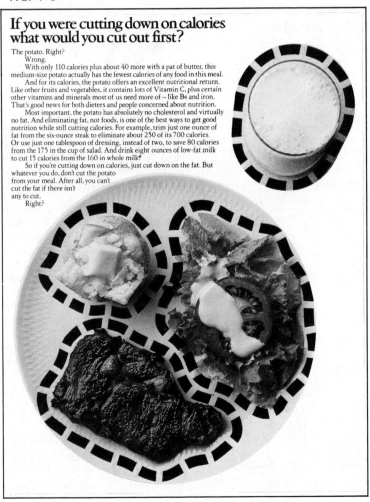

If you were cutting down on calories what would you cut out first?

The potato. Right?
   Wrong.
   With only 110 calories plus about 40 more with a pat of butter, this medium-size potato actually has the fewest calories of any food in this meal.
   And for its calories, the potato offers an excellent nutritional return. Like other fruits and vegetables, it contains lots of Vitamin C, plus certain other vitamins and minerals most of us need more of — like B6 and iron. That's good news for both dieters and people concerned about nutrition.
   Most important, the potato has absolutely no cholesterol and virtually no fat. And eliminating fat, not foods, is one of the best ways to get good nutrition while still cutting calories. For example, trim just one ounce of fat from the six-ounce steak to eliminate about 250 of its 700 calories. Or use just one tablespoon of dressing, instead of two, to save 80 calories from the 175 in the cup of salad. And drink eight ounces of low-fat milk to cut 15 calories from the 160 in whole milk.*
   So if you're cutting down on calories, just cut down on the fat. But whatever you do, don't cut the potato from your meal. After all, you can't cut the fat if there isn't any to cut.
   Right?

Source: The Potato Board.

SUMMARY

Fats, like carbohydrates, are composed of carbon, hydrogen, and oxygen. Carbons bond together to form fatty acids, which are attached to a molecule called glycerol to form a triglyceride. Depending on whether all possible bonds within the carbon chain are filled with hydrogens, the fatty acids can be said to be saturated (all bonds filled with hydrogens), monounsaturated (one double bond), or polyunsaturated (more than one double bond). According to the category into which a fatty acid falls, it will have certain characteristics: saturated fats tend to be solid at room temperature and come from animal sources; unsaturated fats tend to be liquid at room temperature and be found more in plant products.

Cholesterol, a substance best described as a cross between an alcohol and a fat, not only is found in foods, but is actually manufactured by the body. It plays an important role as a component of many tissue structures and acts as a precursor to many body compounds. Because it has been found to accumulate in the tissues and blood vessels leading to the heart, it has been implicated in the development of heart disease.

In order to be digested, fats must combine with a substance called bile. Shorter-chained fatty acids pass into the bloodstream, where they are attached to proteins to enhance their solubility in water. Longer-chained fatty acids are first coated with proteins before they can go through the lymphatic system. From there they enter the bloodstream. Once delivered to body tissues, fats can be converted into energy, become part of tissues, or be stored for future use. Because they are so high in energy, fats provide an ideal long-term store.

Fats are important in the diet because they carry the fat-soluble vitamins and the essential fatty acids (linoleic and linolenic acids); they also give food flavor and satiety value.

Issue

Atherosclerosis

Man is only as old as his arteries.
LEONARDO DA VINCI

Cardiovascular disease (CVD) or coronary heart disease (CHD), as it is commonly called, is not a new phenomenon. Not only have symptoms of heart disease been found in Egyptian mummies, but no human society studied so far has been free of the disease.(4,5) What is shocking to modern researchers is that the disease can begin so early in life. Autopsies performed on American soldiers killed in action during the Korean conflict in the 1950s showed that damage to the coronary arteries is present in early adulthood.(6) One-third of the American soldiers examined had greater than 15 percent narrowing of their coronary arteries due to cholesterol blockages, yet the average age of the soldiers was only 22 years.

TERMS

The cardiovascular system, made up of the heart and blood vessels, is affected by a number of diseases. Arteriosclerosis refers to pathological conditions in which there is a thickening, hardening, and loss of elasticity of the arteries. It progresses slowly, sometimes beginning in childhood and going undetected until middle age or later. The type of arteriosclerosis that most often produces serious consequences, called atherosclerosis, may involve the arteries of the heart, legs, or brain. Atherosclerosis results when the inner lining of the arteries becomes thickened by soft deposits of fat, protein, cholesterol, and cell debris (Figure 4–7). If a deposit, called atherma or *plaque,* impedes or cuts off blood flow, a condition of ischemia results. If the heart artery is only partially blocked, episodes of chest pain or angina pectoris may occur. Angina pectoris does not lead directly to

death, but is a sign of increased risk for heart attack.(7)

When the affected artery is one leading to the heart, the resulting tissue death is called a *heart attack* or *myocardial infarct;* in the brain it is called a *stroke;* in the legs it is called *gangrene.* This combination of heart and blood vessel problems is referred to as cardiovascular disease (CVD). Coronary heart disease or simply heart disease, however, are terms much more commonly used in lay publications referring to this constellation of problems, even though much more than the heart may be involved.

Sudden death from traveling clots is a serious threat in CVD. In one-fourth of the cases, the first sign of CVD is death within minutes to a few hours after the first symptoms. About one-third of those who survive these first few hours and who experience some tissue death will die within a year.(7) With such sudden and severe symptoms, it is important to understand how CVD develops and why it strikes particular people.

INCIDENCE

CVD is the leading cause of death in this country, claiming more deaths than all other causes combined (Figure 4–8).(8) The number one cause is heart attack,

FIG. 4–7

Normal and plaque-filled arteries

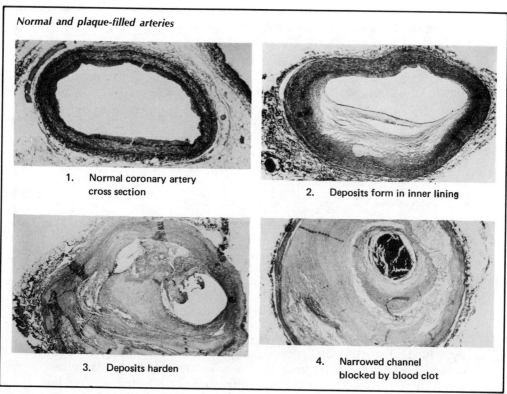

1. Normal coronary artery cross section

2. Deposits form in inner lining

3. Deposits harden

4. Narrowed channel blocked by blood clot

followed by stroke and hypertensive (high blood pressure) disease. Over 40 million Americans have some form of heart and blood vessel disease.(8) At heaviest risk are middle-aged men who have about a 25 percent chance of developing some type of this disease between the ages of 40 and 64.(9)

In the United States, the incidence of CVD increased rapidly between 1920 and 1950. Many factors played a role in this rise, including better diagnosis of the disease, decreases in other causes of death, an aging population, and an actual rise in incidence.(7) Toward the end of the 1960s the rate of increase in coronary deaths began to level off, and by 1977 it was down 23 percent from 1968 (Table 4–4). Since this decrease was not seen worldwide, researchers are trying to determine what factors in the United States might explain this occurrence. Are people more

FIG. 4–8

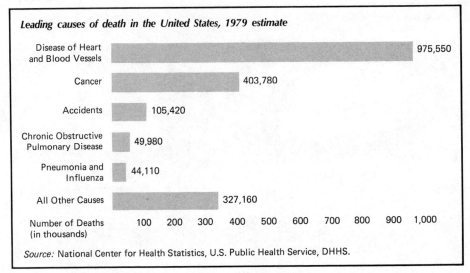

Leading causes of death in the United States, 1979 estimate

Cause	Number of Deaths (in thousands)
Disease of Heart and Blood Vessels	975,550
Cancer	403,780
Accidents	105,420
Chronic Obstructive Pulmonary Disease	49,980
Pneumonia and Influenza	44,110
All Other Causes	327,160

Source: National Center for Health Statistics, U.S. Public Health Service, DHHS.

health conscious? Have diets improved? By examining the process by which atherosclerosis develops, it may be possible to arrive at some answers to these questions.

HOW HEART DISEASE DEVELOPS

Signs of atherosclerosis can begin early in life, in some infants before their first birthday.(10) The

TABLE 4–4   **Worldwide Incidence of CVD, 1970 to 1977***

Country	1970	1977	Change
USA (white)	332.5	266.9	down 19.7%
Israel	194.2	168.3	down 13.3
Australia	297.4	263.0	down 11.6
Japan	34.2	30.3	down 11.4
Netherlands	201.4	184.6	down 8.3
Norway	213.1	203.4	down 4.6
Scotland	343.2	345.0	up 0.5
Switzerland	107.2	108.8	up 1.5
West Germany	147.7	155.1	up 5.0
England/Wales	259.1	272.4	up 5.1
Denmark	176.3	186.4	up 5.7
Northern Ireland	317.2	356.8	up 12.5
Sweden	136.5	156.6	up 14.7
Austria	132.2	168.9	up 27.8
Hungary	145.7	215.0	up 47.6

*Death rate for males aged 45 to 54 per 100,000 population.

Source: World Health Organization.

earliest change in the artery is the formation of yellow-grey fatty streaks composed of cholesterol deposits around the cells near the artery's lining. Since all populations, even those with a low incidence of CVD, show these streaks, many researchers feel they are not a sign of future heart disease. At this stage there is no bump protruding into the artery channel, and blood can flow through unrestricted.

As atherosclerosis progresses, newly formed cells in the muscular artery wall loaded with cholesterol begin to multiply and jut into the channel. These pearly-white plaques spread, harden, and eventually make the artery so stiff it is unable to expand and contract.(11) As the inner surface of the artery becomes more jagged, blood clots begin to form (Figure 4–9).

FIG. 4–9

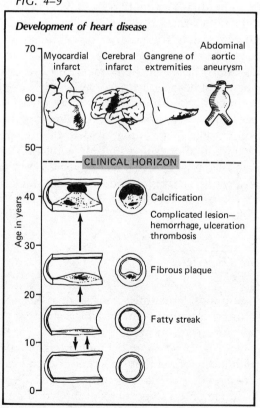

Source: Adapted from H.C. McGill, J.C. Geer and J.P. Strong, "Natural History of Human Atherosclerotic Lesions," in M. Sandler and G.H. Bourne (eds.), *Atherosclerosis and Its Origins* (New York: Academic Press, 1963), p. 42.

Speculation as to why the cells of the artery wall begin to overgrow in the first place has it that the turbulence of the blood flow damages the artery lining. Damage may also be caused by high blood pressure, high blood cholesterol, or injury from a variety of sources. Other theories compare the growth of these cells to a type of cancer or explain it as a result of a viral infection. Blood components called platelets may begin to clump at the points of injury along the artery wall, later breaking loose to form traveling clots.

The rate at which plaque develops varies from one person to the next, and from one artery to the next within a given individual. As many as 15 to 30 years may elapse before the gradual narrowing of the artery becomes noticeable. The vessels must close to one-third of their original size before a clot can obstruct the artery, causing a true heart attack or chest pain.

No one single factor causes CVD. Instead, a number of factors (appropriately called risk factors) increase a person's chances of developing the disease. Risk factors are personal habits and inherited or acquired traits that describe an individual's potential for developing the disease—that is, they correlate with higher rates of heart disease. But a correlation, no matter how strong, does not satisfy the criteria for demonstrating cause and effect. One rather famous epidemiological study showed a very strong relationship (90 percent correlation) between the number of telephone poles in a given region and the incidence of heart attacks. You might deduce that more telephone poles imply environmental conditions that are more stressful and competitive, but you would be hard pressed to assert that telephone poles cause heart attacks. This study and others like it are often cited to demonstrate the fault in assigning cause when the situation suggests only a relationship or association.

The most dangerous risk factors for CVD in the United States are high blood cholesterol levels, high blood pressure, and cigarette smoking. These, plus other known risk factors for the disease, are shown in Table 4–5 and discussed below.

Blood (Serum) Cholesterol

The strongest and most consistent risk factor observed from human studies is serum cholesterol, although it is a stronger predictor in younger rather than older persons.(7) You are at higher risk for a heart attack if your serum cholesterol level is greater than 250 milligrams per 100 milliliters. Serum is the watery portion of the blood that separates out when all clotting factors and cells have been removed; plasma has only the cells removed. Concentrations of cholesterol and fats in these portions of the blood mirror those of whole blood.

Sources of Blood Cholesterol. Two sources of cholesterol exist: cholesterol from the diet and that made by the body itself. The usual American

TABLE 4-5 **Some Risk Factors Associated with Heart Disease**

Eating and drinking too much
Not exercising enough

High total fat consumption
High saturated fat consumption
Low polyunsaturated:saturated fat ratio
High cholesterol consumption

Advancing age
Heredity
Maleness
Postmenopausal state

High salt consumption
Overweight

Personality type
Diabetes
Cigarette smoking

Source: Adapted from *Dietary Goals for the United States,* 2nd ed. Prepared by the staff of the Select Committee on Nutrition and Human Needs, U.S. Senate, December 1977, p. xxiv.

diet supplies about 300 to 800 milligrams cholesterol per day, of which only about 150 to 300 milligrams are absorbed, even with high intakes. All body tissues have the capacity to synthesize cholesterol, and the bodymade variety accounts for much more of the cholesterol in the body than dietary cholesterol.

The liver is able to increase or decrease its synthesis of cholesterol to adjust for the amount in the diet. Some individuals have an inherited defect in this mechanism and synthesize too much cholesterol no matter how little they ingest. Others are able to eat foods high in cholesterol and maintain normal blood levels. This mystery is only now beginning to be solved, and part of the answer lies in the manner in which cholesterol is transported in the blood.

"Good" versus "Bad" Cholesterol.   Since the plaque constricting the arteries is composed largely of cholesterol, it is not surprising that early researchers began to study levels of cholesterol in the blood. Their reasoning was that high levels of blood cholesterol would lead to a greater likelihood of plaque accumulation in the arteries. The only problem was that as researchers looked more closely at cholesterol, they found that it moves through the blood in different "packages." Depending on the type of package, it can worsen or lessen the risk of CVD. How can this happen?

Remember that cholesterol and other fats, because they are not water-soluble, must be carried through the bloodstream piggyback fashion by lipoproteins. Lipoproteins differ in the amount of cholesterol and other fats they carry and are identified by their densities. The ones primarily involved with CVD are the very low-density lipoproteins (VLDLs), low-density lipoproteins (LDLs), and high-density lipoproteins (HDLs).

Most of the time, when you hear that someone's serum cholesterol is high, it refers to LDLs. This is the cholesterol that gets trapped inside arteries and is an important risk factor in the development of heart disease. VLDLs are neutral, neither increasing nor decreasing risk. HDLs interfere with the process of atherosclerosis by competing with LDLs for binding sites on cells, reducing the LDLs that gain entrance into the cells. HDLs also protect against CVD by scavenging excess cholesterol and returning it to the liver for excretion. So the more HDLs you have, the lower your total body cholesterol.

Certain factors affect HDL levels, although individuals vary in their response. Smoking, poor control of diabetes, use of oral contraceptives containing progestin, obesity, and a sedentary life style lower HDL levels, while vigorous exercise and a vegetarian diet, or one that includes fish, tend to raise it. Moderate alcohol consumption raises HDL levels, but at the same time increases LDL levels. As you age, the balance of LDLs to HDLs changes. At birth about half of the total blood cholesterol is carried on HDLs; by adulthood, this figure has dropped to one-fourth. In general, HDLs are higher in women. Since the risk of heart disease is greater for those with high levels of serum cholesterol (LDLs), factors that increase these levels become important. One of the most obvious is the amount of cholesterol in the diet.

The Relationship of Dietary Cholesterol to Blood Cholesterol. When large population groups are compared, there is a strong association among the amount of cholesterol consumed, the amount in the blood, and death rates from heart disease.(9) But if we look at individuals instead of populations, we will find no consistent correlation for any given person between dietary cholesterol and blood cholesterol levels or between either of these and heart disease. People with blood levels over 250 milligrams percent do suffer from higher rates of CVD, but about half of actual heart disease victims have cholesterol levels lower than this. In studies where subjects were placed on low-cholesterol, low-fat diets, their risk of heart disease did not decrease. But these studies have usually involved middle-aged men already showing signs of heart disease and may not be a true indication of what would happen to younger, healthier subjects.(9)

The positive association between dietary cholesterol and blood cholesterol found in population groups is also found in small groups of vegetarians. Well-nourished American vegetarians show lower blood cholesterol levels and lower prevalence of CVD, and do not show the usual gradual rise in blood cholesterol levels with advancing age. Although generally vegetarians eat less fat and cholesterol than meat-eaters, their body weights are also lower, a factor that complicates the interpretation of these data.

Before you jump to the conclusion that dietary cholesterol is the cause of CVD, remember that cholesterol is rarely found in the diet apart from other fats, especially saturated fats. The increased consumption of saturated fats that occurred among Americans in the early twentieth century correlates with an increasing number of heart disease victims. Yet, it is not possible to examine an individual's diet and predict who will suffer a heart attack.(12) If cholesterol and saturated fats were the only villains, this prediction should be possible. But look at some of the complicating factors: low-fat, low-cholesterol diets are the norm in areas of the world where the rate of heart disease is low, but people in these areas also consume fewer kcalories, and are leaner and more physically active. Other cultures, like the East African Masai and the Samburu in Kenya, have low rates of heart disease, but their diets are rich in saturated fat and cholesterol.(7) At the other extreme are those who consume low-cholesterol diets and who have a difficult time maintaining a cholesterol level less than 300 milligrams percent.

The Arguments on Both Sides. The cholesterol issue is so hotly debated today that it is important to take a closer look at the arguments on either side. The "dietary cholesterol causes CVD" arguments run as follows: (1) Cholesterol intake determines, in part, the cholesterol levels in the blood (especially LDLs). (2) The concentration of LDLs is associated with risk of heart disease. (3) Cholesterol is a major component of plaque. (4) Artery damage similar to that found in humans can be induced by feeding cholesterol (along with other dietary components) to several animal species. (5) There is no reason to believe that low-cholesterol diets are harmful or that cholesterol is an essential nutrient for humans.

Those less prone to point the finger at dietary cholesterol are quick to argue that: (1) The link between dietary cholesterol and heart attack is statistical, not one of cause and effect. (2) There are people with high blood cholesterol levels who have never suffered from a heart attack, while some patients with heart disease have low serum cholesterol levels. (3,9) Two major epidemiological studies showed no relationship between blood cholesterol levels and dietary fat and cholesterol intake. (4) It has not been shown that reducing blood cholesterol levels in a given individual will prevent heart disease.

So although a high serum cholesterol level is a risk factor for CHD, the part dietary cholesterol plays in the process is still uncertain. A number of other factors are related to heart disease, and many of them have effects on blood cholesterol levels.

High Blood Pressure (Hypertension)

High blood pressure (HBP) is a symptom, not a disease, but is directly related to risk of CVD. Not only does HBP force the heart to work harder, but it may promote atherosclerosis by mechanically injuring the lining of the artery.

Blood pressure is the force the flowing blood exerts against the artery walls. With extremely high pressure, the lining of the blood vessels and underlying fiber and muscles tear and eventually form scar tissue. The walls of large and medium-sized arteries thicken and harden, becoming clogged with cholesterol and fat deposits. The blood vessels primarily affected are those supplying the kidneys, brain, and heart, which are called *target organs*. Once the damage has occurred, it is often irreversible.

Normal blood pressure in an adult is considered to be 120/80 (written as the systolic/diastolic pressure). "Borderline" hypertension (pressure above 140/90 but less than 160/95) is usually treated by weight reduction and a

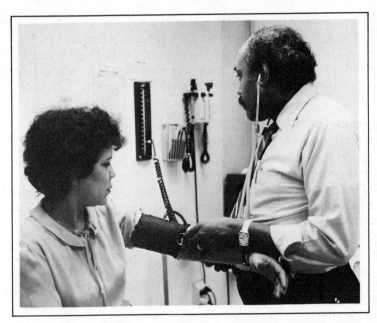

Persons whose families have a history of hypertension should have their blood pressure checked regularly.

restricted salt intake. At this level, the risk of heart attack is 2.5 times normal. Individuals with blood pressure of 160/95 or higher should seek medical treatment. Blood pressure tends to rise with age, but the elderly do not tolerate higher levels any better than the young. HBP elevates the risk of CVD in women as much as it does in men. Hypertension affects about 20 percent of the adult population. It has no early symptoms, but may lead to such severe complications as stroke, heart attack, congestive heart failure, or kidney failure.

Risk factors for HBP include race (blacks have higher rates than whites), age, family history, obesity, excessive sodium or alcohol consumption, kidney disease, psychological stress, and the use of oral contraceptives. For this reason, oral contraceptives are not recommended for women over age 40, those with a family history of premature CVD, and those over 30 who smoke more than a pack of cigarettes a day.

There is no definite proof that sodium intake is the cause of hypertension, but societies that have high sodium diets tend to have higher rates of hypertension. The highest incidence is found in northern Japan,(13) where the average per capita sodium chloride intake is about 26 grams (sodium chloride is another name for salt, the most common source of dietary sodium). Health professionals in the United States recommend an intake of only about 3 grams sodium a day, which would be about 7 to 8 grams of sodium chloride or salt per day.(14) There is a strong genetic component in the body's ability to handle excess salt, but certain people (about 15 to 20 percent of Americans) cannot do so adequately.

Although hypertension can be controlled, there is no known cure. Early detection is important by means of regular checkups. The simplest methods of control are achieving and maintaining ideal weight and restriction of salt intake, but these are not always sufficient in themselves. Moderate degrees of hypertension can be treated with diuretics, which increase the kidney's rate of sodium excretion.

Cigarette Smoking

Cigarette smokers consistently have been found to be at increased risk for CVD. The risk is related to the number of cigarettes smoked per day, so that a two-pack-a-day smoker is at higher risk than someone who smokes one pack a day. Individuals who quit smoking can lower their risk. Over about a 10-year period, an ex-smoker's chance of a heart attack becomes equivalent to that of a nonsmoker.

Cigarette smoking may increase the risk of CVD in a number of ways: nicotine may increase the oxygen needed by the heart and simultaneously constrict the coronary blood vessels. There is a constant level of carbon monoxide in the bloodstream of cigarette smokers that combines with hemoglobin, the substance in red blood cells responsible for transporting oxygen. Thus the level of oxygen the red blood cells can carry is reduced. Platelets become stickier, allowing greater clumping of the blood. Substances entering the blood during smoking may damage the lining of the blood vessels in the heart, allowing cholesterol and other fatty substances to enter the blood vessel wall. These factors speed the development of disease by injuring the artery lining as well as decreasing the blood cells' ability to carry oxygen to the heart muscle. Cigarette smoking also multiplies the effects of other damaging factors. Cigar and pipe smokers, on the other hand, do not show an increased risk of CVD over nonsmokers.

Exercise

Studies indicate that sedentary persons, especially adults, are more likely to have a heart attack than active individuals. One group of researchers found a two to four times higher incidence and greater severity of CVD in bus drivers who sit all day driving than in bus conductors who are required to walk and climb stairs.(15)

A great deal of controversy exists about what type of exercise is most beneficial and the extent to which it should be practiced. Exercise sufficient to produce cardiovascular conditioning (aerobic exercise) causes a slight decrease in LDL and VLDL levels and an increase in HDL levels. Regular, daily exercise is preferred over sporadic heavy workouts, such as shoveling snow, especially for those over 40. Anyone over 40 who has not maintained a regular exercise program for a number of years should first see a physician. Usually the condition of the heart and lungs will be evaluated, followed by an assessment of

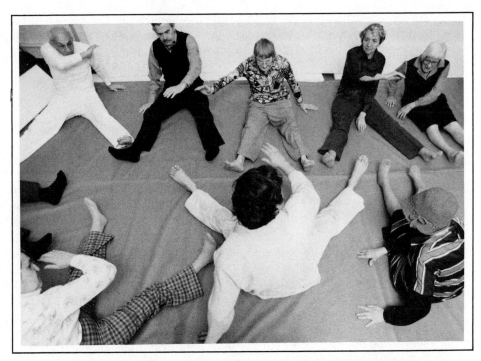

Regular exercise can help lower risk of heart disease. Group exercise classes, such as this one for older persons, can keep motivation and interest high.

coronary risk factors. Some persons may be asked to undergo a bicycle or treadmill exercise (stress) test. If there is any evidence of CVD, the person will have to increase the level of physical activity gradually over a period of weeks and months. Walking is a recommended exercise for beginners.

Other Risk Factors

Diabetes.   Diabetics, both Type I and Type II, have long been known to have higher rates of CVD than nondiabetics. Diabetic men have a 50 percent greater chance of getting the disease than nondiabetic men, while in diabetic women the risk is more than doubled. The most important steps diabetics can take to reduce their risk are to maintain normal weight, follow a prescribed diet faithfully, take medication, exercise regularly, and avoid cigarettes.

Heredity and Sex.   Some researchers say atherosclerosis is due to inherited metabolic abnormalities in the absorption, synthesis, and circulation of blood fats. Though the exact cause is not known, a family history of premature

CVD places a person at higher risk. During the early and middle years, females are at lower risk than males, possibly due to some protective effect provided by higher levels of estrogen, a sex hormone.

Stress and Personality Type.   Everyone experiences stress to some degree, but some people are better able to deal with it than others. The stress theory of CVD was originally introduced in the book *Type A Behavior and Your Heart*, by Meyer Friedman and Ray H. Rosenman. These researchers, after studying over 3500 subjects, consistently found certain personality traits in heart attack victims that were absent or of lesser intensity in those who never experienced CVD. Some of these traits (collectively referred to as Type A behavior) include a competitive striving, a desire for perfection, inability to slow down or relax, compulsiveness over work, and irritation when anyone or anything interferes with goals. The inability to deal effectively with stress can lead to elevations of blood pressure and blood cholesterol. Persons who are relaxed or retiring in nature (Type B) are at lower risk. The relationship between stress and heart disease becomes fuzzy when you try to separate out other related risk factors. For instance, to cope with stress, people may take up smoking cigarettes, overeat, or overindulge in alcohol, practices that may also raise the risk of CVD.

Obesity.   There is conflicting evidence as to whether obesity, without the presence of other risk factors, increases the risk of CVD.(7) (Moderate obesity of 10 to 20 percent over ideal weight does not appear to increase mortality risk.) The obese show certain metabolic changes that may predispose them to the disease: Blood lipids increase, but HDL levels are low (possibly due to decreased physical activity); and there is greater risk of diabetes and hypertension.(16) The obese may be more prone to CVD since they may consume larger amounts of salt, saturated fat, and cholesterol.(18) They also are more likely to develop diabetes.

Fats.   Animal and human studies conducted under carefully controlled laboratory conditions have shown that the type and amount of dietary fat consumed can significantly affect blood cholesterol levels. Saturated fats tend to raise blood cholesterol; polyunsaturates tend to lower it; and monounsaturates tend to have no effect at all. Mediterranean peoples have long been known to use great quantities of oil in cooking, but have usually shown low rates of heart disease. It is now recognized that the oil most often used, olive oil, is one of the richest sources of monounsaturated fats and thus should have little effect on blood cholesterol levels.

The typical proportion of unsaturated to saturated fats (called the P/S ratio) in the American diet is about 2 to 1. Diets of this type are associated with increased blood cholesterol levels. If the total amount of fat is reduced and the proportion of polyunsaturated fats in this new total is increased so that the ratio is closer to 1 to 1, blood cholesterol concentrations tend to decrease. But polyunsaturated fats, even though they tend to lower blood cholesterol levels, should not be consumed in large amounts, since they may be implicated in aging, cancer development, and increased gallstone formation.(7,12) In the last decade, a falling prevalence of CVD has correlated in time with an increased substitution of polyunsaturated for saturated fats, although it is still uncertain whether these changes are the result of other environmental factors.(12) And some foods, even though they may be high in fat, may contain factors that inhibit cholesterol synthesis. For example, some studies indicate that milk may lower rather than raise blood cholesterol levels in humans.(18)

Sugar.   Researchers advocating the theory that sugar increases risk of heart disease claim that high sucrose intakes lead to "sticky" blood platelets (the components of blood involved in blood clotting), which in turn increase the chances of blood clots forming.

In countries where people consume diets high in fats and sugar there are higher rates of CVD, but whenever a relationship between diet and CVD has been reported, it has been more closely linked to the fat intake than to sugar. Among populations or individuals, a consistent and independent relationship between sugar intake and CVD has never been shown.(19) (See Chapter 3 for a detailed discussion of sugar.)

Fiber.   Not only do certain types of dietary fibers lower blood cholesterol levels, but a high-fiber intake may help control obesity and diabetes, both risk factors for heart disease. The mechanisms by which fiber exerts these effects are explained in greater detail in Chapter 3.

Alcohol.   There is no strong association between alcohol and heart disease, but men with greater than average alcohol consumption have about twice the prevalence of hypertension than moderate drinkers. Excess caloric intake may be partly responsible, since heavy drinkers tend toward obesity and often consume one-third to one-fourth of their daily kcalorie intake as alcohol.

Alcohol consumption increases the level of fats in the blood, a known risk factor for heart disease. Ironically, though, alcohol also increases the level of HDLs in the blood. This effect could be a result of the reduction in stress many people experience when they have a social drink after a hard day's work. Researchers still are not sure of the mechanism behind alcohol's effect on HDLs.

Water Hardness.   There is a direct relationship between water softness and mortality from CVD. Although this is still a highly controversial area, the explanation has been offered that soft water may leach toxic minerals like cadmium, cobalt, and lead from plumbing pipes, causing metal intoxication.(7) Also, hard water contains calcium, which may protect against the absorption of lead. Soft water may contain excessive sodium, or too few minerals, such as magnesium, or a combination of these factors. More research needs to be done in this area.

Some of the risk factors mentioned above, such as cigarette smoking, HBP, high blood cholesterol, body weight, stress, diabetes, and diet, are controllable. Others (age, sex, family history) are not. The more risk factors you have, the greater your chances of getting CVD. But the risk is more than cumulative (Figure 4–10). For instance, if you have one risk factor, you may have twice the risk of getting heart disease as someone with no factors. If you have two risk factors, your chances increase not by two, but by three or four times. With three risk factors, your chances may rise by eightfold. Risk factors are fair predictors of heart disease, although not all risk factors are of the same potency. What is not so well understood is whether you can lower your risk by reducing the number of factors you have, and whether modifications in diet really make a difference and how. Let us take a look at the studies that have been done and their results.

Animal Studies.   Experimental animals given high-cholesterol, high-fat diets develop atherosclerosis, while in those given low-fat, low-cholesterol diets the process is reversed. Evidence such as this must be interpreted with care, because animals use cholesterol differently from humans. The laboratory is

FIG. 4–10

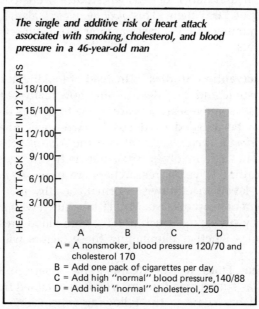

The single and additive risk of heart attack associated with smoking, cholesterol, and blood pressure in a 46-year-old man

A = A nonsmoker, blood pressure 120/70 and cholesterol 170
B = Add one pack of cigarettes per day
C = Add high "normal" blood pressure, 140/88
D = Add high "normal" cholesterol, 250

Source: J.W. Farquhar, *The American Way of Life Need Not Be Hazardous to Your Health* (New York: W.W. Norton & Co., 1978), p. 17.

a vastly different environment (possibly providing more stress and less exercise) than the free-living situation of humans. Also, there is some evidence indicating that the cholesterol in these laboratory diets acts in a different manner than cholesterol found naturally in foods.(18)

Clinical Trials. In clinical trials, human volunteers follow a carefully controlled diet and periodically undergo medical evaluation. These studies have shown that reducing consumption of saturated fats and cholesterol and increasing consumption of polyunsaturated fats resulted in lowered levels of blood cholesterol. Despite this effect, these dietary changes did not decrease the chances of developing CVD.

Population (Epidemiological) Studies. Large epidemiological studies have shown a positive link between blood cholesterol levels and incidence of CVD.

The most extensive epidemiological study of CVD to date is the *Framingham Study*, an effort begun in 1949 and involving more than 5000 men and women, considered typical of the U.S. population, over a 20-year period. Dietary information (kcalories, protein, fat, cholesterol) was collected, as well as results from medical exams. The researchers concluded that if there was any association between diet and serum cholesterol in this study, it was a weak one. They also found *no* relationship between incidence of CVD and diet.

In an effort to test the findings of the Framingham experience, the results from a number of smaller studies were combined to form a single population of 7000 men. This *pooling project* also found no evidence of an increased number of CVD cases among those subjects consuming diets high in saturated fats.

Intervention Studies. Instead of looking at the type of diet groups of people consume and then determining how many of these individuals develop heart disease, some researchers are trying to change dietary habits to see if heart disease can be avoided or delayed. Two such intervention studies are the *Coronary Primary Prevention Trial* and the *Multiple Risk Factor Intervention Trial (MRFIT)*. The first involves 3800 men between ages 35 and 59. In a study designed to run 10 years, researchers are trying to find out if lowering blood cholesterol levels in otherwise normal, healthy men will reduce or slow the development of heart disease. MRFIT takes men who place high on the risk scale because they smoke too much or have high blood pressure or cholesterol levels and examines whether eliminating these factors will prevent or delay CHD.

What Does It All Mean? The American Council on Science and Health(4) has summarized the information obtained from these various types of studies and has come to the following conclusions:

- People suffering from CVD generally exercise less and have higher levels of total blood cholesterol.

- People living in industrialized societies have more heart disease and higher average blood cholesterol than those in less developed areas.

- Consistently high blood cholesterol levels together with other risk factors increase the risk of developing CVD.

- Dietary changes can lead to reduced blood cholesterol levels for some people.

- Atherosclerosis and high blood cholesterol levels are the result of many factors, both genetic and environmental.

- Individual differences in blood cholesterol levels occur in people with the same dietary habits.

RECOMMENDATIONS

We are now forced to examine a crucial question: Can modifying the diet decrease the chances of developing CVD? As pointed out earlier, reducing certain components of the diet can help reduce serum cholesterol, but there is little evidence yet to indicate that this reduction in serum cholesterol will help people avoid death from heart disease.

The General Recommendations Debate

Because of the lack of proof, two different schools of thought have developed over whether diet recommendations should be made for the general population.

The Pro Group. The group that advocates recommendations, comprised of organizations such as the American Heart Association, the USDA, and the Senate Select Committee on Nutrition and Human Needs, believes there is enough evidence to recommend general decreases in consumption of total kcalories, total saturated fats and cholesterol, and a general increase in the proportion of polyunsaturated to saturated fats. The basic premises of this group are that the recent decrease in mortality from CVD is related to changes in American life styles and habits (a decrease in tobacco consumption, a decline in consumption of animal fats and oils, and an improvement in physical fitness; see Table 4–6); that with enough time and money, a proper study could be conducted giving the proof that diet affects CVD. Any dietary changes that decrease serum cholesterol, body weight, or blood pressure are believed to decrease risk of CVD and likely to do no harm.

The USDA, in an attempt to achieve broad changes in the American way of eating, published the *Dietary Guidelines for Americans* (see Chapter 2), seven dietary recommendations calling for a reduction in the consumption of fats, particularly saturated ones, cholesterol, salt, and sugar. Consistent with these guidelines is the *Prudent Diet*, published by the American Heart Association (AHA) and intended for both sexes and all ages (Table 4–7).

TABLE 4–6 **The Nation's Changing Habits**

Change in Per Capita Use or Consumption of Products Affecting Coronary Heart Disease Risks, 1963–77

All tobacco products	down 29.3%
Eggs	down 11.5
Fluid milk and cream	down 22.5
Butter	down 36.2
Animal fats and oils	down 47.4
Vegetable fats and oils	up 57.9

Source: U.S. Department of Agriculture. The 1977 figures used in calculating the percentages are preliminary.

The USDA and AHA recommendations are fairly moderate. Other groups, however, advocate more severe dietary changes. The Pritikin diet was devised by Nathan Pritikin, who is knowledgeable about nutrition though not formally trained in the subject. Pritikin's belief is that a very low-fat, low-cholesterol diet accompanied by a vigorous exercise program will reverse the progress of atherosclerosis, hypertension, and diabetes. This program, administered at the Longevity Institutes in California and Florida, runs 30 days and costs about $3000. To keep the diet as low in fat and cholesterol as Pritikin recommends, all dairy products must be made from skim milk and only 4 to 5 oz of very lean meat, fish, or poultry can be eaten a day. No added fat in the form of butter, margarine, oils, or dressings is allowed. Egg yolks are not permitted. Fruits are limited, and remaining kcalorie needs are met through consumption of vegetables and grain products made without sugar, fat, whole milk, or egg

TABLE 4–7 **The Prudent Diet: Substitutes for Cholesterol-Containing Foods**

Foods High in Cholesterol and/or Saturated Fat	Recommended Substitutes
Egg yolk (275 mg cholesterol per yolk)	Egg white (no cholesterol or fat) Cholesterol-free egg substitute
Dairy products: Whole milk (30 mg cholesterol per 8 oz) Cheeses (30 mg cholesterol per oz) Butter (70 mg cholesterol per oz) Ice cream (35 mg cholesterol per half cup)	Skim milk (7 mg cholesterol per 8 oz) Whey cheeses, noncreamed cottage cheese Soft corn oil or safflower oil margarines (no cholesterol) Sherbets, nonsaturated fat ice milks
Fatty "marbled" red meats, hot dogs, hamburgers, luncheon meats, sausage, bacon (30–35 mg cholesterol per oz)	Limited amounts of lean red meats (30–35 mg cholesterol per oz)
Skin and internal organs, such as liver, kidney, brain (100–600 mg cholesterol per oz)	Fish and chicken (20 mg cholesterol per oz)
Shellfish (40–70 mg cholesterol per oz)	Textured vegetable protein products (no cholesterol)

Source: Adapted from F.J. Stare, ed., *Atherosclerosis*, (New York: Medcom, 1974), p. 67.

yolks. The Pritikin diet, if followed strictly, could lead to possible deficiencies in essential fatty acids and fat-soluble vitamins, continual hunger (since satiety depends to some extent on the fat content of the meal), and continuing weight loss from insufficient kcalories. Such a program should *not* be undertaken without medical supervision.

The Anti Group.   Those who follow the second school of thought do not feel there are enough data to warrant sweeping changes in the American way of eating. Members of this group, like the Food and Nutrition Board (FNB) of the National Academy of Sciences and the American Medical Association, recommend dietary changes for those individuals found to be at risk of CVD, as evidenced by studying their medical history and measuring their blood lipids. This group believes that certain dietary goals, such as maintaining ideal body weight, are fine, but that no one specific dietary recommendation is likely to be appropriate for everyone. For instance, where the other group advocates a general reduction of fats, this second group feels that the fat content of the diet should be adjusted to the kcalorie needs of each individual, with infants, adolescent boys, pregnant teenage girls, and adults performing heavy labor requiring a higher percentage.

In 1980 the Food and Nutrition Board released a highly controversial publication called *Toward Healthful Diets.* In it, the FNB reviewed scientific studies concerning the relationship between diet and heart disease and other chronic degenerative diseases. One part of the report, the section on dietary cholesterol, created much disagreement in the nutrition community. Although many nutritionists had for years been telling people to cut down on cholesterol intake, the FNB did not find enough evidence to caution Americans to reduce cholesterol intake unless they had been diagnosed by their physicians as being at risk of CVD. In general, members of this second school of thought feel that limiting cholesterol may be protective for some people, but may give others a false sense of security. Since high blood cholesterol levels are now known to result from both genetic and environmental factors, individuals at risk may require more than dietary therapy.

They also believe that certain people should *not* reduce cholesterol intake. For example, it may be hazardous to give infants low-cholesterol diets. Normal levels may be important to help the infant's body develop the enzyme systems necessary to break down cholesterol. Dietary cholesterol may be needed for brain development; rats deprived of cholesterol early in life failed to develop a complete nervous system and became deficient in sex hormones. A shift to formulas high in corn, coconut, or soybean oil (remember vegetable oils contain no cholesterol) may decrease the cholesterol levels of infants below that found in infants fed human or cow's milk. Breast milk, by the way, contains a substantial amount of cholesterol. There is little evidence indicating that modifying the fat or cholesterol content of the diets of children after the first year of life will produce harmful effects.

Another problem cited by this second group is that animal product substitutes (margarine, egg, and meat substitutes) have been pushed so much by their manufacturers and the media that people are beginning to consider all animal products deadly and all substitutes medicinal.(20) Across-the-board dietary changes may themselves produce some adverse effects. For example, changes in the food growing and processing industries may pose some unknown hazards. Intakes of some of the most nutritious and popular foods, such as meats, dairy products, and eggs, would be reduced, possibly to the detriment of people already on barely adequate diets.(9) There may be an increased incidence of gallstones and gall bladder disease due to increased consumption of polyunsaturated fats.

Some Practical Guidelines

Even though this debate seems confusing, there are some recommendations that would be agreed upon by both groups:

- Reach and maintain ideal weight.
- If excessively sedentary, begin a sensible exercise program.
- If you smoke, cut down or quit.
- If you use alcohol, do so in moderation.
- If you have high blood pressure, consult your physician on ways to lower it.
- Anyone with one or more risk factors should see a doctor in order to take measures to lower the risk.
- Eat a variety of foods to ensure adequate intake of all nutrients, especially magnesium, folacin, niacin, biotin, pantothenic acid, and vitamin E, all required for a healthy heart.

In short, the best diet recommendations to date are moderation, variety, and balance. Many problems can arise from cutting out all dietary fat, or increasing enormously the amount of polyunsaturates, or overindulging in fiber and vitamins and minerals. The primary objective should be to maintain ideal weight. Although egg orgies are not recommended, the consumption of eggs periodically should not give you cause for alarm.

You should have a plasma lipid examination done when you go for a physical, especially if there is a history of CVD in your family. Anyone with a cholesterol level above a range of 200 to 210 milligrams per 100 milliliters of blood should consider changing some dietary practices. Above 250 milligrams per 100 milliliters, a diet should be prescribed; and above 300 milligrams per 100 milliliters the diet should be followed strictly. For those of you who would like to eat more prudently, the following suggestions may help you in altering your diet.

Cut Down on Cholesterol. Moderate your intake of foods high in cholesterol. This includes organ meats, shrimp, butter, and cream. Eat only two or three eggs a week.

Cut Down on Fats, but Increase the Proportion of Polyunsaturates.
Saturated fats are found primarily in animal products. To avoid a high intake of saturated fats, choose lean meat, fish, poultry, dry beans, and peas as your protein sources; limit your intake of butter, cream, hydrogenated margarines, shortenings, and foods made from such products. Instead, use more polyunsaturated vegetable oils, such as safflower, corn, sunflower, soybean, and cottonseed. Trim excess fat off meats, and broil, bake, or boil rather than fry.

A few fats of vegetable origin are saturated; they include coconut oil, palm kernel oil, and chocolate. The first two are used commercially in nondairy coffee creamers, nondairy whipped toppings, nondairy sour creams, cake mixes, and cookies. Any type of chocolate product is high in saturated fat, except those made with cocoa powder, which is chocolate with the fat removed.

In dairy foods, the fat is saturated. To avoid the fat yet still get all the vitamins, minerals, and protein, use skim milk and skim-milk products fortified with vitamins A and D. Buttermilk is frequently nonfat. Low-fat plain yogurt is a good substitute for recipes calling for sour cream. If you switch from butter to margarine, check to see that the first ingredient is a liquid polyunsaturated vegetable oil that has not been hardened or hydrogenated. When margarines are hydrogenated, the bonds produced are slightly different from the bonds found in foods naturally saturated with hydrogens. The resulting products are called *trans-fatty acids*. When fed to pigs, these have been shown to create greater atherosclerosis and lead to higher cholesterol levels than diets rich in saturated fats. Most nutritionists would still recommend margarine over butter for those who need to cut down on saturated fats, but they agree that more research needs to be conducted in this area. Cheeses are usually high in fat, but some cheeses, like uncreamed cottage cheese, farmer cheese, and part skim-milk mozarella or ricotta, have a lower fat content. Table 4–8 gives the percentage of fat in foods.

Cut Down on Sodium. Although it is the sodium content of foods that is a health concern, the most popular form of sodium in the food supply is table salt. Sodium intake is more and more being determined by food processors. Because people are devoting less time to cooking from scratch, they rely more on convenience foods, many of which are high in salt (Table 4–9). Large quantities of sodium can be found in canned or dried soups, canned vegetables, cheese, tomato juice, dill pickles, olives, canned tuna and crab, sauerkraut, frozen dinners, condiments (soy sauce, catsup, salad dressings), instant pudding, breakfast cereals, ice cream, cookies, cakes, bread, kosher foods, some toothpaste, monosodium glutamate, and chemically softened water. One way to cut down on sodium intake is to start making greater use of spices and herbs. Table 4–10 provides some suggestions for spices that are low in sodium. Another way is to keep the salt shaker off the table.

Increase Fiber. Try using whole grain products instead of refined white, and eat more fruits and vegetables. Begin to replace simple carbohydrates (candy and soft drinks) with complex carbohydrates (breads, potatoes, vegetables).

TABLE 4–8 Percentage of Fat in Foods

	Dairy	Poultry	Fish	Beef	Pork	Lamb	Vegetables
VERY LOW FAT (less than 21% of kcalories from fat)	Buttermilk, if made from skim milk only Low fat cottage cheese Low fat milk (½ to 1% milkfat by wt) Skim milk Skim milk cheeses	Light meat chicken without skin (baked, boiled, roasted) Light meat turkey without skin	Most fish fillets, including cod, flounder, haddock, perch, pollock, sole Most shellfish, including crab, lobster, shrimp, scallops Tuna in water				
LOW FAT (21–40% of kcalories from fat)	Ice milk Low fat milk (2% fat by wt) Low fat yogurt, plain Regular cottage cheese (4% fat by wt)	Chicken liver (not fried) Dark meat chicken, without skin (baked, boiled, roasted) Dark meat turkey, without skin	Salmon, pink or chum-canned	*Roasts: rump, armbone, round *Steaks: flank, round, and wedge or round-bone cut of sirloin Beef liver (not fried)		*Leg *Loin	

MEDIUM FAT (41–60% of kcalories from fat)	Ice cream, regular Part-skim mozzarella Part-skim ricotta Whole milk Whole milk yogurt	Fried chicken, most cuts	Herring Sardines Salmon, red, Atlantic or King	*Roasts: rib or blade *Steaks: porter-house, T-bone, club, or hipbone sirloin	*Ham *Pork loin or shoulder	Untrimmed leg *Lamb chops	
HIGH FAT (more than 60% of kcalories from fat)	Ice cream, rich Whole milk cheeses, including blue, brick, Camembert, cheddar, Swiss, most processed cheeses			Corned beef Ground beef Untrimmed meats, except round steak	Bacon Processed meats: bologna, deviled ham, frankfurters, liverwurst, salami Spareribs Untrimmed ham, pork loin or shoulder	Untrimmed lamb chops Untrimmed loin	Avocado Margarines Nuts and nut butters Olives Shortenings Vegetable oils

*Denotes cuts that have been trimmed of *all* outside fat.

Note: Values for meat products reflect averages of samples studied by U.S. Dept. of Agriculture. Due to variation in fat content of meats, cuts will sometimes be leaner or fatter than listed.

follow none of them. The recommendations, however, are good ones, if for no other reason than they promote good general nutrition. You have little to lose and possibly a lot to gain by adopting them.

REFERENCES

1. *Cholesterol and Diet: A Brief Review.* United Fresh Fruit and Vegetable Association, March 1977.

2. C. Chandler and R. Marston, "Fat in the U.S. Diet," Consumer and Food Economics Institute, USDA, *Nutrition Program News,* May–August 1976, pp. 1–8.

3. E.M. Pao, "Nutrient Consumption Patterns of Individuals, 1977 and 1965," *Family Economics Review,* SEA, USDA (Spring 1980), pp. 16–20.

4. American Council on Science and Health, *Diet Modification—Can It Reduce the Risk of Heart Disease?* New York, 1980.

5. H.C. McGill, Jr., "The Geographic Pathology of Atherosclerosis," *Lab Investigation* 18(1968):463–653.

6. J.W. Farquhar, *The American Way of Life Need Not Be Hazardous to Your Health* (New York: Norton, 1978).

7. H.C. McGill and G.E. Mott, "Diet and Coronary Heart Disease." In *Present Knowledge in Nutrition,* 4th ed., (Washington, D.C.: The Nutrition Foundation, 1976).

8. E.H. Ahrens, "Introduction, Symposium, The Evidence Relating Six Dietary Factors to the Nation's Health: Consensus Statements," *American Journal of Clinical Nutrition* 32(1979):2627–31.

9. H.C. McGill, "Appraisal of Cholesterol as a Causative Factor in Atherogenesis," *American Journal of Clinical Nutrition* 32(1979):2632–36.

10. E.M. Hamilton and E. Whitney, *Nutrition: Concepts and Controversies* (St. Paul, Minn.: West Publishing Company, 1979).

11. "Hardening of the Arteries—1980," *The Harvard Medical School Health Letter* 5 (February 1980).

12. C.J. Glueck, "Appraisal of Dietary Fat as a Causative Factor in Atherogenesis," *American Journal of Clinical Nutrition* 32(1979):2637–43.

13. L.K. Dahl, "Sodium and Hypertension," *American Journal of Clinical Nutrition* 25 (1972):231–244.

14. FASEB (Federation of American Societies for Experimental Biology), *Tentative Evaluation of the Health Aspects of Sodium Chloride and Potassium Chloride as Food Ingredients.* Contract with FDA #223-75-2004, 1978.

15. J.N. Morris, J.A. Heady, P.A. Raffle, C.G. Roberts, J.W. Parks, "Coronary Heart Disease and Physical Activity of Work," *Lancet* II (1953):1053–1111.

16. T.B. Van Itallie, "Appraisal of Excess Calories as a Factor in the Causation of Disease," *American Journal of Clinical Nutrition* 32(1979):2648–53.

17. R.E. Olson, "Is There an Optimum Diet for the Prevention of Coronary Heart Disease?" in *Nutrition, Lipids, and Coronary Heart Disease,* R. Levy, B. Rifkind, B. Dennis, and N. Ernst, eds. (New York: Raven Press, 1979).

18. R. Reiser, "Diet and Blood Lipids: An Overview." *Food and Nutrition News* 51(December 1979–January 1980):1–4.

19. E.L. Bierman, "Carbohydrate and Sucrose Intake in the Causation of Atherosclerotic Heart Disease, Diabetes Mellitus, and Dental Caries," *American Journal of Clinical Nutrition* 32(1979):2644–47.

20. R. Reiser, "Oversimplification of Diet: Coronary Heart Disease Relationships and Exaggerated Diet Recommendations." In *Controversies in Clinical Nutrition,* J.J. Cunningham, ed. (Philadelphia: George F. Stickley Company, 1980), pp. 65–75.

Proteins
5

With slightly different genes, you could have ended up as a turnip or beagle, but as it happened, your genetic inheritance read "human." Considering the importance of genetics in passing characteristics from one generation to the next and in making each person unique, you may be surprised to learn that your entire genetic machinery is designed to direct the creation of one special class of nutrients, the proteins.

The importance of proteins has not been lost upon the American public, though sometimes it is greatly exaggerated. Misconceptions about protein have led to some unusual eating practices. Take the athlete who dumps a couple of tablespoons of powdered protein supplement into milk in hopes of building extra muscle tissue. Or the crash dieter who trades in food for a nonfood product like liquid protein. Protein food choices can be good indicators of your life style. Many teenagers subsist on fast-food burgers, while members of certain religious sects avoid meat altogether and rely on legumes, seeds, nuts, and grains for protein. But not all proteins are alike, so before you can evaluate the soundness of these choices, you must first understand the different properties of proteins.

THE STRUCTURE OF PROTEINS

Proteins differ from carbohydrates and fats primarily because they contain nitrogen. Just as carbohydrates have glucose units and fats fatty acids, proteins are formed by linkages of smaller units called amino acids. These differ from the repetitive units of glucose in complex carbohydrates because amino acids can differ from each other.

An amino acid is composed of an acid group, an amino group (containing nitrogen), and a side chain (Figure 5–1). The side chain, which can vary in size and shape, distinguishes one amino acid from another. For instance, the side chain on some amino acids contains a sulfur group; on others a ring-type structure is attached. Each amino acid may be positively or negatively charged or neutral. As the amino acids are strung together in long, unbranched chains, the attraction and repulsion of charges bend the protein into twisted and tangled shapes. The type and arrangement of amino acids determine the characteristics of the protein. Some proteins are long, stringy fibers, such as those in hair, skin, nails, and bones. Others can be soft and globular, such as those in blood. Various agents, such as heat and alcohol, can break or unwind proteins. When this happens, the protein is *denatured*. Cooking an egg denatures the proteins and results in a firmer product that is more palatable than a raw one. Some proteins are more easily digested once denatured.

Essential versus Nonessential Amino Acids

Plants not only make their own proteins, but can also make the necessary amino acids first. Humans can make protein only if they are provided with certain amino acids and nitrogen. Both are found conveniently packaged together in the protein obtained from food. (Technically, humans do not require dietary protein, only amino acids and nitrogen.) The body can manufacture certain amino acids if it has the necessary ingredients. These amino acids, called nonessential or dispensable amino acids, are made from available oxygen, hydrogen, carbon, and nitrogen. The first three elements are obtained from the breakdown of nutrients in the diet and from general body pools; the nitrogen is

FIG. 5–1

The structure of an amino acid

C– Carbon
O– Oxygen
H– Hydrogen
N– Nitrogen (the
    component unique
    to proteins)

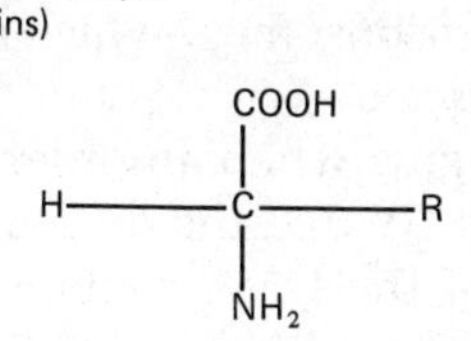

$$\text{H}-\!\!\!-\!\!\!-\overset{\textstyle \text{COOH}}{\underset{\textstyle \text{NH}_2}{\text{C}}}-\!\!\!-\!\!\!-\text{R}$$

The R represents different groups that can attach here. This group makes each amino acid different.

broken off other amino acids that may have come from the dietary proteins or body pools. Essential or indispensable amino acids are those the body cannot synthesize and must obtain through the diet. Of the 20 naturally occurring amino acids, 8 are essential for adults and 9 for infants. There is some indication that the ninth one may also be essential for adults, but research is not yet definitive.

THE 20 NATURALLY OCCURRING AMINO ACIDS

Glycine	Tryptophan*
Alanine	Cysteine
Valine*	Cystine
Leucine*	Proline
Isoleucine*	Aspartic acid
Serine	Glutamic acid
Methionine*	Glutamine
Threonine*	Histidine†
Phenylalanine*	Arginine
Tyrosine	Lysine*

*Essential for adults and infants.
†Known to be essential for infants, but not certain
    for adults.

Coding for Proteins

In order to make a protein, cells must line up amino acids in a specific sequence. There is only one correct sequence for each protein, and the genetic information stored in the nucleus of each cell directs this process. The task of constructing a specific protein belongs to two nucleic acids: deoxyribonucleic acid (DNA) and ribonucleic acid (RNA). DNA, concentrated in the cell nucleus and identical in every cell, contains the master plan or blueprint for all genetic information. DNA tells the cell what proteins to produce. RNA is chemically related to DNA and is responsible for carrying out these instructions. Although the blueprint for protein synthesis is found in the cell nucleus, the proteins are actually constructed on ribosomes, which are small particles located within the cell but outside the nucleus.

The process begins when an order arrives for a specific protein needed somewhere in the body. Within the nucleus a messenger RNA (mRNA) forms a complementary copy of the DNA containing the amino acid requirements for this particular protein. The mRNA leaves the nucleus and attaches to a ribosome elsewhere in the cell. From this position, the mRNA is ready to direct the synthesis of the protein.

At the same time, within the cell fluid, thousands of transfer RNA (tRNA) molecules are picking up amino acids, one amino acid to each tRNA. The mRNA directs each tRNA to deposit its amino acid in a specific order, forming a chain of amino acids along the ribosome. Once the protein strand is completed, the mRNA is broken down and the tRNAs return to the cell fluid until called upon to round up their amino acids again (Figure 5–2). Even though only about 20 amino acids are found in nature, they can link together in an almost infinite number of sequences, allowing for an incredible number of potential proteins.

Because of their sequencing, proteins can code and relay information and instructions to the cells, a feat carbohydrates and fats are unable to duplicate. As beautifully designed as this system appears, there are two

FIG. 5–2

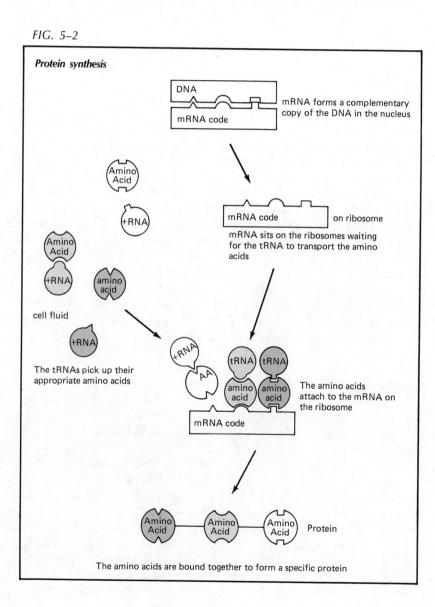

Protein synthesis

DNA

mRNA code

mRNA forms a complementary copy of the DNA in the nucleus

Amino Acid

+RNA

mRNA code   on ribosome

mRNA sits on the ribosomes waiting for the tRNA to transport the amino acids

Amino Acid

+RNA

amino acid

cell fluid

+RNA

The tRNAs pick up their appropriate amino acids

+RNA

AA

tRNA tRNA

amino acid amino acid

mRNA code

The amino acids attach to the mRNA on the ribosome

Amino Acid ⎯ Amino Acid ⎯ Amino Acid Protein

The amino acids are bound together to form a specific protein

potential problems. First, if for some reason the wrong amino acid is incorporated into a protein chain, serious consequences can result. This is the case with sickle-cell anemia. An incorrect amino acid is incorporated into the sixth position of a hemoglobin protein chain, resulting in hemoglobin that cannot carry and release oxygen. A second problem is that each specified amino acid must be available in the quantity needed at the time of protein synthesis. The absence of any single one halts the process. If the missing amino acid is nonessential, the body can gather the necessary ingredients to manufacture it on the spot. If the amino acid is essential, the body cannot synthesize it and is forced to stop the protein synthesis. Whatever function that protein was destined for will remain unfilled.

PROTEIN DIGESTION

Saliva contains no digestive enzymes for protein, but chewing thoroughly helps to break up the morsels of food into smaller pieces. Protein digestion begins in the stomach, where acid smoothes out the coiled proteins. Digestive enzymes, called pepsins, can then break the chains into shorter units containing varying numbers of amino acids. Upon entering the small intestine, alkaline juices neutralize the acid from the stomach. In the small intestine, the protein fragments are broken up into even shorter chains of amino acids by a group of enzymes from the pancreas called peptidases. Some single amino acids are freed by this process. Other peptidases are located on the surface and inside of the cells lining the intestinal tract. These enzymes complete protein digestion by breaking the short amino acid chains into individual amino acids.

The intestinal cell wall absorbs amino acids at specific sites. Carriers must transport amino acids across cell membranes and, at any given point in time, a number of amino acids compete for the same carrier. (A current fad is the practice of taking supplements of individual amino acids. This may cause an amino acid imbalance since the excess of one amino acid can overwhelm a carrier, creating too much competition for other amino acids.) Once in the bloodstream, the liver regulates the incoming amino acids. If they are needed to build tissue, they are sent to the cells. Inside the cell, the amino acids can be picked up by the tRNAs for use in constructing proteins. If they are not needed to build tissues, the nitrogen is taken off and the remaining portion is converted into a molecule that can be broken down to yield energy. If there is no immediate need for energy, it is converted into fat and stored. With a diet very low in kcalories, the amino acids are used for energy whether or not they are needed for tissue synthesis. (This is why strict reducing diets can lead to sagging muscles.) Figure 5–3 shows the digestion of proteins.

The nitrogen released from the breakdown of amino acids can be reused to make nonessential amino acids, or it may be excreted in urine, mainly as urea. All the nitrogen lost from the body (in skin, hair, nails, urine, feces, sweat, and other body secretions), must be replaced daily through the diet, primarily from protein, because there is no storage to cover periods of shortage. The end

FIG. 5–3

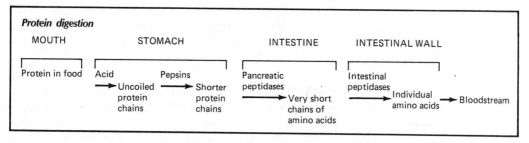

Protein digestion

MOUTH	STOMACH	INTESTINE	INTESTINAL WALL

Protein in food | Acid ⟶ Uncoiled protein chains | Pepsins ⟶ Shorter protein chains ⟶ | Pancreatic peptidases ⟶ Very short chains of amino acids | Intestinal peptidases ⟶ Individual amino acids ⟶ Bloodstream

products of protein breakdown in the body are carbon dioxide, water, energy, and nitrogen.

FUNCTIONS OF PROTEINS

During starvation, the body adapts in a way that preserves protein for as long as possible. It is not surprising that the body chooses to protect its protein supply, considering the crucial functions proteins perform.

FUNCTIONS OF PROTEIN

Primary function:	Component of body tissues (cells, enzymes, hormones, antibodies)
Secondary functions:	Regulator of fluid and salt balance Maintenance of body neutrality Nonpreferred energy source

Component of Body Tissues. Every cell is partly composed of proteins. Next to water, protein is the most abundant substance in the body. In fact, half of the dry weight and about 20 percent of the total wet weight of adults is protein. (If you weigh 150 pounds, about 30 pounds of that weight is protein.) Particular tissues are composed in large part of specific proteins, such as the keratin of hair and nails; the collagen and elastin of cartilage, ligaments, and tendons; hemoglobin, the oxygen-carrying component of red blood cells; and fibrin, a blood-clotting factor.

As much as 90 percent of the proteins in cells are enzymes. Enzymes speed up the rate at which specific reactions take place. Over 2000 known enzymes work to break down food for energy, synthesize compounds, and regulate biological reactions. Hormones, sometimes made of protein, help regulate the body's general physiological condition. Antibodies are proteins that provide disease resistance by forming when the body is under attack from foreign substances such as bacteria and viruses.

Since proteins are part of the structure of so many tissues, they are needed for growth and maintenance. Pregnant women and their unborn babies, infants, and children require protein to form new tissue. A lactating woman's diet must replace the protein present in the milk she secretes. Full-grown adults need protein to replace old, worn-out cells like those of the digestive tract, which slough off every three days, and for tissues such as nails and hair that continue to grow throughout life.

Regulator of Fluid Balance. The body contains many fluid compartments that must be maintained at a certain volume. Water diffuses freely across membranes, but proteins, because of their large size, are blocked. Proteins, however, attract water. The cells keep a certain amount of protein both within and outside cell walls so the surrounding fluid remains at the appropriate level. The proteins in the blood help maintain blood volume because they are unable to cross the blood vessel wall. One of the signs of protein malnutrition is edema, a condition in which water seeps into the spaces surrounding cells because there is an inadequate amount of protein in the blood.

Proteins within the membranes of the cells are finely tuned to respond to changes in fluids within and outside the cells. They control substances passing through the membrane. This is particularly important in the transmission of nerve and muscle impulses, which depend on the movement of sodium and potassium into and out of cells.

Maintenance of Body Neutrality. Proteins are buffers; that is, they can neutralize both acids and bases. The acidity or alkalinity of the blood changes as various reactions in the body produce excess acid or base that must be excreted. Proteins are able to pick up excess acid (by taking on hydrogens) or can correct a situation of too much base by releasing acid (giving up hydrogens).

Nonpreferred Energy Source. Amino acids from protein in excess of needs are broken down to yield energy or converted into fat once the nitrogen is removed. This process is not only inefficient, but protein is a relatively expensive source of energy compared to the other two fuel nutrients.

PROTEIN REQUIREMENTS AND CONSUMPTION

Nutritionists recommend protein intakes based on the amount of nitrogen (protein quantity) and kind of amino acids (protein quality) needed.

Protein Quantity

Protein quantity refers to the nitrogen concentration of a given food in relation to the nitrogen needs of humans. The nitrogen, of course, is derived from the protein in the food. Requirements differ by age, sex, and physiological

TABLE 5–1 **Protein Needs by Age, Sex, and Physiological State**

Group	(age)	Protein (grams)
Infants	0.0–0.5	Weight in kg × 2.2
	0.5–1.0	Weight in kg × 2.0
Children	1–3	23
	4–6	30
	7–10	34
Males	11–14	45
	15 +	56
Females	11–18	46
	19 +	44
Pregnant		+ 30
Lactating		+ 20

Source: Recommended Dietary Allowances, Food and Nutrition Board, National Academy of Sciences, 1980.

state (Table 5–1). The quantitative protein value of food can be determined by comparing the amount of protein in a serving of the food to the amount required by humans. The percentage of the food made up of protein is measured as grams of protein per 100 grams of food (Table 5–2). Generally animal protein sources are more concentrated than plant sources. Exceptions include bacon (which is low) and soy flour (which is high). Bread has 2 grams of protein per slice, which becomes significant for those who consume several slices a day. Even if you consume the recommended number of grams of protein daily, you may still not be getting a sufficient proportion of essential amino acids; much depends on the quality of the protein you get.

TABLE 5–2 **Protein Concentration of Some Common Foods**

Food	g Protein/Serving
3 oz serving of cooked, lean beef	20 g
1 cup cooked soy beans	
mature	20 g
immature	15 g
1 cup cooked navy beans	15 g
1 cup noodles	7 g
1 cup milk	9 g
1 oz cheddar cheese	7 g
1 egg	6 g
1 tablespoon peanut butter	4 g
½ cup lima beans	7 g
½ cup peas	5 g
1 slice bread	2 g

Source: Based on data from C.F. Adams, *Nutritive Value of American Foods in Common Units, Agriculture Handbook 456* (Washington, D.C.: ARS, USDA, 1975).

Protein quality refers to the essential amino acids in a protein as compared to the essential amino acid needs of the body. The better the match, the more efficient the body's use of the protein. If proteins are inefficiently used, many of the amino acids will be broken down and the nitrogen will show up in the urine. One way to determine the quality of a protein is to measure its *biological value (BV)*. BV is a figure based on the amount of nitrogen from a protein that is retained and used by the body.

Before a protein can be used in the body, it first has to be digested and the amino acids absorbed. Digestibility is the term used to express the amount of protein digested. This figure, combined with the BV gives the *net protein utilization (NPU)*, the actual measure of the efficiency with which the body uses a particular protein. Figure 5–4 gives the NPU values for some sample foods.

A third way to judge protein quality is to determine the *protein efficiency ratio (PER)*, which represents the weight gain (in grams) of a growing animal per gram of food eaten. If a protein is unable to support growth, it will have a PER of 0. Milk protein which is often used as a standard has a PER of 2.5.

On the basis of their quality, proteins have been classified as complete, incomplete, and partially complete. These terms can be misleading because "incomplete protein" implies to many people that one or more of the essential amino acids is lacking. In fact, nearly all protein foods contain some amount of all the essential amino acids. But if one or more is limited or present in a much smaller quantity than humans require, the protein food is not adequate for growth and/or maintenance of the body.

Proteins with all eight essential amino acids in the proper proportions to support growth and maintenance are called *high-quality proteins. Low-quality proteins,* though they contain all the essential amino acids, do not have sufficient amounts of one or more to meet the daily needs of the body. In order for body proteins to be synthesized and tissues formed or repaired, all eight essential amino acids must be present in the right amounts in the diet. If one essential amino acid is in short supply it is as if all were. So the quality of the protein is determined by the essential amino acid present in the smallest amount in relation to human requirements. This is the *limiting amino acid* (Table 5–3).

Protein RDA

The RDA for protein is set through use of *nitrogen balance studies.* By measuring how much nitrogen is lost in the urine, feces, and sweat, the amount of nitrogen needed to replace these losses can be determined. Normally, a healthy adult should be in nitrogen balance. A positive nitrogen balance occurs when the body is building up tissues so it retains more nitrogen than it excretes, as happens during periods of growth (childhood, pregnancy). A negative

FIG. 5–4

Net protein utilization values for various food

FOOD	ESSENTIAL AMINO ACIDS		NET PROTEIN UTILIZATION (PERCENT) 0 25 50 75 100
	POOR	ADEQUATE	
DAIRY			
EGGS	—	Trp, Lys, Met, Cys	
COW'S MILK	—	Trp, Lys	
COTTAGE CHEESE	—	Lys	
SWISS CHEESE	—	Lys	
MEATS			
FISH	—	Lys	
TURKEY	—	Lys	
PORK	—	Lys	
BEEF	—	Lys	
CHICKEN	—	Lys	
LAMB	—	Lys	
VEGETABLES			
CORN	Trp, Lys	—	
ASPARAGUS	Met, Cys	—	
BROCCOLI	Met, Cys	—	
CAULIFLOWER	Met, Cys	Trp, Lys	
POTATO	Met, Cys	Trp	
KALE	Lys, Met, Cys	—	
GREEN PEAS	Met, Cys	Lys	
GRAINS AND CEREALS			
BROWN RICE	Lys	—	
WHEAT GERM	Trp	Lys	
OATMEAL	Lys	—	
WHEAT GRAIN	Lys	—	
RYE	Trp, Lys	—	
POLISHED RICE	Lys, Thr	Trp	
MILLET	Lys	Trp, Met, Cys	
PASTA	Lys, Met, Cys	—	
LEGUMES			
SOYBEANS	Met, Cys, Val	Lys, Trp	
LIMA BEANS	Met, Cys	Trp, Lys	
KIDNEY BEANS	Trp, Met, Cys	Lys	
LENTILS	Trp, Met, Cys	Lys	
NUTS AND SEEDS			
SUNFLOWER SEEDS	Lys	Trp	
SESAME SEEDS	Lys	Trp, Met, Cys	
PEANUTS	Lys, Met, Cys, Thr	—	

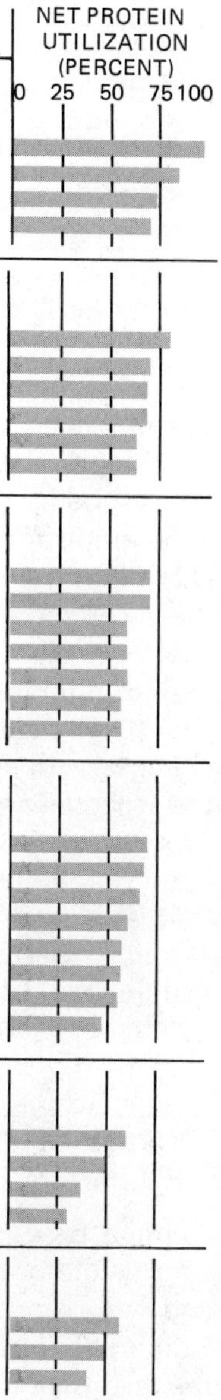

Source: N.S. Scrimshaw and V.R. Young, "The Requirements of Human Nutrition," *Scientific American* 235 (1976): 51–64.

TABLE 5–3   The Limiting Amino Acids in Various Vegetables and Grains*

Food	Limiting Amino Acid
Corn	Tryptophan, lysine
Wheat	Threonine, lysine, methionine
Rice	Lysine
Potato	Methionine
Soy	Methionine (close enough to milk so that soy milk formulas fortified with methionine can support normal growth in infants)

*As compared to milk.
Source: G.B. Forbes, "Food Fads: Safe Feeding of Children," *Pediatrics in Review,* 1 (1980): 207–10.

nitrogen balance results when muscles are breaking down, as happens with bedridden patients. In these cases, more nitrogen is excreted than is taken in.

Using these data, the Food and Nutrition Board set the RDA for protein at 56 grams for a 70 kilogram (154 pound) man and 44 grams for a 55 kilogram (121 pound) woman. The RDA is generous, and in all likelihood two-thirds of the recommended level would satisfy the protein needs of most individuals. Another way to calculate protein need is to multiply ideal weight (in kilograms) by 0.8 grams of protein.

The amount of total protein and of each essential amino acid required changes with age. The proportion of total protein that should be furnished by the essential amino acids also varies with age. Approximately 40 percent of the protein required by infants must be from essential amino acids, while in the adult only 20 percent must come from essential amino acids. This means a food that is an adequate protein source for adults may be inadequate for infants or young children. Protein requirements may also increase for those who are ill or malnourished.

FOOD SOURCES OF PROTEIN

Animals produce proteins that contain all the essential amino acids in amounts similar to those needed by humans, so the protein from meat, fowl, fish, milk, and eggs tends to be of high quality. Vegetable proteins tend to be low in quality, although brown rice, wheat germ, dried yeast, and soybeans approach the quality of animal proteins. Gelatin, an animal protein, is unusual because it is low in a number of essential amino acids. Protein from vegetable sources can be improved by combining foods so that all essential amino acids are present (see Issue: Vegetarianism).

The total protein value of a food depends on both the quantity and the quality of the protein present. Foods can have generous amounts of low-quality protein, small amounts of high-quality protein, or any combination of the two:

High quantity, high quality	Meat, fish, poultry
High quantity, low quality	Beans
Low quantity, high quality	Brown rice, bacon
Low quantity, low quality	Most fruits, leafy vegetables

Foods can be compared according to how much protein they contain and the quality of this protein based on their NPU values. In Figure 5–5 the foods on the left of the "food protein continuum" are ranked according to percentage of protein; foods on the right are ranked by NPU values.

FIG. 5–5

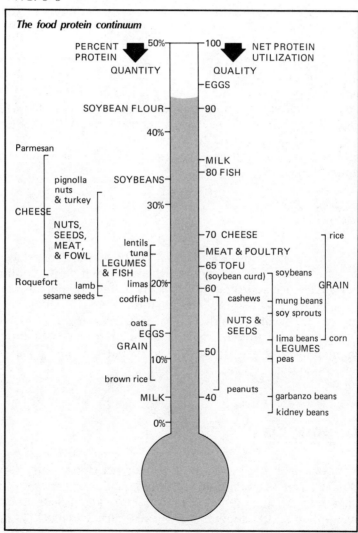

Source: F.M. Lappé, *Diet for a Small Planet* (New York: Ballantine Books, 1975), p. 78.

Protein Conversion Efficiency

Eating meat and other animal products is not always the most efficient way of meeting protein requirements. Animals can convert plant products into human food with an efficiency that ranges from 2 to 18 percent,(1) which means that the animal must consume more energy and protein than it is able to produce for human consumption. Eggs and milk have the highest efficiencies. The practice of consuming diets high in animal products would be fairly wasteful except for one unusual characteristic of ruminant animals (cows, sheep, goats). These animals can transform products of little use to humans into nutritious food. Instead of competing with humans for grain, they can live on grasses that humans cannot digest and on by-products from different food processes (meal from cottonseed and peanuts, beet pulp, molasses), slaughterhouse wastes, even the manures of cattle and poultry.

In poor countries, grain is reserved for animals like chickens and pigs that are somewhat efficient at converting kcalories into tissue. Ruminants must graze on unproductive land or eat wastes. In developed countries, though, most animals are fed diets supplemented with grain in order to increase their rate of weight gain (as in beef cattle) or to increase their milk production (as in dairy cows). Grain is also used to fatten cattle prior to slaughter, since it is the marbling in meat that gives it the taste and tenderness to which most Americans are accustomed.

Costs of Protein

The costs of protein foods vary. The most inexpensive sources are dried beans and peas. Certain types of fish and low-fat dairy products, because they are relatively rich sources of high-quality protein, do not need to be consumed in large quantities and so can provide a day's protein allowance cheaply. Other foods (steak, bacon, nuts) have a larger percentage of fat, which reduces their concentration of protein, making them more expensive sources. The costs presented in Table 5–4 are shown for comparison only; actual prices for specific items, of course, constantly fluctuate.

PROTEIN CONSUMPTION

Americans, with the exception of some strict vegetarians, have little to worry about in terms of getting enough high-quality protein. The RDA for protein ranges from 44 to 56 grams for adult females and males, yet per capita food consumption figures show that we have available to us 117 grams of protein per person per day. (These figures are determined by estimating the total amount of protein-containing foods produced or imported minus what is wasted, divided

TABLE 5–4 Protein Cost Chart

Cost (per gram of protein): Lowest → Highest

Dairy Products	Legumes	Grains and Flour	Seafood	Nuts and Seeds	Meats
Dried nonfat milk	Soy beans	Whole wheat flour			
	Blackeyed peas	Rye flour (dark)			
Cottage cheese	Split peas	Roman meal/wheat germ			
		Oatmeal	Turbot		
Buttermilk	Chick peas	Spaghetti	Herring		
Whole egg	Kidney beans	Brown rice	Swordfish		
	Lentils	Gluten flour	Perch		Hamburger
Whole milk	Black beans	Wheat bran			
		Egg noodles	Canned tuna	Peanut butter	
Swiss cheese			Catfish		
			Sardines	Raw peanuts	Chicken
Cheddar cheese		Millet		Sunflower seeds	
			Salmon		
Ricotta cheese		Cornmeal		Roasted peanuts	
		Whole wheat bread	Oysters		
Blue mold cheese		Rye bread			
Parmesan cheese			Crab (in shell)	Pumpkin seeds	Pork
Yogurt			Clams (in shell)	Raw cashews	
				Brazil nuts	Steak
Camembert				Black walnuts	Lamb chops
				Cashew nuts	
			Shrimp (canned)	Pignolia nuts	

Source: Adapted from F.M. Lappé, *Diet for a Small Planet* (New York: Ballantine Books, 1971).

by the number of people.) The results of the most recent food consumption survey (1977) revealed that average protein consumption among adults in the United States was 102 grams daily, with a range from about 99 to 113 grams for the various income groups. By these measures, most Americans are consuming slightly less than two times the RDA and, as we pointed out earlier, the RDA already exceeds the physiological needs of a large percentage of the population.

Americans tend to undervalue the protein contribution that can be made by foods other than flesh or animal products. Over two-thirds of the protein consumed in the United States comes from animal foods. In 1977, total protein consumption was as follows:(2)

Red meats	30.2 percent
Poultry	8.6 percent
Dairy products	21.8 percent
Eggs	4.8 percent
Fish	4.1 percent
Flour and cereal products, nuts, legumes	23.0 percent

In America, too little protein is hardly a problem. Not only is the American diet rich in terms of protein quantity, but many foods are of animal origin, providing high-quality protein as well. In fact, Americans may be consuming too much protein, and questions have now been raised about the risks involved in excess protein consumption. First, the excess nitrogen must be cleared by the kidney, which presents a risk for individuals with kidney malfunction. Recent research suggests that very high protein consumption may be associated with demineralization of bone, particularly if calcium consumption is low. Current research reports have also called attention to the possibility that high protein consumption may alter the internal environment and the microorganisms of the colon. This has raised the question of whether high-protein diets are associated with a greater incidence of colon cancer (see Chapter 3, Fiber). As yet these reports are speculative, but they cannot be dismissed altogether.

SUMMARY

Proteins are the nitrogen-containing components of food. Each protein is composed of a number of amino acids; the type and arrangement of amino acids determine the characteristics of the protein. The genetic information that directs what protein will be synthesized is contained in the cell nucleus. Deoxyribonucleic acid (DNA) carries the genetic code, which is transcribed onto the messenger ribonucleic acid (mRNA). The mRNA carries the genetic information to the ribosomes, the sites of protein synthesis. The amino acids required to form a particular protein are delivered to the site by transfer ribonucleic acid (tRNA). By joining the acids in the proper sequence, individual proteins are synthesized.

Some of these amino acids can be made by the body and are called nonessential amino acids. Eight (9 for infants) of the 20 naturally occurring amino acids cannot be made by the human body and must be supplied in the diet. These are the essential amino acids. All the amino acids to be included in a specific body protein must be available simultaneously for protein synthesis to proceed. This means that all eight essential amino acids should be available in the same meal and in the proportions needed for human protein synthesis.

Dietary protein is evaluated in terms of protein quantity and protein quality. The former is an index of the concentration of protein in a food (grams of protein per 100 grams of food). The latter evaluates protein in foods according to the amount of each essential amino acid present in relation to human requirements. Food sources of high-quality protein generally come from animals, while those of low-quality proteins are most often derived from plants.

Protein is required by the body primarily for the synthesis of body compounds, regulation of fluid and electrolyte balance, and maintenance of acid-base balance. If there is an excess of dietary protein, it will be converted into fat and stored.

Issue

Vegetarianism

In 1965 a young woman, weak from malnutrition, was admitted to a hospital in Passaic, New Jersey. She suffered from bleeding gums and small hemorrhages under the skin. After an interview, it was found that the woman had been following strictly the highest level of the Zen macrobiotic diet, and had consumed over a period of nine months nothing but brown rice and small amounts of fluid. The woman refused any other food from the hospital staff and insisted that she would be "purified" if she remained on the diet for just a few days longer. Two days later she died.

Sarah has been a vegetarian for 10 years, ever since she decided that eating meat was harmful to her health. Now it is quite natural for her to sit down to a meal of miso onion soup, humus with cashew nut sauce, whole wheat pita bread, and fresh salad hidden under a mound of sprouts, followed by a cup of peppermint tea and, of course, ice cream. She appears to be in good health.

Several million Americans consider themselves vegetarians, but their diets can range anywhere from all fruit to everything but "red" meat (beef, pork, and lamb).(3) Although the first written recommendation for a vegetarian diet is found in the Rig-Veda (second millenium B.C.), it was not until 1842 that a group of Britons coined the word "vegetarian" to describe their practice of avoiding meat.(3)

WHY VEGETARIANISM?

There are many reasons for choosing to eliminate meat from the diet. People have often been forced to adopt vegetarian practices when there was a shortage of animal foods, though voluntary vegetarian groups have always existed despite the availability of meat and animal products.(4) Trappist monks, under vow to live simply, consider meat a luxury and therefore to be avoided. Hindus believe the murder of an animal is the same as that of a human, since the soul transmigrates from one body to another. Some Seventh-Day Adventists refrain from eating meat for reasons of compassion and self-discipline.(4) Buddha is said to have lived on nuts and seeds for religious and ethical reasons, while George Bernard Shaw considered the consumption of meat the same as "eating corpses."(3) Although Americans cite these as well as other reasons, such as ecology, food preferences, economics, political beliefs, and curiosity, overriding motivation today for turning to vegetarianism appears to be health-related.

According to the subjects in one study,(5) eating meat made them feel tired and dull; others felt that meat contained too many "hormones," "chemicals," saturated fat, uric acid, and bacteria. The second most often stated reason was ethical; subjects felt that humans should adopt a nonviolent code toward animals and respect the dignity of life. Others held that a vegetarian diet was more conducive to meditation. Ecological concerns centered around the wastefulness of meat in light of current population and environmental problems. A smaller number of subjects responded that they disliked the taste of meat, felt it was too expensive, or had eliminated meat as a form of political protest against agribusiness.

THE VARIETIES OF VEGETARIANISM

Strictly speaking, a vegetarian is a person who abstains from the consumption of meat, fowl, and fish as food, with or without allowances for eggs and/or dairy products. Yet even this definition has some very liberal interpretations. The different types of vegetarians can be organized according to degree of dietary restrictions. One of the most extreme types is *fruitarianism*, the practice of restricting food intake to raw or dried fruits and nuts, and sometimes honey. Next would be the *vegan* or *strict vegetarian*, who eats no flesh foods or other animal food such as eggs or dairy products. *Lacto-vegetarians* allow dairy products and *ovo-vegetarians* permit eggs; *lacto-ovo-vegetarians* consume both. At the most liberal end are the *semi-vegetarians*, who eat fish and/or poultry, with or without restriction of dairy foods and eggs. So to say you are a "vegetarian" does not say anything except that you do not eat red meat.

In recent years, many Americans, particularly the young, have adopted vegetarian practices. These "new" vegetarians typically ate meat during childhood but chose to abstain as adults. Often their food restrictions are dictated by the rules of a group that has a spiritual or philosophical basis.

One diet that was very popular in the 1960s was the Zen macrobiotic diet. Originated by George Ohsawa, a Japanese born in 1893, the macrobiotic diet is intended to guide its followers to the path of longevity and peace of mind.(6) The regimen was first described in two books: *Zen Macrobiotics* and *Philosophy of Oriental Medicine*. It involves ten diets: the lowest level (−3) is composed of 10 percent cereals, 30 percent vegetables, 10 percent soup, 30 percent animal products, 15 percent salads and fruits, and 5 percent desserts; diets higher than this become increasingly more restrictive. The highest level (+7) is composed of 100 percent cereals. Fluids are restricted. At all levels, the diet is based on a mixture of antagonistic yet complementary forces (*yin* and *yang*). *Yin* foods include sugar, oil, yeast, honey, fruit, water, nuts, sea vegetables, and beans; *yang* foods include fish, soy sauce, crude salt, fowl, meat, and eggs. The perfect balance of *yin* and *yang* is found in grains.(6) Followers hold that all diseases can be treated by proper natural food, with no medicines, no surgery, and no inactivity.(7)

Although the original macrobiotic rules have been liberalized, they still veer from sound nutritional practices. Followers interpret the dietary rules differently, so that some may obtain a nutritious diet by staying with the lower levels of the regimen; others, like the overzealous woman from New Jersey, try to exist at the highest level for periods of time that even the most devout follower would not recommend. At this level, over prolonged time periods, a follower would be at risk of scurvy, anemia, protein, and calcium deficiencies, emaciation, loss of kidney function due to fluid restriction, and death. The Zen Buddhist Church does not recognize or recommend the macrobiotic system.

EVALUATING VEGETARIANISM

Nutritional Considerations

In general, the more restrictive the diet, the greater the chance a deficiency will develop. Vegetarian diets may contain so much bulk that young children have a difficult time obtaining enough kcalories before they become

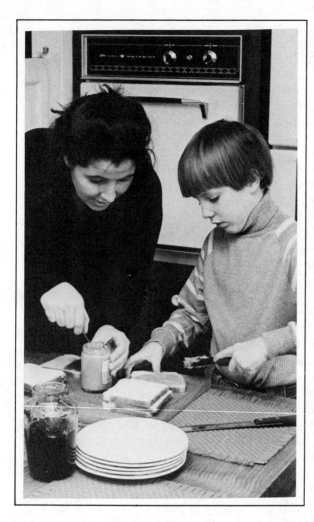

Peanut butter sandwiches provide the basis for many a vegetarian's lunch. The amino acids in the peanuts are complemented by the amino acids in the wheat.

full. With fewer kcalories, protein may be inefficiently used to provide energy instead of building tissues.(4) Cases have been reported of vegetarian children with rickets (vitamin D deficiency disease), vitamin B-12 deficiency, calcium imbalances, and general undernutrition.(9) Potential deficiencies differ depending on the foods eliminated from the diet.

The Zen Macrobiotic Diet. Adults following the macrobiotic diet show low intakes of kcalories, calcium and riboflavin and, among women, iron.(10) In order for the body to use calcium efficiently, vitamin D is required. Yet the macrobiotic diet is limited in vitamin D, since this vitamin is present almost entirely in animal products. Vitamin D can be formed by the body if the person is exposed to sunlight, so individuals at risk of a deficiency are those, particularly children, who are rarely out in the sun. Infants on this diet can receive sufficient energy and protein from the macrobiotic infant cereal Kokoh if enough kcalories are provided from other sources.(4)

Vegans. The strict vegetarian (vegan) diet tends to be low in calcium, vitamin D, vitamin B-12, riboflavin, and zinc. Dairy foods are the major sources for calcium and riboflavin. None of the vegetable sources of calcium (collards, turnip greens, mustard greens, broccoli, spinach, chard, blackstrap molasses, kale, beans, maple syrup, rhubarb, flour, figs, nuts) is equal to dairy products.(9) Also, although some vegetables like spinach and chard may be high in calcium, the calcium may be poorly absorbed due to the vegetable's high fiber content or the presence of a calcium-binding substance called oxalic acid. Absorption of calcium from grain products may be hindered by another mineral-binding substance, phytic acid. As with those who follow the macrobiotic diet, vegans may compound their calcium problem by having low intakes of vitamin D. Some cases of rickets have been reported in breastfed babies of vegan mothers.(8)

Problems can arise from using vegetables and cereals as the only sources of protein.(9) The amount and quality of protein is often low. Some nonmeat protein sources are not well digested because of their high fiber content. Young children do not digest beans well.(4) And certain legumes contain "antinutritive" factors; soybeans, for instance, contain an inhibitor of trypsin, an enzyme necessary for protein digestion.

Vegan preschool children consume less protein, fat, calcium, and riboflavin than children who consume some dairy or flesh foods.(4) Infants weaned onto vegan diets may not be able to consume enough kcalories because of the small capacity of their stomachs, the large amounts of food they must eat, and the limits on the kinds of food and the frequency of meals.(8) Children should not be put on a strict vegetarian diet unless medical and nutritional expertise is available to supervise the diet and monitor the child's health. If the diet is carefully planned, however, and if energy needs are met by a variety of unprocessed foods, protein requirements can be met. To ensure this, the use of properly fortified soy milk is recommended.(8)

Vitamin B-12 is usually present only in foods of animal origin, and the vitamin is actually synthesized by microorganisms. Meat, dairy products, and eggs contain B-12 because the diets of the animals producing them are contaminated with dirt containing microorganisms and because bacteria in their digestive tracts synthesize the vitamin.(3) Unfortunately, in humans the vitamin is synthesized in the colon, beyond the point where absorption occurs. Much controversy surrounds human dietary requirements for B-12, because if we cannot get the vitamin from plants, the implication is that humans should not be vegetarians. Few vegans have ever shown deficiency signs of this vitamin, however, and those who did generally had other accompanying medical problems, such as malabsorption of the vitamin.

A number of reasons have been suggested for why so few vegans show a B-12 deficiency. The human liver, and to a lesser extent the lungs, kidney, and spleen, can store enough B-12 to last up to five years. Little B-12 is used daily, and when stores become depleted, the body is more efficient at reabsorbing any of the vitamin that would normally be excreted.(3) Individuals vary tremendously in how low their serum levels must drop before deficiency signs show, as well as in how long they can maintain normal body function on these low levels.(4) A deficiency of B-12 may be "masked" by high intakes of folic acid, a vitamin often present in large amounts in vegetarian diets.

Some foods not of animal origin do contain B-12, which may be the reason people in other cultures (such as Zen monks in Japan) have lived healthfully for years on strict vegetarian diets. Certain foods may be grown with a lot of manure and then not be thoroughly washed. Fermented soybean foods such as *tempeh* (an Indonesian bean cake), *natto,* and *miso* (Japanese bean pastes) are contaminated by a B-12-producing bacteria. Researchers at Cornell University found the B-12 levels in *tempeh* sold in North America to range from 1.5 to 6.3 micrograms for 3½ ounces of a dried portion (the RDA for B-12 is about 3 micrograms).(3) If *tempeh* is prepared with Klebsiella bacteria, its B-12 content increases remarkably. Sea vegetables contaminated by plankton also contain B-12. These include *kombu, wakame, nori, hijiki, dulse, arame,* kelp, *alaria,* green *nori* flakes, and unprocessed agar. Few of these, however, are reliable sources, since their B-12 content varies considerably.(8) Nonbacterial sources include the yeasts, although in their natural state only those grown on a medium rich in B-12 contain the vitamin. Other yeasts (nutritional, brewer's, torula) usually have B-12 added. Although nonanimal sources of B-12 exist, vegans may not choose to eat any of these foods. For these individuals vitamin B-12 supplements or B-12 fortified foods are recommended.

The vegan may also have difficulty obtaining sufficient zinc because zinc from plants is not as well absorbed as that from animals. In addition, the fiber found in grains and vegetables inhibits zinc absorption, as does phytic acid, a mineral-binding compound.(3) (Yeast fermentation, like that which occurs during breadmaking, helps to lower the phytic acid in whole wheat flour and aid zinc absorption.)

Lacto-ovo-vegetarians. A lacto-ovo-vegetarian diet offers no risk to children or adults in regard to protein. Iron may present a problem if care is not taken routinely to include rich sources of the mineral. When the nutrient intakes of lacto-ovo-vegetarians, fish eaters, and meat eaters were compared, the results were surprising.(11) The fish eaters and lacto-ovo-vegetarians consumed many foods of high nutrient density. The vegetarians had higher intakes of carbohydrate, vitamins A and C, thiamin, calcium, phosphorus, and iron.

The higher iron intake of vegetarian women was due to a generous intake of legumes, seeds, nuts, and grains. Since milk and eggs are poor iron sources, the vegan may have a higher iron intake than the lacto-ovo-vegetarian.(3) The kcalorie intake was similar for all three groups, but the meat eaters had more obesity, a result of less daily exercise.

"Casual vegetarians" are those who are not completely committed to a vegetarian diet. They do not eat fish or shellfish or take the time to prepare beans or rice. Because they rely primarily on eggs and cheese, they are at risk of low intakes of iron.(12)

Vegetarianism, if practiced intelligently, can be a healthful way to eat. But there are certain issues to be considered. Young children on strict vegetarian diets may grow at rates below established norms. Slowed growth (measured in terms of weight and length) has occurred in children under 2 years of age,(4) and in 3- to 5-year-olds (measured in weight and height).(8) These children often fail to grow because they are fed nut and seed milks after weaning. Many vegan mothers are now beginning to switch to soy milks fortified with all the vitamins and calcium,(6) and some with added iron.

Some followers of vegetarian diets believe that all medical problems can be prevented and/or cured by diet and may fail to seek medical advice when necessary. On the other hand, vegetarianism can promote health in a number of ways. Vegetarians tend to have a lower incidence of obesity, a risk factor for a number of disorders. The high fiber content of most vegetarian diets may prevent constipation and certain digestive tract disorders. The breast milk of mothers who eat little animal fat contains fewer pesticide residues.(3). Osteoporosis, a condition affecting four out of five elderly women in the United States, results from a loss of bone density.(8) Although many factors affect the loss of bone mineral, research suggests that high intake of protein over a lifetime may contribute to the problem. Lacto-ovo-vegetarians have only about half the bone loss seen in 60- to 90-year-old meat eaters.(8)

Several researchers have advanced the hypothesis that vegetarians may be at less risk of coronary heart disease and colon cancer than nonvegetarians. Certainly most vegetarian diets, except those that include a lot of cheese, butter, and whole milk, are generally high in fiber and complex carbohydrates and low in saturated fats. Leguminous seeds (chick peas) have a cholesterol-lowering effect. The evidence supporting this hypothesis, though, is epidemiological, and conflicting data also exist.(4)

A number of religious groups that have unusual eating patterns as well as lowered rates of certain diseases have been studied. About half of Seventh Day Adventists (SDA) follow a lacto-ovo-vegetarian diet, along with avoidance of alcohol and tobacco. SDAs have a mortality from certain cancers 50 to 70 percent lower than that of the general population. These cancers (of the gastrointestinal tract and reproductive organs) are not related to smoking or drinking.(13) The link between diet and cancer among this group, however, is still speculative.

A study on California SDAs found a lower rate of coronary heart disease mortality among vegetarian males over 65 and among all females.(14) This finding may result in part from the prohibition on smoking. Strict vegetarian women, of all the SDA vegetarians, had the highest risk for coronary heart disease deaths, although their rate was comparable with that of the general population. Other studies have found lower serum cholesterol levels in vegetarians.(15)

The population of Utah, more than 70 percent Mormon, has a cancer mortality rate less than the United States average.(4) The residents of Utah do not restrict themselves to vegetarian diets, but the Mormon Church does call for moderation in the use of meat. What part this plays in reduced cancer mortality is still open to question. The answer may lie in the better overall health habits found among both SDAs and Mormons. Since the most frequently stated reason for a vegetarian diet is health, any positive effect resulting from consuming such a diet is as likely to come from the accompanying changes in life style people often adopt, such as giving up cigarettes, cutting down on alcohol, or increasing exercise, as it is from the diet itself.

PLANNING A VEGETARIAN DIET

Meat Alternatives

A major concern in planning a vegetarian diet is to allow for enough high-quality protein. There are several alternatives to meat protein, but in order to replace meat adequately, they must meet two criteria.

First, the quantity (grams) of protein provided by the substitute should be close to the amount provided in an average serving of meat (20 grams). Any amount over half this is acceptable, so the substitute must contain at least 10 grams of protein per serving. Second, the pattern of the eight essential amino acids must be present in proportions similar to those required by humans.

Three general types of meat alternatives meet these criteria. Direct substitution of flesh foods (meat, fish, poultry) with other high-quality protein products (milk, cheese, and eggs) gives a product with excellent protein quality. In fact, on a per gram basis this protein is better used than meat. It is, however, not as concentrated in protein on a per serving basis as meat.

A second type of meat alternative extends high-quality proteins by combining small quantities of high-quality protein (eggs, dairy products) with larger quantities of plant proteins such as beans, noodles, and other grain products. Although these plant products are fairly concentrated in protein, certain essential amino acids are limiting. The large quantities of essential amino acids even in small portions of meat, eggs, or cheese, supplement the amino acids of the plant foods so that the combination is well utilized. For example, dairy products are good sources of lysine, whereas cereal grains are low in lysine. By combining the two, the result is a food with good protein quality. At the same time, the quantity of protein provided by the small amount of dairy product is increased by that in the larger quantity of grains—this is why macaroni and cheese is such a good protein source.

Mutual complementation, the third type of meat alternative, is the combination of different plant proteins with mutually complementary amino acid patterns. A particular plant protein may be deficient in one or two specific amino acids but be adequate in all the others. A second plant protein, which "complements" the first, provides adequate amounts of these deficient amino acids. In turn, the first source provides what is limiting in the second. For instance, legumes are limited in the sulfur-containing amino acids (methionine, cystine). Nuts, seeds, and grains are limited in lysine. If legumes are served with grains or nuts, the legumes furnish the lysine, while the grains and nuts supply the sulfur-containing amino acids. Together they provide a good amino acid pattern. Other examples of complementary proteins are legumes plus rice; soybeans plus rice and wheat; beans plus wheat; beans plus corn; and soybeans plus wheat and sesame (Table 5–5.)

Complementary protein mixes do not give a perfect amino acid pattern fully usable by the body, but combinations can increase the protein quality as much as 50 percent above the average of the items if they are eaten separately.

Some common examples of meat alternatives and the quantity of protein contained in an average serving are shown in Table 5–6. As these samples show, meat alternatives often do not contain as much protein per serving as 3 ounces of meat, so if you rely on these alternatives, you may need larger or more frequent servings.

In recent years, vegetable protein products have become available in the United States. The marketplace has been the testing ground for a new type of

---

TABLE 5–5 **Complementary Proteins**

Protein	Food
Legumes plus grains	Hopping John (blackeyed peas and rice) Frijoles and corn tortillas Tofu (soy bean curd) and rice Peanut butter and whole wheat bread sandwich Baked beans and Boston brown bread
Legumes plus seeds	Tahini (garbanzo and sesame seed spread) Split pea soup with sesame seed crackers Peanut and sunflower seed snacks
Legumes plus nuts	Lentil casserole with nut topping

The proteins in dairy products and eggs also complement the proteins in plant foods and increase their value:

Grains plus dairy products	Hot or cold cereal and milk Macaroni and cheese Cheese and whole wheat bread sandwich
Grains and eggs	Egg salad sandwich Rice custard
Legumes plus dairy products	Peanuts and cheese cubes Lentil soup made with milk
Legumes and eggs	Cooked blackeyed peas with egg salad
Seeds or nuts with dairy products	Sesame seeds mixed with cottage cheese Cheese ball rolled in chopped nuts
Seeds or nuts with egg	Omelet sprinkled with sesame seeds

TABLE 5–6	Meat Alternatives		
Alternative		Protein/Serving	Type
Cheese soufflé:			
cheese and milk		11 g	Direct substitution
eggs		4	with high-quality
		—	protein
		15g/serving	
Macaroni and cheese			
macaroni		6 g	Extended high-quality
cheese and milk		8	protein
		—	
		14 g/serving	
Chicken and noodles			
chicken (1 oz)		7 g	Extended high-quality
noodles		8	protein
		—	
		15 g/serving	
Navy beans and cornbread			
¾ cup beans		11 g	Mutual complementation
2 cornbread muffins		6	
		—	
		17 g/serving	

meat alternative. Called *meat analogs, textured vegetable protein (TVP),* or *extended protein products (EPP),* these foods are composed of a variety of ingredients that simulate meat. Available in frozen, canned, or dried form, these substitutes are made from grain (wheat, oats, barley, millet), legumes (soybeans, peas, lentils), nuts, or a combination of all these. Sometimes egg is added, and dehydrated vegetables are used for flavoring.(3)

The advantage of meat analogs is that they can be formulated to contain any level of protein, fat, or carbohydrate desired. They can even be combined to complement amino acids, though this is not always done. In general, these analogs are lower in fat and protein than the meats they replace, and they are convenience foods because they require little preparation time.(3) The disadvantages of these products are that they may lack many of the trace minerals and other nutrients available from meat; the processing of the products can destroy the B-vitamins (some are fortified with B-12); they may lead to flatulence; they are often tasteless and have poor texture; and they cost more than meat. Even so, meat analogs should reach 10 percent of all domestic meat consumption by the year 2000.(16)

Daily Food Guides for Vegetarians

Meat is an excellent source of nutrients other than protein, particularly iron and certain B-vitamins. To assure that these plus other nutrients are consumed in adequate amounts, vegetarians should give careful attention to eating a variety of foods from the groups allowed in their particular regimen.

Lacto-Ovo-Vegetarian. Table 5–7 shows a dietary guide with suggested number of servings from the four food groups available to the lacto-ovo-vegetarian. Care should be taken to avoid "empty kcalorie" foods (fats, oils, sweets) that are low in nutrient density. A lacto-ovo-vegetarian can be better nourished than a meat eater if the latter eats a lot of fats, sugars, and muscle meats and limits whole grains, fruits, and vegetables.(15)

Meats are replaced with legumes, nuts, and meat analogs from wheat and/or soy proteins. Most of these are good sources of iron and a number of B-vitamins. Nonfat or lowfat dairy products (milk, cottage cheese) are preferable to whole because they contain more protein and calcium per serving. Individuals who have lactose intolerance may be able to drink small amounts of milk. For those who cannot, the use of Lact-aid in milk breaks down the lactose, so that there are no uncomfortable side effects.(8) Soy milk does not contain lactose.

Whole grains and cereals are preferred to refined. A variety of dark green vegetables and fresh and dried fruits should be eaten for their vitamins A and C and mineral content. A vitamin C source should be included with each meal to aid in iron absorption.

Vegan. A dietary guide for the vegan is shown in Table 5–8. Vegan diets rely on mutual complementation for adequate essential amino acids. Combining proteins of vegetable origin to provide a good balance among the essential amino acids requires special knowledge. Also, foods of vegetable origin are not generally concentrated in protein, so larger portion sizes are required.

The milk group for the lacto-ovo-vegetarian supplies 75 percent of calcium, 43 percent of riboflavin, 22 percent of protein, and 100 percent of vitamin B-12 requirements.(15) The vegan should increase quantities of foods that provide nutrients normally supplied by the deleted milk group. For instance, a fortified soy milk drink could be used. Most, but not all, commercial

---

TABLE 5–7   **A Dietary Guide for Lacto-Ovo-Vegetarians**

Grains, legumes, nuts, seeds: protein, carbohydrates, fat, thiamin, niacin, folic acid, vitamin E, zinc, magnesium, fiber
6 servings or more. Include several slices of yeast-raised, whole-grain bread, a serving of beans, a few nuts and seeds.

Vegetables: vitamin A, folacin, riboflavin, vitamin C, calcium
3 servings or more. Include one or more servings of dark leafy greens.

Fruits: vitamins C, A
1–4 pieces. Include a raw source of vitamin C.

Milk and eggs: protein, vitamin B-12, riboflavin, calcium
2 or more glasses of fresh milk for adults
3 or more for children (children under 9 use smaller glasses)
Other dairy products or eggs can meet part of milk requirement.

Source: L. Robertson, C. Flanders, and B. Godfrey, *Laurel's Kitchen* (Berkeley: Nilgiri Press, 1976), p. 67.

TABLE 5–8 **A Dietary Guide for Vegans**

Grains
4 slices of bread
3–5 servings of grain
1 serving of nuts or seeds daily

Legumes
⅓ cup beans and 2 cups fortified soybean milk, or 1¼ cups beans plus other sources of vitamin B-12 and calcium every day.

Vegetables
4 or more servings of good-quality vegetables every day (3 grams of protein).
Include 2 substantial servings of dark leafy greens for calcium and riboflavin.

Fruit
1–4 servings daily. Include a raw source of vitamin C.

Good sources of some limited nutrients
B-12: 2 cups fortified soy milk, fortified nutritional yeast, or a vitamin pill.
Calcium: fortified soy milk, leafy greens without oxalates, sunflower seeds, unhulled sesame seeds, blackstrap molasses.
Riboflavin: beans, green leaves, certain nuts, nutritional yeasts, wheat germ.

Source: L. Robertson, C. Flanders, and B. Godfrey, *Laurel's Kitchen* (Berkeley: Nilgiri Press, 1976), p. 322.

soy or sesame seed milks are fortified with calcium and vitamins A, D, and B-12. Those developed for infants also include vitamin K. Homemade infant formulas based on soy are rarely fortified with either vitamins or calcium and may not be heated to destroy the trypsin inhibitor. As compared to breast milk or other commercial formulas, these homemade varieties contain less calcium, zinc, vitamins A, B-12, D, K, and thiamin.(8)

A moderate amount of yeast can be used. Yeast contains a relatively large amount of nucleic acids compared with other foods, so excessive use should be avoided.(8) Calcium and riboflavin will be reduced, since milk and milk products are deleted, so increased quantities of dark green leafy vegetables, broccoli, dandelion greens, kale, turnip greens, legumes, soybeans, nuts, and winter squash are recommended.

Adequate kcalories should be consumed, since vegan diets are high in fiber, which dilutes the kcalorie content. Increased use of breads, cereals, legumes, nuts, and seeds is recommended. A vitamin B-12 supplement may be advisable, or commercially fortified products. Some sample menus are shown in Table 5–9.

Recommended Cookbooks

- J. Hewitt, *The New York Times Natural Foods Cookbook* (New York: Avon Books, 1971).(contains some nonvegetarian recipes)
- E.B. Ewald, *Recipes for a Small Planet* (New York: Ballantine Books, 1973).

TABLE 5–9 Sample Vegetarian Menus	
Vegan	*Lacto-Ovo-Vegetarian*
Breakfast	
orange juice	cheese omelet with onion, mushrooms,
oatmeal with soy milk	green peppers, tomato
2 tbsp soy grits	1 slice whole wheat toast
1 slice whole wheat toast	low-fat or skim milk
tea	½ grapefruit
Lunch	
pita bread	2 slices whole grain bread
humus (chick-pea spread)	ricotta cheese mixed with nuts and raisins
tahini (sesame seed paste)	tomato juice
cut-up vegetables	
1 orange	
almonds	
Dinner	
vegetable soup	eggplant parmesan
salad with seeds and nuts sprinkled	salad
on top	whole grain bread
soybean croquettes served with a	yogurt with orange slices or strawberries
cashew nut sauce	tea
orange muffins	
soybean milk	

- L. Robertson, C. Flanders, and B. Godfrey, *Laurel's Kitchen* (Berkeley: Nilgiri Press, 1976).

- M. Katzen, *The Moosewood Cookbook* (Berkeley: Ten Speed Press, 1977).

- A. Thomas, *The Vegetarian Epicure*, Book 1 (New York: Vintage, 1972).

- A. Thomas, *The Vegetarian Epicure*, Book 2 (New York: Knopf, 1980).

- J. Larson and R. McLin, *The Vegetable Protein and Vegetarian Cookbook* (New York: Arco, 1977).

REFERENCES

1. J. Janick, C.H. Noller, and C.L. Rhykerd, "The Cycles of Plant and Animal Nutrition," *Scientific American* 235(1976):75–86.

2. A.O. Johnson, *Food Consumption Prices and Expenditures*. USDA Agriculture Economics Report 138, Suppl. 1977.

3. "Vegetarianism: Can You Get By without Meat?" *Consumer Reports,* June 1980, pp. 357–65.

4. "Nutrition and Vegetarianism," *Dairy Council Digest* 50, January–February 1979, pp. 1–6.

5. J.T. Dwyer, L. Mayer, K. Dowd, R.F. Kandel, and J. Mayer, "The New Vegetarians: The Natural High?" *Journal of the American Dietetic Association* 65(1974):529–36.

6. D. Erhard, "The New Vegetarians," *Nutrition Today,* January–February 1974, pp. 20–27.

7. Council on Foods and Nutrition, "Zen Macrobiotic Diets," *Journal of the American Medical Association* 218(1971):397.

8. "Position Paper on the Vegetarian Approach to Eating: American Dietetic Association Reports," *Journal of the American Dietetic Association* 77(1980):61–69.

9. Committee on Nutritional Misinformation, Food and Nutrition Board, *Vegetarian Diets.* (Washington, D.C.: National Academy of Sciences, May 1974).

10. P.T. Brown and J.G. Bergan, "The Dietary Status of "New" Vegetarians," *Journal of the American Dietetic Association* 67(1975):455.

11. L.A. Taber and R.A. Cook, "Dietary and Anthropometric Assessment of Adult Omnivores, Fish-Eaters, and Lacto-Ovo-Vegetarians," *Journal of the American Dietetic Association* 76(1980):21–29.

12. J. Wurtman, "Vitamin and Mineral Supplements," *The Harvard Medical School Health Letter VI* (November 1980):3–4.

13. R.L. Phillips and F.R. Lemon, "Role of Life-Style and Dietary Habits in Risk of Cancer among Seventh-Day Adventists," *Cancer Research* 35(1975):3513.

14. R.L. Phillips, F.R. Lemon, W.L. Beeson, and J.W. Kuzma, "Coronary Heart Disease Mortality among Seventh-Day Adventists with Differing Dietary Habits: A Preliminary Report," *American Journal of Clinical Nutrition* 31(1978):S191.

15. U.D. Register and L.M. Sonnenberg, "The Vegetarian Diet," *Journal of the American Dietetic Association* 62(1973):253–61.

16. T.M. Hammonds and D.L. Call, *Utilization of Protein Ingredients in the U.S. Food Industry.* (Ithaca, New York: Cornell University, Department of Agriculture Economics Research 320 and 321, 1970).

Energy

6

Each year close to 5000 runners, decked out in T shirts, shorts, running shoes, and an occasional Superman outfit, charge from Hopkinton, Massachusetts, to the Prudential Center Plaza in Boston in the annual Boston marathon. The amount of energy that keeps all those legs moving and hearts pumping is enormous. As an estimate, if a participant were to complete the 26-mile, 385-yard race (given a rough calculation of 660 kcalories per hour with an average finish time of 3 hours), the total energy requirement would be about 2000 kcalories. This is equivalent to 28 oranges, 16 beers, or 3½ Big Macs. And if you trace the energy expended by these marathoners back to its source, you would eventually find the sun.

PHOTOSYNTHESIS AND BIOLOGICAL OXIDATION

According to one law of physics, energy can neither be created nor destroyed. It can, however, be transformed from one state to another. This is true for both living and nonliving things.

The sun's radiant energy, for instance, can be converted into chemical energy, which in turn can be used for mechanical work. Participants in the Boston marathon were running (mechanical work) on energy from food (chemical energy) that had been transferred to plants as they matured in fields (radiant energy). These energy conversions involve two major biological processes: photosynthesis and biological oxidation.

One aspect of living organisms that sets them apart from nonliving matter is their need and capability for breaking down nutrients from the environment for use as materials in manufacturing structural components. Some organisms depend more on these outside nutrients than others.

The most self-sufficient are plants and certain bacteria that can "self-feed." By using light-sensitive pigments (such as chlorophyll) located in special cells, they trap the sun's energy and use it to convert carbon dioxide (from the air) and water (from the air and soil) into complex forms of carbon, hydrogen, and oxygen. Plants also require certain minerals, such as nitrogen, phosphorus and potassium, which they obtain from the soil. By reshuffling the carbon, hydrogen, and oxygen atoms, they create simple carbohydrates or sugars like glucose. Some oxygen is released into the air. This process, known as photosynthesis, is represented by the following equation:

$$\underset{\underset{\text{from air}}{\uparrow}}{\text{carbon dioxide}} + \underset{\underset{\underset{\text{from soil}}{\uparrow}}{\text{from air}}}{\text{water}} + \text{solar energy} \longrightarrow \text{carbohydrates} + \underset{\underset{\text{to air}}{\uparrow}}{\underset{\text{released}}{\text{oxygen}}}$$

Once the plant makes the sugars, it chains them together to form more complex carbohydrates, known as starches and cellulose. Each plant differs in how much sugar it converts into complex carbohydrates.

Some plants, such as potatoes and rice, are not sweet because the starch predominates. In others, such as sugar beets and sweet peas, there are larger amounts of sugar than starch, so the plant tastes sweet. The sugar-to-starch ratio within a plant changes over time. Bananas become sweeter as they ripen because the starch is converted to sugar during ripening. The blacker the banana, the sweeter the fruit. Other vegetables like corn are initially sweet but become starchy as they mature. Figure 6–1 shows the photosynthetic process and lists the different types of carbohydrates produced according to their predominance in particular plants.

In the initial steps of photosynthesis, the plant forms sugars, starches, and cellulose. Plants can then rearrange the carbon, hydrogen, and oxygen from these compounds and forms fatty acids, along with a molecule called glycerol. When three fatty acids join with a glycerol molecule, the result is a fat. Fats are found mainly in seeds and nuts that act as long-term energy stores for the young seedling. But another compound, protein, remains to be synthesized. Proteins contain not only carbon, hydrogen, and oxygen, but also nitrogen. So, in order to make them, plants must have a nitrogen source. Nitrogen in the air is relatively useless to most living organisms. The exceptions are the nitrogen-fixing bacteria, such as those of the genus Rhizobium. These bacteria colonize in root nodules on certain types of plants called legumes (peas, beans, alfalfa),

FIG. 6-1

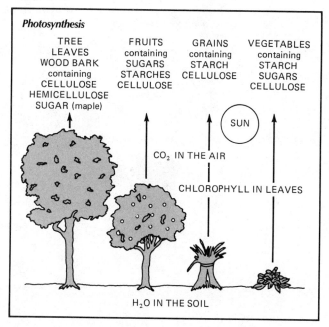

Photosynthesis

TREE	FRUITS	GRAINS	VEGETABLES
LEAVES	containing	containing	containing
WOOD BARK	SUGARS	STARCH	STARCH
containing	STARCHES	CELLULOSE	SUGARS
CELLULOSE	CELLULOSE		CELLULOSE
HEMICELLULOSE			
SUGAR (maple)			

SUN

CO_2 IN THE AIR

CHLOROPHYLL IN LEAVES

H_2O IN THE SOIL

where they extract and use nitrogen from the air. The legumes can use this nitrogen to make proteins. Other plants must have a different nitrogen source.

These other plants obtain nitrogen through a cycle that involves three players: plants, animals, and soil microorganisms. First plants take nitrogen from the soil in the form of nitrate and put together the amino acids. Recall that amino acids are combinations of carbon, hydrogen, nitrogen, and oxygen linked together to form proteins.

Animals consume these plant proteins and break them down into amino acids to use as nutrients for their own needs. They can reconnect the amino acids to make body proteins or use them for other biochemical processes. To use the amino acids for these other processes, the body must first detach the nitrogen from the carbon, hydrogen, and oxygen structure and excrete it as waste onto the soil. If the amino acids are used to make body proteins, the nitrogen remains attached and is returned to the soil as decay matter after the animal's death. Some of the plant proteins consumed by animals are not absorbed and these are excreted as waste in the feces. Whether as waste or decay, this nitrogen must be converted into nitrate before plants can use it again. This is the function of soil microorganisms. By converting the nitrogen back into nitrate, they complete the nitrogen cycle (Figure 6-2).

The plant has now taken carbon dioxide from the air along with water from both air and soil and, powered by sunlight, has created carbohydrates and fats. In addition, it has extracted nitrogen from the soil (or air via the Rhizobium bacteria) and created proteins. These three complex forms of carbon, hydrogen,

FIG. 6–2

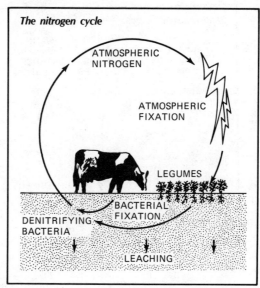

The nitrogen cycle

and oxygen (and nitrogen for proteins) compose the stems, roots, leaves, flowers, fruits, and seeds of the plant. Plants thus provide animals, including humans, with a dietary source of the fuel nutrients.

Biological Oxidation

This flow of nutrients from plants to animals is called a food chain. You can meet your nutritional needs by eating low on the chain and consuming only plant products; or you can, and probably do, eat higher up on the chain and consume animal products as well as plants. At various levels on the chain, the nutrients differ. Recall that proteins from plants are usually of lower quality than protein from animals, and fats from plants tend to be more unsaturated than fats from animals. For conversion to useful energy, however, all these complex forms of nutrients must be broken down to their basic components and degraded to carbon dioxide and water. This process is called biological oxidation.

Biological oxidation involves a series of reactions by which energy stored in food is converted to chemical energy usable by the body. During biological oxidation, the body cells use oxygen in a process that converts carbohydrates, fats, and proteins to carbon dioxide and water. This particular aspect is called respiration. Respiration is the opposite of photosynthesis; oxygen is used to

FIG. 6–3

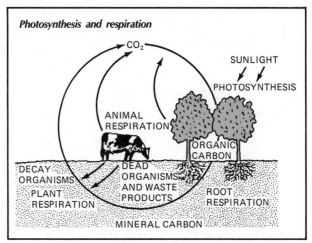

Photosynthesis and respiration

release food energy, with carbon dioxide and water being the end products. The balance between photosynthesis and respiration is shown in Figure 6–3.

Through photosynthesis, plants trap the sun's energy in the chemical bonds of carbohydrates, fats, and proteins. Humans cannot use this energy until it is converted into a different form of chemical energy, adenosine triphosphate (ATP).

MEASURING ENERGY INPUTS

Energy leaves the body as heat, so food energy is measured in terms of the physicists' unit for heat energy, the calorie. A calorie is not a nutrient; it is defined as the amount of heat necessary to raise one gram (1 milliliter) of water by 1 degree Centigrade. The energy released from food is too enormous to be described by these units, so nutritionists refer to the calorie or kilocalorie (kcalorie) equivalent to 1000 of these small calories, in measuring the energy from carbohydrates, fats, and proteins. Though not technically correct, most consumer literature calls these units "calories."

Carbohydrates, fats, and proteins provide different amounts of energy. (Alcohol also provides energy and is discussed in more detail in Chapter 2.) The number of kcalories a food has depends on its composition and on how well you digest and absorb the food.

Recall that carbohydrates and protein both yield 4 kcalories per gram. Fat is a more concentrated source of fuel. Fats provide 9 kcalories per gram, or more than twice the amount produced by carbohydrates and proteins. Alcohol provides 7 kcalories per gram.

You can estimate the energy value of a food by knowing its composition of carbohydrates, fats, and proteins. If a given food, say a small bag (3.5 ounces) of peanuts, contains 20 grams of carbohydrate, 40 grams of fat, and 25 grams of protein, the total amount of energy (kcalories) released upon oxidation can be calculated as follows:

Carbohydrates
20 grams × 4 kcalories/gram = 80 kcalories

Fats
40 grams × 9 kcalories/gram = 360 kcalories

Protein
25 grams × 4 kcalories/gram = 100 kcalories
Total   540 kcalories

This small bag of peanuts provides about 540 kcalories. (Notice how quickly kcalories add up in foods high in fat.)

MEASURING ENERGY OUTPUTS

Your body uses the energy from ATP to fuel a wide variety of processes from the mental concentration required for chess to the movement of individual ions across a cell membrane. These energy-requiring processes are divided into three categories:

- Basal metabolism
- Thermogenic effect of food
- Voluntary (physical) activity

Basal Metabolism

The first, basal metabolism, is the energy used for internal or cellular work (respiration, circulation, glandular activity, and maintenance of body temperature) while the body is at rest. It includes all the activities, except food digestion and absorption, that go on without conscious effort, such as the heart beating. This is the least or "basal" amount of energy required for living.

The amount of energy needed for basal metabolism is influenced by body size. The larger the body, the more cells there are which require nourishment, and the more extensive the respiratory, circulatory, and glandular systems. These all lead to a higher basal metabolism. Since men are usually larger than women, they generally have a higher metabolism. The following formula gives a rough estimate of basal needs:

For women:	Take your present weight and add a zero to it. To that new number add your present weight.

Example:	If you weigh 120 pounds	
	Add zero to weight	1200
	Add present weight	120
		1320
		kcalories

For men:	Take your present weight and add a zero to it. To that new number add twice your present weight.

Example:	If you weigh 160 pounds	
	Add zero to weight	1600
	Add twice present weight	320
		1920
		kcalories

A 160-pound man expends about 2000 kcalories daily for maintaining internal processes. These derived figures give only an approximation of basal energy needs, but even so you can see that your internal processes require quite a large expenditure of energy.

Basal metabolic rate (BMR) is the least amount of energy required for a given length of time per unit of body surface area or body weight. Basal metabolic rate differs from basal metabolism in that BMR measurements are expressed per unit of body surface area or body weight, so that total body size plays a smaller role, and is also measured over a given unit of time (one hour). The best time to measure BMR is immediately upon rising in the morning, before events such as breakfast have a chance to exert an effect. Since it involves units of surface area or body weight and is measured over time, the BMR of each individual is affected by factors such as body composition, sex, age, emotional state, body size, and activity of the thyroid gland.

Body Composition and Sex. Muscle tissue needs more energy than fat in order to maintain tone. Since men generally have a larger proportion of muscle to fat tissue than women, they typically have a higher BMR. Physically active people also have a higher BMR than those who are sedentary because they develop more muscle tissue and maintain its tone.

Age. BMR always increases during periods of rapid growth (infancy, adolescence, last trimester of pregnancy). Infants up to 18 months of age show rapid growth in cell number and cell size, and demand large amounts of energy. Although they require fewer total kcalories than adults, the proportion per unit of body weight demanded for basal needs is higher than for adults. BMR decreases slightly with age due to the usual decrease in physical activity accompanying advancing years. Reduced activity leads to loss of muscle tissue, which in turn reduces the body's energy needs.

Emotional State. People under emotional strain have increased muscle tension, which raises BMR.

Body Size. The body produces heat in proportion to the surface area of the skin because heat is continually lost through the skin. Taller, thinner persons have greater surface areas and higher BMRs than shorter, fatter persons of the same weight.

Thyroid Secretion. The most direct controllers of BMR are the hormones secreted by the thyroid gland. An elevated or depressed secretion of these hormones alters energy needs. An undersecretion, called hypothyroidism, lowers BMR and leads to weight gain. Hyperthyroidism, an oversecretion of the thyroid hormones, elevates BMR and results in weight loss. But although many people blame an underactive thyroid gland for their weight problems, few are overweight for this reason.

Thermogenic Effect

The second category of energy expenditure is the thermogenic effect of foods. This is the energy used solely for digestion of foods and absorption of nutrients, and it accounts for only 6 to 10 percent of the body's total energy expenditure. This category is set apart from basal metabolism, even though it uses involuntary processes, because it is a periodic activity. It occurs only for the duration of digestion and the time required to absorb the last of the ingested nutrients. You can remember it as a separate category from basal metabolism if you note that during sleep, when all the basal activities are occurring, you are not usually eating, so energy is not diverted to digest and absorb nutrients. (This precludes any subconscious raids on the refrigerator or napping after meals.)

Physical Activity

Physical activity, defined as movement of the body in the environment, is the third and last category of energy expenditure. Energy expenditure varies with type of activity, length of time involved in the activity, and size of the participant. A larger person requires more energy to perform the same job in the same amount of time as a smaller person, since the former has to move more mass.

This is the only energy-expenditure category you can manipulate to any great extent. An individual's BMR is fairly constant, although major changes in physical activity can alter body composition by increasing muscle and decreasing fat, causing a slight rise in metabolic rate. The thermogenic effect of foods can only be minimally changed by diet, since proteins require slightly more energy for digestion than do fats and carbohydrates. This increase is insignificant compared to the total energy output. Physical activity, on the other hand, accounts for wide fluctuations in energy needs. The following chart provides a set of factors for estimating total energy needs (basal metabolism + thermogenic effect + physical activity), based on current body weight and activity level.

Activity Level	Men	Women
Sedentary	16	14
Moderately active	21	18
Very active	26	22

The sedentary classification represents most office workers and students. Moderately active includes those following a regular exercise program. Very active includes lumberjacks and Olympic contenders. To estimate your energy needs, choose the factor under the column corresponding to your sex and next to the line with your activity level. Multiply this factor by your current weight to give kcalories of daily energy expenditure. This figure represents your daily energy needs, but it is only an approximation.

Example: If you are a 120-pound sedentary woman (you manage to walk to class from the bus stop):

Factor		Weight	Energy expenditure
14	X	120	1680 kcalories

If you are a 120-pound very active woman (you are a member of a gymnastics team):

Factor		Weight	Energy expenditure
22	X	120	2640 kcalories

The difference in these energy levels, a result of different levels of physical activity, is close to 1000 kcalories. Appendix E shows the number of minutes you must engage in various activities in order to "use up" the kcalories from different foods.

SUMMARY

In nature, matter is continuously used and released by one group of organisms only to be picked up by another group for its survival needs. Photosynthesis and biological oxidation represent two such cycles. Plants, by taking up carbon dioxide and water, create carbohydrates that in turn can be converted to fats. Animals consume these nutrients, break them down by the process of biological oxidation, and return them as end products (carbon dioxide and water) into the environment. By means of a third cycle, plants take nitrogen from the soil (and air via nitrogen-fixing bacteria) and make amino acids, later to become proteins. Once animals consume the proteins, the nitrogen may be removed from the amino acids (basic units of protein) and excreted as waste or the amino acids may be incorporated as part of body protein and returned to the soil upon the animal's death.

Plants capture solar energy in the chemical bonds of the carbohydrates, fats, and proteins they create. When animals and humans consume these nutrients, the energy is transferred to the compound adenosine triphosphate (ATP). More precisely, the energy is captured in the bond between the second and third phosphate groups on this molecule.

Energy available for work is measured by kilocalories, (kcalories) or Calories (more popularly called "calories"). The three fuel nutrients, plus alcohol, release different amounts of energy; carbohydrates and proteins provide 4 kcalories per gram; fats provide 9 kcalories per gram; and alcohol, 7 kcalories. The body uses this energy to fuel three types of processes: basal metabolism, thermogenic effect of food, and physical activity. Basal metabolism is influenced by body composition, sex, body size, age, emotional state, and thyroid secretions. The thermogenic effects of food account for the energy needed for digesting foods and absorbing nutrients. Physical activity is the movement of the body in the environment. All three added together give the total energy requirement. Proportionately greater amounts of energy are required for growth, and lesser amounts for maintenance of the body once growth is completed. Large people need more energy than small people; boys and men usually need more than girls and women. Active people require more energy than inactive people.

Office workers and students are prone to sedentary lifestyles.

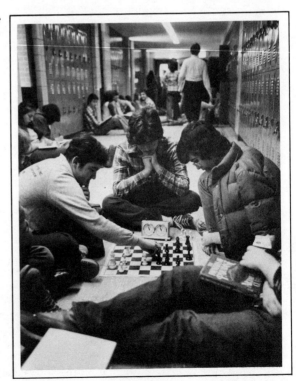

Issue

Weight Control

"But wait a bit," the Oyster cried
"Before we have our chat
"For some of us are out of breath
"And all of us are fat."
From Lewis Carroll, "The Walrus and the Carpenter"

Maybe not all of us are fat, but at least 79 million Americans are overweight, and 40 million are obese or overfat.(1) At any one time an estimated 9.5 million Americans are dieting,(2) spending about 10 billion per year, and most will fail to achieve a permanent loss. And the situation seems to be getting worse.

Military records of Civil War recruits entering the Union Army in 1863 show the average weight for a 5-foot 10-inch man, aged 30 to 34 years, to be about 147 pounds. In 1960–62, American men in this height and age category weighed about 23 pounds more, averaging 170 pounds. Today they are heavier still.(3) The good news is that average weights of young women are decreasing,(4,5) probably a result of the social pressure to be thin. The incidence of obesity increases as the population ages. Men show a trend toward obesity in their late twenties and thirties, while women are affected more in their forties and fifties.(6) Overall, those in their fifties show the highest rates of gain (Table 6–1). Between 65 and 74, average weight tends to plateau, and declines thereafter.(7) This decline is probably due to the decreased life expectancy of the very obese.

TABLE 6–1 **Prevalence of Overweight and Obesity**

Age	Men		Women	
	Overweight	Obese	Overweight	Obese
20–74	18.1%	14.0%	12.6%	23.8%
20–24	11.1	7.4	9.8	9.6
25–34	16.7	13.6	8.1	17.1
35–44	22.1	17.0	12.3	24.3
45–54	19.9	15.8	15.1	27.8
55–64	18.9	15.1	15.5	34.7
65–74	19.1	13.4	17.5	31.5

Source: S. Abraham and C. L. Johnson, *Overweight Adults 20–74 Years of Age: United States, 1971–74.* Vital and Health Statistics, Advance Data No. 51, National Center for Health Statistics (Hyattsville, Md.: Public Health Service, Department of Health, Education and Welfare).

OVERWEIGHT AND OBESITY

Most people think of obesity as overweight that has gotten out of control. Although often used interchangeably, these two terms are not identical. Rather they are different points on a continuum.(4)

Obesity is excessive storage of fat and indicates body composition. Overweight is weight in excess of some arbitrary standard. Since total body weight measures bone structure and muscles as well as fat tissue, it does not indicate anything about degree of fatness. If weight were to be used as the only measure of obesity, two problems would arise. Athletes, like college football linemen, who have little body fat, would be classified as overweight because they have extra muscle tissue; others, particularly the elderly and those who are sedentary, might have too much body fat but weigh within the normal range for their age and sex.

Weight can vary for reasons other than differences in body muscle and fat. A large accumulation of water in the body, called edema, can account for extra weight, as it does for people with protein-energy malnutrition. Also the minerals of the body skeleton, making up approximately 6 percent of the normal adult body weight, can vary from a low of 4 percent to a high of 9 percent.(8)

A certain percentage of body fat is necessary for life. Fat is an asset during periods of prolonged food shortage, such as famine or war. As insulation from extremes of temperature and as protection from shock, fat is necessary for survival. Adolescent girls must have a certain proportion of body fat before they can reach menarche.(9) The ideal range of body fat for a given individual varies with survival needs. An early Polynesian embarking on a 2- to 3-month canoe trip who was forced to consume his own body fat for fuel would have had a greater chance of surviving at a weight of 250 pounds than at 150. By contrast, African hunters who run down their prey would never capture their dinners if they had to carry around extra fat.(10)

Ideally, adult men in Western societies should have about 15 to 20 percent body fat. If they have more than 20 percent they are considered obese;(11) a 5 percent body fat content provides enough energy for 1 to 2 weeks without food.(12) Adult women should have a body fat content of between 20 and 25 percent, with greater than 28 percent defined as obesity. When measured in terms of weight, obesity is defined as greater than 20 percent above ideal weight; overweight is greater than 10 percent.

Determining Ideal Body Weight

To find your ideal body weight, refer to a height-weight table such as that shown in Table 6–2. But be careful when you interpret these tables. The standards are not derived from scientific studies of weight and longevity, but are norms for the U.S. population as a whole based on insurance company statistics. If everyone was overweight, the charts would use higher figures as standards.

TABLE 6–2 Guidelines for Body Weight*

Height (ft., in.)	Men Average Weight (lb)	Men Acceptable Weight (lb)	Women Average Weight (lb)	Women Acceptable Weight (lb)
4 10			102	
4 11			102	92 119
5 0			104	94 122
5 1			107	95 125
5 2	123	112 141	110	99 128
5 3	127	115 144	113	102 131
5 4	130	118 148	116	105 134
5 5	133	121 152	120	108 138
5 6	136	124 156	123	111 142
5 7	140	128 161	128	114 146
5 8	145	132 166	132	118 150
5 9	149	136 170	136	122 154
5 10	153	140 174	140	126 158
5 11	158	144 179	144	130 163
6 0	162	148 184	148	134 168
6 1	166	152 189	152	138 173
6 2	171	156 194		
6 3	176	160 199		
6 4	181	164 204		

*Height without shoes, weight without clothes.

Source: Adapted from the recommendations of the Fogarty Center Conference on Obesity, 1973. In G. Bray, ed., *Obesity in America* (NIH Publ. No. 79–359, November 1979), p. 7.

As you might have guessed, ideal weight is the weight at which an individual will live the longest and be a good insurance risk.

Some height-weight tables require you to estimate your body frame size. The best way is to compare wrist size with a number of other people. Other tables do not indicate whether height is measured with or without shoes. To use these charts, you must also have access to a good scale. Scales differ slightly, so be sure to weigh yourself on the same scale each time, keeping it on a similar type of surface (carpet versus floor).

A simple, quick method of obtaining an estimate of ideal weight is given in the following formulas:(13)

For women: Allow 100 pounds for your first 5 feet of height. For each additional inch over this, add 5 pounds. For each under, subtract 5 pounds.

For example: at 5'5": 100 pounds (for first 5 feet)
+ 25 pounds (for remaining 5 inches)
___
125 pounds

For men: Allow 105 pounds for your first 5 feet of height. For each additional inch over this, add 6 pounds. For each inch under, subtract 6 pounds.

For example: at 6': 105 pounds (for first 5 feet)
+ 72 pounds (for remaining 12 inches)
___
177 pounds

(For either sex, subtract 10 percent if you are small-boned; add 10 percent if you are large-boned.)

This method is as imprecise as the height-weight tables because it also ignores variations in body composition. Yet it is useful for giving a general indication of ideal weight. Both methods focus on weight, but some measures determine the percentage of body fat in a given individual. Some of these are impractical for routine office use. Measuring body density, for example, requires weighing subjects underwater. One possible future method may be the electromagnetic technique for measuring the fat content of live hogs.(4)

At present, the most practical method is to measure the fat directly under the skin, which is called subcutaneous fat, at particular sites on the body. Common areas to measure are the back of the arm, beneath the shoulder blade, and on the abdomen. A caliper is used to pinch a fold of skin with a fixed amount of pressure, giving a reading that can be inserted into a formula to obtain percentage of body fat. Correct use of this technique requires training and practice. Though it is useful for diagnosing degree of fatness, it has some limitations. Usually only a small number of sites are measured. Readings may not accurately reflect total body fat, since the distribution of fat varies with each individual. Some people have excess fat on their legs and upper arms, no matter how much weight they lose. Another problem with skinfold measurements involves finding enough loose skin on the arms and legs of very obese persons to make a fold to measure. Children and the aged are particularly difficult to measure.(14)

Health Risks from Obesity

Obesity can be dangerous. A number of serious disorders stem from, or are worsened by, excess fat. Obesity does not always cause these disturbances, but it can make the symptoms of existing conditions more pronounced or cause them to appear at an earlier age.

Physically, the human body is not designed to carry an extra load of fat. Pressure of excess pounds on the weight-bearing joints can cause osteoarthritis of the knees, hips, and spine as well as flat feet. Muscles in the abdomen and legs can be so overloaded with fat that their normal mechanical action is hindered, resulting in abdominal hernias and varicose veins. Fat surrounding the chest and diaphragm can obstruct free breathing, a factor related to winter coughing and bronchitis.(15) It is harder to keep the body oxygenated, resulting in a decreased tolerance for exercise.(16)

Metabolic disorders are also more common in the obese. Obesity is associated with higher levels of fats and cholesterol in the blood (13) and with stones in the gall bladder. Higher rates of four types of cancer (breast, pancreas, uterus, and gall bladder) are linked to obesity, as are higher rates of kidney disease. Diabetes, a disease characterized by the body's inability to use carbohydrates properly, can be promoted in obese persons who have an inherited tendency toward this condition. In fact, the degree and duration of obesity is the factor most strongly associated with Type II diabetes in the United States.(17)

Mild obesity is not a major risk factor in heart disease, but the circulatory system is stressed if ideal weight is exceeded by 30 pounds or more. High blood pressure (hypertension) is more common among the obese.(18) In order to move an overweight body, the heart has to do extra work, raising the possibility of a premature heart attack. If other complications already exist, like diabetes, high blood pressure, or cigarette smoking, the risk of heart disease is intensified even with a mild degree of overweight. Lean and obese individuals with similar blood pressure and levels of fats in the blood have the same risk of heart disease; it is just that the obese usually have higher blood pressure and fat levels.(19) Life expectancy is unaffected until weight exceeds 30 percent of the ideal.(20)

Fat below the skin of an obese person prevents heat from escaping from the body. Folds of fatty tissue around the scrotum, causing high temperatures, can lead to infertility in males.(16) Skin irritation, caused by the heat, friction, and moisture of overlapping layers of skin, often occurs below the breasts and near the abdomen. Obese women suffer more menstrual disorders than women of normal weight.

A well-planned program of diet and exercise for obese persons can help reduce these risks. In mild cases of diabetes and high blood pressure, weight reduction can lower blood pressure and improve the body's ability to handle blood sugar. Figure 6–4 shows some of the health risks of obesity.

The obese also suffer from social and psychological problems. Insensitivity, discrimination, and prejudice toward the obese are found in every segment of society (school, sports, jobs, and social activities). The obese are often viewed as sloppy, unreliable, and undisciplined. Obese children and adolescents are less accepted by their peers, have poorer self-images, and often have disturbed personalities.

The Fat Cell and Obesity

The fat cell is not like other cells. It is the largest of body cells, and within it the nucleus and other components are squeezed into a small area. Remaining space is filled with lipid, which at body temperature is an oil.(21) Figure 6–5 shows the fat cell.

Fat (or adipose) tissue is about 72 percent lipid and 23 percent water, with small amounts of protein and mineral salts. For a long time nutritionists believed this fat was inactive, moving only if a person gained or lost weight. Now we know that the fat cell is very active, constantly recycling its lipids. The total amount of fat in the body depends on two factors: the number and size of fat cells. Fat cells are laid down during certain periods of life. Two researchers, Hirsch and Knittle,(22) found that during critical phases of growth the body has the potential to accumulate too many fat cells. These periods are the last three months of fetal development, the first three years of life, and adolescence. To recognize the significance of these critical periods, we need to understand how

FIG. 6–4

Health risks of obesity

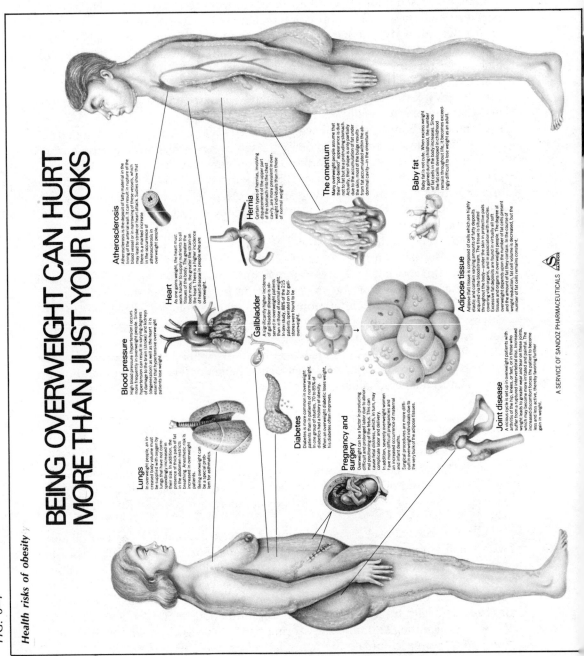

BEING OVERWEIGHT CAN HURT MORE THAN JUST YOUR LOOKS

Atherosclerosis
Atherosclerosis is the deposit of fatty material in the lining of the arterial wall. It can result in rupture of the blood vessel or in narrowing of these vessels, which may lead to stroke or heart attack. Studies show that there is a marked increase in the occurrence of atherosclerosis in overweight people.

Heart
As one gains weight, the heart must work harder to supply nutrients to all tissues of the body. The greater the body mass, the greater the strain on the heart. There is a higher incidence of heart disease in people who are overweight.

Blood pressure
High blood pressure (hypertension) occurs more frequently in overweight people. Since hypertension can result in varying degrees of damage to the brain (stroke) and kidneys (degeneration) as well as the heart, it is essential that hypertensive overweight patients lose weight.

Lungs
In overweight people, an increased body volume must be supplied with oxygen by lungs that have not correspondingly increased in their size. In addition, the presence of thick pads of fat in the abdomen restricts breathing. Anesthetic risk is increased in overweight patients.
Being overweight can be a special problem for asthmatics.

Gallbladder
A significantly higher incidence of gallbladder disease is observed in overweight patients than in those of normal weight. In one study, 88% of the 215 patients operated on for gallstones were found to be overweight.

Diabetes
Diabetes is more common in overweight patients than in patients of normal weight. In one group of studies, 70 to 85% of diabetics had a history of obesity.
When an overweight diabetic loses weight, his diabetes often improves.

Pregnancy and surgery
Overweight can be a factor in producing difficult and prolonged labor due to abnormal positioning of the fetus. This can cause fetal distress, which, in turn, may complicate labor and delivery.
In addition, severely overweight women have more difficult pregnancies and an increased occurrence of maternal and infant deaths.
Surgical procedures are more difficult in overweight individuals due to the very bulk of the adipose tissues.

Hernia
Certain types of hernia, involving displacement of the upper part of the stomach, are more prevalent in overweight individuals than in those of normal weight.

The omentum
Many overweight people assume that their "pot-bellied" appearance is due not to fat but to a protruding stomach. Actually, their shape is only partially due to the accumulation of fat under the skin; most of the bulge results from fat accumulated within the abdominal cavity—in the omentum.

Baby fat
Baby fat is not cute. When excess weight is gained during childhood, the number of fat cells in the body increases. Since the fat cells developed in childhood remain throughout life, it becomes exceedingly difficult to lose weight as an adult.

Joint disease
A vicious cycle is set up in overweight patients with arthritis of the knees, or feet, or those who suffer from a ruptured intervertebral disc. Increased weight leads to greater wear and tear on these joints, which may become more irritated and painful. The increased discomfort forces the patient to become less and less active, thereby favoring further gain in weight.

Adipose tissue
Adipose (fat) tissue is composed of cells which are highly elastic and contain varying amounts of fatty deposits acquired via the bloodstream. The tissue is situated throughout the body—under the skin or between organs covering vital organs, and in association with muscles. Excessive fat deposits are found in virtually all soft tissues and organs in overweight people. The degree of overweight depends upon the number of fat cells present and the amount of fat they contain. In the course of weight reduction, fat cell volume is decreased, but the number of fat cells remains constant.

A SERVICE OF SANDOZ PHARMACEUTICALS

FIG. 6-5

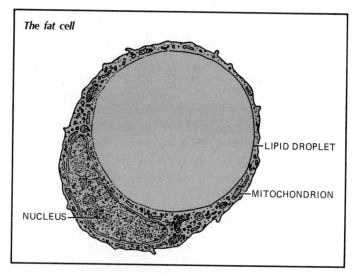

growth occurs. During different periods of life, three kinds of growth take place:

1. The number of cells increases (*hyperplasia*).
2. The number of cells increases (*hyperplasia*) and the size of cells increases (*hypertrophy*).
3. The size of cells increases (*hypertrophy*).

From the moment of conception, the fetus grows by rapid cell division and differentiation into the different systems of the body. Rapid cell division continues to be the major form of growth through the first 12 to 18 months of life. When cells are dividing rapidly, the infant is vulnerable to excess accumulation of fat cells (hyperplasia). If too many cells accumulate, they are permanent unless weight loss occurs before age 6.(11) Though genetics can play a part, overnutrition is mainly responsible for the excess fat cells during this period.

After 18 months the cells are also increasing in size (hypertrophy) until a point at which they stop multiplying in number and increase only in size. Obese children show an accelerated growth in total body size. They generally have more muscle tissue, advanced bone ages, and mature sexually at an earlier age than other children.(23,24) During the growth spurt of adolescence, cells once again begin to divide rapidly. This is the third phase during which a person is vulnerable to accumulating too many fat cells. Obesity beginning during any of these three phases (fetal development, early childhood, or the growth spurt of adolescence) is called *juvenile-onset obesity* and presents a different physiological picture than obesity beginning in adulthood. In *adult-onset obesity*, growth is mainly a result of an increase in the size of cells in the fat compartments of the body.(25) In cases of extreme obesity (greater than 170 percent of ideal body weight), cells may start to increase in number again.(11,26)

Unfortunately, the body does not have any limits on the amount of fat it can store. In order to lose fat, those who have become obese as adults must reduce the size of their fat cells, unless they are extremely obese and have added new fat cells as adults. Those who became obese during childhood generally have a harder time losing weight because, even if they reduce the size of their fat cells, they will always have too many of these cells, making weight gain much easier. The number of fat cells, to some extent, regulates appetite; those people with a larger number of cells may feel hungry more often than lean individuals. The differences in number and size of fat cells among people are just two of the factors determining who will be predisposed to weight gain and obesity. So many factors play a role in the onset of obesity that it is easy to understand why so few dieters are successful at losing weight permanently.

CAUSES OF OBESITY

Obesity is a symptom, not a disease, and it is far more complex than most people suppose. Even the word itself oversimplifies the nature of the problem: *obesity* comes from *ob* (over) and *edere* (to eat).(4) Obesity is a problem of energy balance—the relationship between the number of kcalories consumed and the number expended. The energy equations are expressed as follows:

- *Energy equilibrium:* The same number of kcalories are consumed as expended; body weight remains stable.
- *Negative energy balance:* Fewer kcalories are consumed than expended, resulting in weight loss.
- *Positive energy balance:* More kcalories are consumed than expended, resulting in the storage of fat and weight gain.

The question is then: Why do some people overeat? Gluttony is not the answer. In recent decades researchers in obesity have tried to identify factors involved in regulating food intake in both obese and normal weight people. The findings show that obesity is not a single disorder. Instead, there are many "obesities" that result from different factors, including life style (eating and exercise habits), cultural norms, economics, and physiology. These factors fall into two categories: those internal to the person (genetic, physiological, and metabolic) and those external or related to the environment (psychological, social, and cultural).

Internal Factors

The *internality theory* identifies the physical and chemical regulators of food intake. It pools many different findings into a complex model. Among the internal factors are genetic relationships. Studies with animals have shown that genetic defects can restrict the ability of the animal's body to produce heat so that energy is more efficiently stored or can predispose the animal to shunt kcalories into fat tissue before meeting energy needs. The animal has to eat more food in order to meet these needs. Through an inherited mechanism, there can be too many fat cells or too many hormones that enhance fat absorption, causing energy to be stored. Genetic obesity exists in laboratory animals. The Zucker rat is a strain of laboratory rat that has a greatly increased number of fat cells and remains obese in spite of a regular diet.

Researchers have not shown a genetic link for obesity in humans except through the use of statistics. A child has a 7 percent chance of being obese if both parents are of normal weight; a child with one obese parent has a 40 percent chance of becoming obese; but 80 percent of children with both parents obese become obese themselves.(24) This may happen for the same reason that fat pet owners have fat pets;(27) that is, parents may overfeed their children or pass on poor eating habits.

Identical twin studies are useful in separating the effects of genetics from eating habits. In studies of 57 pairs of identical twins, twins usually had similar weights, even those who had been raised in different environments. Unrelated children adopted by obese parents, however, also had similar weights, as did adopted brothers and sisters of obese children.(28)

Hypothalmic or physiological obesity results when the body is unable to tell hunger and appetite from satiety, a feeling of fullness. Hunger is a physiological response to the body's need for food. Appetite is a learned response initiated for reasons other than need for food. The smell of freshly baked bread or the sight of chocolate immediately after a meal can make you want to eat even though your body does not need any more energy.

A few years ago, researchers believed that an area at the base of the brain, called the hypothalamus, controlled feelings of hunger and satiety. The hypothalamus was supposed to have a hunger and a satiety center that dictated whether the person should eat or not. Any interference with or damage to these centers by chemical, surgical, or electrical means would cause animals to eat compulsively and become obese or stop eating and starve to death. Now scientists believe there are no specific centers for hunger and satiety, but that nerve tracts leading from particular points in the body to the hypothalamus transmit information on the current status of the body's energy needs. Consistent with this theory of a monitoring system are two other theories of obesity: the *glucostatic and lipostatic theories*. The glucostatic theory states that blood sugar levels in the body are being measured. If these levels are high, you feel full; if they are low, you feel hungry. The obese may have a defective monitoring system, causing the wrong messages to be sent to the brain. The lipostatic theory states that tissues, particularly the fat tissues, signal the brain when they are "full." People with more fat cells may require more food before they experience satiety. There is an important difference between the glucostatic and lipostatic theories. Blood sugar differences change within a short time after eating, so that a "glucostat" monitors short-term needs. The lipostatic theory involves long-term regulation because the content of fat cells changes slowly.

Another theory is based on the possibility that the body is programmed to have a set amount of fat. According to this *set point theory*, the body has a constant number of fat cells, and the obese have more than normal. If the lipid in some of these extra cells is depleted (as in weight loss), the cells signal the body to eat so that the set point is maintained. If weight loss is achieved, the body will spontaneously work to regain that loss.(27)

Internal factors associated with obesity also include hormonal disorders. Insulin is the hormone secreted by the pancreas that stimulates the conversion of blood glucose to fat. The abnormally large fat cells of the obese show varying degrees of insensitivity to insulin. Glucose is not converted immediately into fat but remains in the bloodstream where it triggers more insulin release, which in turn causes excessive fat storage.(29) Insulin also stimulates appetite so, to avoid gaining weight, the obese may have to resist more intense hunger sensations than lean persons. Once fat cells shrink, as in weight loss, their insulin sensitivity returns, but until that time, weight loss is difficult.

An undersecretion of thyroid hormone, the regulator of basal metabolism, causes energy needs to be low and easily exceeded by food intake. This is responsible for a small percentage of cases of obesity.

External Factors

Certain life styles can promote obesity. Research on the *externality theory* compares the eating and exercise habits of the obese to those of lean individuals. External factors involved in the onset and maintenance of the obese state include psychological, social, and cultural variables, and attitudes toward exercise.

During the 1960s, experimental psychologists conducted several experiments to identify and explain psychological factors involved in eating behavior.(30) They studied how obese and normal-weight individuals respond to the availability of food after receiving internal hunger cues versus external cues such as social events, time of day, sight, smell, taste, and texture of food. You might logically assume that a hungry person will eat more than a full one. In these studies, normal-weight subjects ate less food when it was offered after a meal than those who were hungry. Obese individuals, however, did not distinguish between hunger and satiety. "Fed" and "fasted" obese subjects ate the same amount. Since the obese were unresponsive to internal states of hunger and satiety, researchers looked at external cues.

In one experiment, as a reward for performing a task subjects were told to help themselves to sandwiches already prepared or to fix their own from a supply of ingredients in a refrigerator. The number of sandwiches on the plate varied. Normal-weight subjects took sandwiches from the plate and then went to the refrigerator to fix more if they were still hungry. Obese subjects ate the sandwiches on the plate (up to three sandwiches) but never went to the refrigerator to make more. The explanation might seem too simple, yet time after time in similar situations the obese were motivated to eat by the presence of food or food cues. They cleaned the plate, and when the immediate cue (available food) was gone, so was the eating response.

Another type of environmentally prompted eating behavior is seen in laboratory animals. Rats fed an ordinary, well-balanced, but monotonous diet will eat enough kcalories to maintain weight. When supermarket snack foods such as chocolate cookies, peanut butter, and marshmallows are offered, the rats ignore the lab food, overindulge in the snack foods, and become obese. When returned to the ordinary lab diet, the rats cut back on their intake and lose weight. They begin to eat enough food to maintain weight only when they have reached their original lean weights. This type of environmentally prompted weight gain is aptly called "supermarket obesity."(31)

Humans show similar behavior. In one experiment, both lean and obese subjects were fed a monotonous but nutritionally balanced liquid formula diet from a feeding machine. They could drink as much of the liquid as they desired. Lean subjects consumed enough of the formula to maintain their weights; the obese cut back intake to 100 to 700 kcalories daily and rapidly lost weight. The formula diet was then diluted, followed by overconcentration, without the subjects' knowledge, to see if they would change their intake based on the concentration of kcalories rather than quantity of fluid. Lean subjects compensated for the changes in the formula and continued to maintain their weights. Obese subjects did not. The researchers speculated that the monotony of the diet and the drabness of the setting reduced the obese person's desire to eat, again indicating the importance of external cues.

People may overeat to fulfill emotional needs. Children with few social contacts may find refuge from insecurity and loneliness in eating. Others may react to an early emotional crisis such as illness, homesickness, or the death of a family member by seeking solace in food. Adults may overeat to relieve depression(32) or to cope with problems.

Children learn eating habits at a young age. It is still controversial whether infant feeding practices such as bottle-feeding and the early introduction of high-kcalorie pureed baby foods lead to obese youngsters.(24) Behaviors during childhood that may lead to overeating in adulthood include "cleaning the plate," hurried meals, frequent snacking on high-kcalorie foods, and use of food as a reward. Social and cultural habits can create an environment conducive for both children and adults to become obese. Some cultures view an overweight baby as healthy and see body fat as a sign of wealth. (A fat baby was probably healthier than a lean one during times when infectious diseases were common.) Cultural norms determine the proper composition and size of meals.(11) Socioeconomic factors also play a part. The poor are leaner than the rich as children, although the reverse is true with adults. Black women have a higher rate of obesity than white women, yet black men have lower rates than white men.(33)

Perhaps the most important factor leading to general overweight in this society is the decrease in physical activity. According to the most recent food consumption data, people are consuming fewer kcalories today than a few years ago.(34) At the same time, they are getting heavier. One explanation for this inconsistency is that people are less physically active. The use of convenience appliances and modern transportation has created a situation in which people have to make a conscious decision to exercise.(35)

Studies on adolescents indicate that the obese consume fewer kcalories than their leaner counterparts, but participate in one-sixth to one-third the physical activity. By using motion pictures, researchers monitored the activity levels of obese and normal-weight teenage girls at two summer camps. Film footage showed that the obese were less active than the nonobese even during supervised sports activities.(36)

TREATMENT: DIETS, DRUGS, FASTING, SURGERY

According to one writer, there are 2876 different ways to lose weight with 2000 diets, and more than 50 percent of them are unsafe.(2) Ideally, a weight reduction diet should restrict kcalories to achieve negative energy balance and at the same time include a balance of all other nutrients. The energy deficit forces the body to break down its own energy stores, such as fat deposits.

Each pound of adipose tissue represents the storage of about 3500 kcalories. Take an individual who consumes an amount of food daily that provides 100 kcalories in excess of energy requirements. In one month, the excess of 3000 kcalories would result in a weight gain of 0.8 pound; in a year, the gain would be about 10 pounds. If you were to overeat consistently by this small amount (equivalent to 2 teaspoons of jam), the gain over a 5- to 10-year period would be substantial. Conversely, to lose 1 pound of adipose tissue, the diet should be deficient in 3500 kcalories for the total time period of the weight loss. Suppose a young woman requires 2000 kcalories a day to meet her energy needs, but consumes a diet that supplies only 1200 kcalories. The weekly deficit would be 5600 kcalories, and the adipose tissue loss would be 5600 divided by 3500, or 1.6 pounds.

Weight gain and loss do not always follow the predicted straight line because of variations in water balance. With weight loss, the fat in the adipose tissue is temporarily replaced with water. Weight will often plateau for a period of time until the cell shrinks and the water is excreted. Also, weight gain and loss are not only the result of changes in adipose tissue; some changes in lean tissues are also taking place. The weight you lose on crash diets is often 5 or more pounds during the first week, much of it water or lean tissue or both. Recommended reducing diets that provide a variety of foods result in a loss of only 1 to 2 pounds per week, most of which is fat.

Considering today's emphasis on leanness, it is not surprising that most people in this country are either on a weight reduction diet, have been on and off several diets, or have a guilty conscience about not dieting. Unfortunately, many people who are not overweight go on strenuous diets. This is particularly common among young women and adolescent girls who, impressed by the appearance of models in women's magazines, go on semi-starvation diets to "improve" their figures. Or there is the middle-aged woman who wistfully hopes to squeeze into her wedding dress, and her husband who cannot convince his World War II Army fatigues to see their way clear of his belly.

Many adults who were normal weight when reaching maturity allow themselves to gain weight steadily and become obese by middle age. They are particularly susceptible to the many fad diets that promise to take weight off fast with no effort or sacrifice on the part of the dieter.

The major difference between fad diets and recommended weight-reduction diets is that fad diets limit food choices and often emphasize only one or two foods. Some are intentionally unbalanced to restrict or eliminate one of the major nutrients. Such a diet will almost always be inadequate in vitamins and minerals. Most fad reducing diets have the following characteristics:

- Promise quick and dramatic weight loss
- Severely restrict and limit food choices
- Restrict or eliminate one of the major nutrients, such as carbohydrates or fats
- Generally are inadequate in minerals and vitamins
- Do not mention exercise
- Cite claims supported by personal testimonials only
- Do not recommend moderation and variety in eating

Such diets include starvation regimens; supplemented fasting; formulas, sometimes accompanied by the use of drugs; hormones; jaw wiring; and other attempts at controlling food intake. There is a vast difference between restrictive diets used under the supervision of a doctor and those embarked upon by the general public after a quick glance at a diet book.

Low Carbohydrate Diets.   Although the low carbohydrate diets have been popular since the 1960s, they are not new. In fact, over a century ago Dr. Harvey developed the prototype of today's diets and promoted it as the Banting Diet. (Banting was the name of one of Harvey's overweight patients.)

All low-carbohydrate diets are based on distorted concepts of metabolism. None require counting kcalories, and all are high in protein. They do vary in the amount of fat allowed and in the degree of carbohydrate restriction. One popular low carbohydrate diet is Dr. Atkin's Diet Revolution. This diet progresses from no carbohydrate to about 40 grams per day and recommends eating all the fat you want. It has been severely criticized by the American Medical Association's Council on Foods and Nutrition.

Two more versions of low carbohydrate diets have recently gained ground on the older versions. These are the Scarsdale diet and the fructose diet. The Scarsdale diet is a 14-day plan containing about 1000 kcalories. It allows large amounts of protein and little carbohydrate and fat. The fructose diet is also low in kcalories (900 to 1000), with a high percentage of protein. The new twist is that a certain amount of the sugar fructose is allowed. These are two versions of the same diet: one allows only 36 to 42 grams of fructose daily and another allows 75 to 100 grams daily. Fructose is used in this diet because promoters claim it can be used by body cells without relying on insulin. Thus the dieter can enjoy some sweetness without having insulin stimulate the appetite. The fallacy in this line of reasoning is that most of the fructose ingested is converted to glucose in the body. Glucose, of course, requires insulin to be used by most cells.

A major criticism of low carbohydrate diets (as with semi-starvation and starvation diets) is that they cause a condition called ketosis, an abnormal and undesirable metabolic state. During World War II the Canadian Army used pemmican as an emergency ration for infantry troops. Pemmican is dried beef with added suet and contains no carbohydrate. After three to four days on this ration, the troops could no longer function. By the fourth day, they were restless, fatigued, and dehydrated. Many were nauseous. Dieters who eat very little carbohydrate also experience these symptoms.

A series of events that occurs during ketosis explains these symptoms. Only three nutrients, carbohydrates, fats, proteins (and alcohol), provide energy, and the body needs a constant source of glucose. Carbohydrate and protein can be broken down and converted into glucose. Fats cannot because humans lack an enzyme necessary for this conversion. Normally, if fats are needed to fill energy requirements, they are broken down into energy. Sometimes the breakdown of fats is too fast for the body to handle through the regular processes. Some of the fats are incompletely broken down and form products called *ketone bodies* or just *ketones*. Ketones are usually produced at the same rate as they are oxidized. During unusual circumstances, such as in fasting or on low carbohydrate diets, ketones are produced at such a high rate that they accumulate in the blood and spill into the urine. When this happens, ketosis has developed. (On some low carbohydrate diets the dieter is supposed to measure the levels of ketones in the urine using colored strips of paper.) Not only are ketones excreted in the urine, but some are exhaled through the mouth, giving a "sweet" breath by the fourth day of the diet. The simplest way to reverse ketosis is to eat some carbohydrate.

All cells can use ketones for energy, except the nerve, muscle, and red blood cells. These require glucose. On a carbohydrate-restricted diet, too little carbohydrate is eaten to nourish these glucose-requiring cells. Fats cannot be broken down to glucose, and the only other source is protein. Protein, when broken down to glucose, produces the waste products urea, uric acid, and ammonia. These wastes, along with the ketones from fats, are filtered through the kidneys and excreted in the urine. Excessive fat and protein breakdown stresses the kidneys and can lead to serious problems with losses of water and sodium, an important element in body fluids (Figure 6–6). The rapid excretion of water explains the sudden initial weight loss on these diets. But the loss is not from fat and will be regained once normal eating patterns are resumed.

The reason for inducing ketosis on a weight-reducing scheme is for its appetite-depressing effect, although there is some controversy over whether this effect really exists.(37) The possible depression of appetite, however, is offset by the potentially dangerous side effects. A summary of the possible effects of low carbohydrate diets is listed below:

- Increased blood uric acid concentrations (may lead to gout)
- Increased uric acid secretion (may aid in the formation of kidney stones)
- Abnormally low blood pressure
- Dehydration due to loss of water and sodium which accompanies the excreted ketones

FIG. 6–6

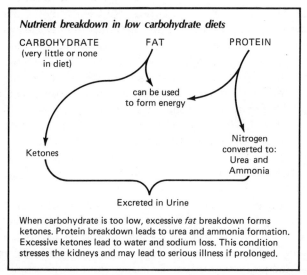

Nutrient breakdown in low carbohydrate diets

CARBOHYDRATE (very little or none in diet)　　FAT　　　PROTEIN

can be used to form energy

Ketones

Nitrogen converted to: Urea and Ammonia

Excreted in Urine

When carbohydrate is too low, excessive *fat* breakdown forms ketones. Protein breakdown leads to urea and ammonia formation. Excessive ketones lead to water and sodium loss. This condition stresses the kidneys and may lead to serious illness if prolonged.

- Possible nausea
- Initial weight loss attributed to water loss
- High fat intake, which is considered a risk factor in the development of coronary heart disease
- Only temporary weight loss; problems with adherence to diet

Supplemented Fasts.　In the late 1970s, the liquid protein diet became popular. The diet advocates the use of predigested liquid protein, sometimes called a protein supplement. Most of these products are either modified proteins or derivatives of the protein collagen. Some are fortified with a limited number of essential amino acids, vitamins, and minerals, but most are nutritionally incomplete.

The diet was initially developed for use in hospitals in treating severely obese patients. Rather than being placed on a complete fast, which depletes lean tissue, patients could ingest about 300 to 500 kcalories a day in the form of protein. The method succeeded in reducing the loss of lean tissue. But this is a rigorous treatment that was never meant to be used outside a clinical setting. Nevertheless, Dr. Robert Linn, an osteopath in Philadelphia, developed a liquid protein called Prolinn that he began using in treating overweight patients. Once he described the treatment in his book *The Last Chance Diet*, the liquid protein dieting craze was launched.

In all there were 40 deaths reported, 15 in which the patients had no other underlying medical problems that could have caused the death. Speculations about the factors causing these 15 deaths ran from mineral deficiencies to lowered resistance to infection. Other reported side effects include nausea, vomiting, diarrhea, constipation, faintness, muscle cramps, fatigue, irritability, cold intolerance, hair loss, and skin dryness.

A slightly different approach to the supplemented fast is the Cambridge Plan developed by Dr. Allen Howard of Cambridge University in England. The plan focuses on a powdered formula that provides 330 kcalories per day from 31 grams of milk protein, 44 grams of carbohydrate (as sugars), and two grams of fat plus vitamins and minerals at RDA levels. Depending on the amount of weight loss desired, the formula is recommended for one to four weeks. Then a period of adding a meal a day is recommended for seven to ten days, and then back to the formula for four weeks if further weight loss is desired.

Although the quality of the protein in the Cambridge Diet is higher than in most of the liquid protein diets, the kcalorie level is dangerously low for anyone not under continuous medical supervision. Also, the amount of protein in the diet is less than that recommended for physician-supervised, supplemented fasts.(38)

At present, the Food and Drug Administration requires warning labels on all the liquid protein products intended for use in weight-reduction diets or weight maintenance. Certain people should be particularly careful to avoid the supplemented fasts: those taking prescribed medications, those with liver or heart ailments, pregnant or lactating women, psychiatric patients, preschool and school-age children, and the elderly.

Diets Emphasizing Single Foods or Single Food Groups. A number of fad diets that were in vogue several years ago emphasized one food, in some instances forbidding all other foods. There was the rice diet, the prune diet, the banana diet, the hard-cooked egg diet, the grapefruit diet (advocates asserted that the organic acid in grapefruit eliminated kcalories because it burned up fat), the all-meat diet. These are all highly desirable foods; but no single food is complete nutritionally, and any one consumed in excess and to the exclusion of other foods can create serious deficiencies. Happily, the monotony of these diets often means people do not stay on them more than one week.

A recent diet which emphasizes a single food group is the Beverly Hills Diet developed by Judy Mazel. It emphasizes fruit; in fact, for the first eleven days of the diet fruits are the only foods allowed. The diet is based on the erroneous notion that undigested food makes fat. Undigested food supposedly gets "stuck" in your body, accumulates and turns to fat. The bizarre reason given for food not being digested is that some foods cancel the action of digestive enzymes on other foods. So great care must be taken not to combine the wrong foods. Fruits are said to digest the fastest of all foods, thus are emphasized. Dairy products, salt, sugar, and refined carbohydrates are to be avoided by users of the diet if at all possible.(39)

There are definite dangers associated with the Beverly Hills Diet if it is adhered to for more than a few days. It can cause severe diarrhea which can lead to potassium deficiency and irregular heart beat.(40) A possible side effect is loss of hair because the diet is deficient in protein at least during the first six weeks.

Formula Diets. There are several liquid diets designed to furnish about 800 kcalories daily. They offer the advantage of eliminating food choices and meal planning, as well as the need to count kcalories. But prolonged use should be undertaken only under medical supervision. Use for a short period of time, or as a substitute for an occasional meal, will probably cause few problems. The disadvantages of this approach are the monotony and expense of the formula. Also, dieters do not learn to change their eating patterns, and so will regain any weight lost once they return to their regular habits.

A variation of this diet is the practice of wiring the jaws shut, allowing only liquids sipped through a straw. There seem to be few serious side effects from this practice, but again the weight lost tends to be regained.

Fiber and Mineral Oil. Some diets are designed to allow the consumption of large quantities of food, but prevent the absorption of the nutrients once the food is ingested. These diets recommend the intake of foods high in fiber, since fiber is not totally digested but passes through the intestines, or suggest that a tablespoon of mineral oil be taken with meals. Mineral oil also is not digested but coats the lining of the digestive tract, interfering with the absorption of nutrients. The problem with this type of approach to weight reduction is that necessary vitamins and minerals also pass through the intestine without being absorbed, leading to the possibility of deficiencies.

Anti-Cellulite Diet. Cellulite (pronounced *cell-u-leet*) is claimed to be a special kind of fat composed of fat, water, and toxic wastes that the body has failed to eliminate. Strangely enough, scientists have yet to discover cellulite.

The cellulite program that purports to rid the body of this lumpy, dimply-looking fat combines diet, elimination, breathing, massage, exercise, and relaxation. The anti-cellulite diet contains about 1000 kcalories, and does not allow table sugar, salt, alcohol, or artificial sweeteners. Fresh fruits and vegetables are allowed, but no frozen or canned ones. Dieters consume brewer's yeast dissolved in fruit juice before meals to reduce appetite.

No studies to date have found any difference between cellulite and fat or established any beneficial effects from the cellulite program. The average cost of the cellulite treatment in a salon is $200 to $500, but the only successful way to lose the fat lumps that usually appear around the hips and thighs is to lose weight, preferably before age 35 to 40, while the skin is still elastic enough to shrink once the fat depot is reduced.(41)

Drugs

Diuretics. Medical conditions resulting in water retention can account for extra body weight. If this is the problem, a doctor can prescribe a diuretic, a substance that helps the body to excrete more fluid. Sometimes it is better simply to reduce salt intake.(16) Since most people's weight problems are caused by excess fat, diuretics will usually be useless. What few pounds may be lost by this method will be regained once water is consumed, as with the temporary weight loss experienced after a sauna or steam bath. Diuretics do not have any effect on appetite or fat stores.

Appetite Suppressants (Anorectics). Diet pills have always been popular among those searching for a quick and easy way to lose weight. They can be nonprescription (over-the-counter) or prescription products. The nonprescription ones are sold under such names as Dexatrim, Prolamine, Appedrine, and Dietac. The ingredients that supposedly depress appetite and deaden taste are phenylpropanolamine and oral benzocaine, or both. These same substances are commonly used in decongestant medications for colds, except that the level used for repressing appetite is higher. Along with suppressing appetite, they can increase blood pressure and metabolism. Caffeine is included in many of these products and also increases blood pressure. Sold in candy, gum, tablet, capsule, liquid, and powder form, the products are marked up 30 to 45 percent and are rarely discounted.(42)

The appetite suppressants in prescription products are chiefly amphetamines and amphetaminelike substances. Most have undesirable side effects ranging from insomnia to nervousness, increased pulse rate, heart palpitations, dry mouth, depression, diarrhea, and a temporary rise in blood pressure. They can be particularly dangerous for persons who are nervous or suffer from heart disease or high blood pressure. To offset these side effects, some amphetamines are combined with barbiturates and other tranquilizing drugs. These reduce some of the unpleasant effects but do not help in the weight-reduction process. A physician prescribing anorectic drugs must decide whether their use is justified for an individual patient. Diet pills help weight reduction over a short period of time. Over an extended period, however, there is no advantage to taking the pills, and problems with addiction can develop.

Other Techniques

Acupuncture. Proponents of the use of acupuncture in the treatment of the obese believe that needles inserted in the earlobes, when pressed a half-hour before meals or when the dieter is hungry, will help reduce appetite.(20) Few studies have been conducted to date on the effectiveness of this technique.

Fasting. Some diets should not be started unless a doctor believes the threat of obesity outweighs the risks. One of these is the zero kcalorie diet, otherwise known as fasting. Complete fasting is often a last resort for the grossly obese and should be conducted in a hospital setting. It is not recommended for individuals whose weight problems are minor, because about 65 percent of the weight loss represents loss of lean tissue, not fat.

In the second or third day of the fast, glycogen reserves are depleted, leading to a state of ketosis. Potassium and other body minerals are lost, so that vitamin and mineral supplements become essential. Blood pressure falls. Since fainting spells may occur, the patient should not drive. Patients lose about 2000 to 2500 kcalories daily depending on their initial weights and activity levels during the fast.(43) Problems with the heart, blood pressure, and acute gout can occur. As with other unusual eating regimens, the dieter does not learn new food habits and frequently gains weight once the fast is over. Ironically, fasting is also expensive if undertaken, as it should be, under medical supervision.

RECOMMENDED APPROACHES TO WEIGHT CONTROL

As the American Medical Association put it: "No matter how much you huff and puff, you can't just shake it off, roll it off, knock it off or bake it off."(44) The only way to lose weight is to eat less and exercise more.

Eating Less

Recommended diets encourage a wide selection of foods to maintain a balance of nutrients, although the quantities of fuel nutrients, particularly carbohydrates and fats, are reduced. Diets must allow for adequate protein, vitamins, and minerals. Some characteristics of a good reducing diet are these:(45)

- It contains fewer kcalories than you need.
- The kcalorie restriction is not so severe as to make it impossible to obtain adequate amounts of protein, vitamins, and minerals.
- It contains one or more servings per day from each of the four food groups within kcalorie limitations.
- Some fat is included in each meal, and the diet emphasizes large quantities of low kcalorie foods. Both increase satiety value.
- It is reasonable in cost.
- It is readily adapted to family meals or public eating places.
- It is easily adhered to for long periods of time because, where possible, it conforms to the tastes and habits of the dieter.
- It changes the eating habits of the dieter.

A daily deficit of about 500 kcalories below maintenance needs allows a loss of about 1 pound per week. Diets extremely low in kcalories, such as those that are less than 1000 kcalories per day, can result in malnutrition because the intakes of protein, vitamins, and minerals are directly related to kcalorie intake. Diets with too few kcalories lead to the breakdown of body protein as well as fat.

A reducing diet includes foods high in nutrients compared to kcalories and cuts down on those, such as fats, sugar, and alcohol, that provide few nutrients compared to number of kcalories. Diets should be tailored to each person; no foods are inherently good or bad, and all that matters is that the diet is varied and nutritionally adequate.

The exchange system allows you to design a personal eating plan, one you are more likely to follow. Appendix D provides a list of foods contained within each exchange group. The foods within each exchange group have a similar number of kcalories and nutrients. Table 6–3 gives sample exchange plans for different kcalorie-restricted diets and one sample menu plan. By determining your daily energy needs and subtracting 500 to 1000 kcalories daily to allow a 1- to 2-pound weekly loss, you can decide which food plan is best for

TABLE 6–3 Exchange Lists for Reducing Diets and Sample Meal Plan

1000 kcalorie Diet

Exchange	Number of Exchanges	kcalories/Exchange	Total kcalories
Milk	2	80	160
Meat	5	55	275
Vegetable	4	25	100
Fruit	3	40	120
Bread	3	70	210
Fats	3	45	135
			1000

1200 kcalorie Diet

Exchange	Number of Exchanges	kcalories/Exchange	Total kcalories
Milk	2	80	160
Meat	7	55	385
Vegetable	4	25	100
Fruit	3	40	120
Bread	4	70	280
Fats	3	45	135
			1180

1350 kcalorie Diet

Exchange	Number of Exchanges	kcalories/Exchange	Total kcalories
Milk	2	80	160
Meat	7	55	385
Vegetable	4	25	100
Fruit	3	40	120
Bread	6	70	420
Fats	4	45	180
			1365

1500 kcalorie Diet

Exchange	Number of Exchanges	kcalories/Exchange	Total kcalories
Milk	2	80	160
Meat	8	55	440
Vegetable	4	25	100
Fruit	3	40	120
Bread	7	70	490
Fats	4	45	180
			1490

1700 kcalorie Diet

Exchange	Number of Exchanges	kcalories/Exchange	Total kcalories
Milk	2	80	160
Meat	8	55	440
Vegetable	5	25	125
Fruit	3	40	120
Bread	9	70	630
Fats	5	45	225
			2085

TABLE 6–3   **(Continued)**

1900 kcalorie Diet

Exchange	Number of Exchanges	kcalories/Exchange	Total kcalories
Milk	3	80	240
Meat	8	55	440
Vegetable	5	25	125
Fruit	4	40	160
Bread	10	70	700
Fats	5	45	225
			1890

2100 kcalorie Diet

Exchange	Number of Exchanges	kcalories/Exchange	Total kcalories
Milk	3	80	240
Meat	10	55	550
Vegetable	5	25	125
Fruit	5	40	200
Bread	10	70	700
Fats	6	45	270
			2085

Sample Meal Plan for 1500 kcalorie Diet

	Exchange	kcalories/ Exchange	Total kcalories
Breakfast:			
Skim milk, 1 cup	1 milk	80	80
Eggs, 2	2 meat + 1 fat	110, 45	155
Orange juice, ½ cup	1 fruit	40	40
Bagel, 1	2 bread	70	140
Margarine, 1 teaspoon	1 fat	45	45
Coffee/tea	free	0	0
Lunch:			
Tuna, ½ cup	2 meat	55	110
Onions, celery, ½ cup	1 vegetable	25	25
Mayonnaise, 1 teaspoon	1 fat	45	45
Rye bread, 2 slices	2 bread	70	140
Lettuce, pickle	free	0	0
Peach, medium	1 fruit	40	40
Tea	free	0	0
Snack:			
Yogurt,2% milk, 1 cup	1 milk + 1 fat	80 + 45	125
Banana, small, ½	1 fruit	40	40
Dinner:			
Chicken, baked, no skin, 4 ounces	4 meat	55	220
Green beans, 1 cup	1 vegetable	25	25
Salad: tomatoes, onions, celery, radishes, ½ cup total	1 vegetable	25	25
Lettuce, wine vinegar	free	0	0
Corn, ⅓ cup	1 vegetable	25	25
Potato, small	1 bread	70	70
Wine, dry white, 3 ounces	1 bread	70	70
Total kcalories for day:			1490

you. Suppose you are a 150-pound, sedentary woman and wish to lose 20 pounds. Your daily energy needs are about 150 × 14, or 2100 kcalories. Subtract 500 kcalories (for a 1 pound weekly loss), and you have a 1600-kcalorie diet. By using the exchange system you can eat the kinds of food you like, within limits, and still lose weight. Table 6–4 suggests ways to prepare appetizing meals that are low in kcalories.(6)

Weight-loss programs are generally not recommended for children and teenagers until after the growth spurt is completed. These individuals are still growing, and weight gain due to increases in muscle and skeletal tissue should be expected. Reducing diets for these age groups result in loss of lean body tissue as well as fat and may retard their growth. Instead, it is better to prevent weight gain from excess fat and to control dietary habits so that growth of skeleton and muscle continues but no more fat accumulates. With this approach the fat will be redistributed, except in extreme cases. Excessive kcalories should be eliminated, but energy intake should not be reduced below expenditure in these age groups.

TABLE 6–4 **Suggestions for Preparing Low kcalorie Meals with the Exchange System**

Milk Exchanges

1. Use milk products that have had the milk fat removed (skim milk), for the kcalorie value is halved. Because the fat-soluble vitamins A and D are removed with the milk fat, use fluid or dry skim milk fortified with both vitamins A and D. The use of dried skim milk powder in cooking and as a beverage is an economical measure. If mixed well in advance and allowed to become thoroughly chilled, the flavor is comparable to fluid skim milk.
2. Milk exchanges may also be used in soups, eggnogs, and custards, and on cereals.
3. Find recipes that substitute low-kcalorie milk products for the kcalorie-rich creams commonly used in desserts, toppings, and dips. Whipped evaporated skim milk can replace whipped creams in some desserts; whipped cottage cheese or yogurt can replace sour cream or mayonnaise in salad and fruit dressings and dips; and flavored skim milk powder can be whipped and used instead of whipped cream.
4. Try plain yogurt and unsweetened fruit, or plain yogurt sprinkled lightly with brown sugar and cinnamon. The kcalorie value of commercially flavored yogurt will vary with the brand, but in general will be twice as high as plain yogurt.

Meat Exchanges

1. Select leaner meats, seafoods, cottage cheese, and skim milk cheeses.
2. Cut all visible fat from meat before cooking and cook without adding extra fat.
3. Remove skin from poultry before eating, as a layer of fat lies attached to this skin. White meat has less natural fat than the moister dark meat.
4. Buy water-packed canned fish or rinse oil from fish with hot water before using.
5. Use lemon juice, herbs, or onion flakes with seafood dishes to add flavor. Fish is an economical and low-fat meat exchange.
6. Use seasoned tomato juice or bouillon in meat, fish, and poultry recipes instead of creamed gravies and rich sauces.
7. Try cooking with dry wines. Most of the kcalorie-rich alcohol evaporates in the cooking but leaves a flavorful sauce. Sweet wine, however, contains more sugar and has more kcalories than dry.
8. Combine meat and fruit for flavor variations, such as pineapple with chicken or apples with ham.

TABLE 6–4 (Continued)

Vegetable Exchanges

1. Experiment with herbs, spices, seasoned salts, vinegar, or lemon juice for added flavor.
2. Try interesting combinations of cooked vegetables, such as cauliflower and peas, peppers and onions, or broccoli and mushrooms.
3. Use combinations of raw vegetables as salads, snacks, and appetizers. Serve vegetables like cauliflower and mushrooms raw and add herbed vinegar for flavor. Use vegetable dips of herbed whipped cottage cheese as an appetizer. Raw vegetables, due to their bulk, are eaten in less quantity than when cooked.

Fruit Exchanges

1. Use a variety of fruits and try them as appetizers, with a main course, or as a dessert.
2. Avoid both canned and frozen fruits that have sugar added. Both water-packed canned and sugar-free frozen fruits are quite sweet.
3. Canned fruit juices should be purchased without added sugar. Read the labels on the cans carefully.

Bread Exchanges

1. Try a variety of breads—herb, whole wheat, rye, cheese, cinnamon, and spiced. A slice of cinnamon toast and fruit can substitute for a rich dessert.
2. Make homemade bread instead of a kcalorie-rich dessert.
3. Carbohydrate-rich vegetables are included in the bread exchanges. Dried peas, beans, and lentils, when combined with small amounts of meat, are good sources of protein and can be used to extend meat dishes for economy.

Fat Exchanges

1. Fat has over twice as many kcalories per gram as carbohydrates or protein. Measure accurately when using butter, margarine, and oils.
2. Margarines and vegetable oils contain polyunsaturated fatty acids that are essential. It is wise not to exclude such foods from a diet altogether.
3. Low-kcalorie cookbooks have a variety of suggestions for salad dressings. Wine vinegar or lemon juice can substitute for regular salad dressings. Packaged mixes can be combined with plain yogurt instead of mayonnaise.

Free Exchanges

1. Experiment with herbs, spices, vinegars, and seasoning to add flavor and interest to foods.
2. Use hot herbed teas, iced tea, coffee, decaffeinated coffee, and hot boullions when you are not really hungry but feel like eating or drinking something.
3. Limited amounts of sugar substitutes may be used as flavoring. You should not use substitutes indiscriminately, as a change in the desire for concentrated sweets is needed. Besides, little is known about the long-term effects of such substitutes. For the same reason, the drinking of diet sodas should be limited, and it is always necessary to read the labels of beverages for kcalorie content.

Alcohol

1. When choosing wine, use light, dry wines instead of the more kcalorie-rich sweet, heavy wines.
2. Use club soda, water, or ice as a mixer with alcoholic beverages.
3. On social occasions substitute low-kcalorie beverages for alcoholic drinks but drink them from regular wine, cocktail, or liquor glasses.
4. Avoid all the high-kcalorie appetizers that frequently accompany alcoholic beverages.

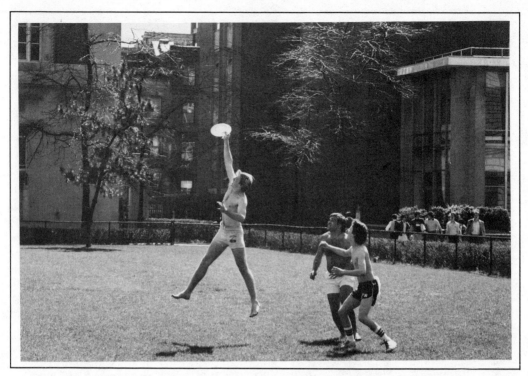

Exercise should be incorporated into daily activities. People who do not maintain a certain level of activity can miss internal cues for hunger and satiety.

Exercise

Exercise should not be an afterthought on a weight-reduction program; it plays too large a role to take a back seat to the diet itself. Consider this: In order to lose 1 pound of body fat, you would have to climb the stairs to the top of the Empire State Building and back down for four hours.(6) If it takes this much effort to lose a pound, you might wonder why you should even bother taking the first step. The reason is that exercise does more than just use up a few kcalories.

Exercise keeps the body's appetite-control mechanisms functioning properly. People who do not maintain a certain level of physical activity are more likely to miss internal cues for hunger and satiety. And 98 percent of the weight lost through diet plus exercise is likely to be fat, while only 75 percent of the weight lost by diet only is fat.(6) Physiologically, exercise offers quite a few benefits to the heart, lungs, and muscles.

Some prescriptions for diet and exercise programs use behavior modification techniques to help the dieter become aware of unhealthful habits and begin to learn constructive behaviors.

Behavioral therapists try to design a special kind of environment for the dieter, since environmental cues often prompt the obese to eat. Some of the environmental factors include physical and social situations (advertisements, people offering food, parties), thoughts about particular foods, watching TV, and sitting in the kitchen. By changing such variables in the immediate surroundings, eating behaviors can be changed. Some techniques used to do this are restricting meals to certain rooms, at certain times, and not while the dieter is engaged in other activities (no eating while reading or watching TV); requiring the dieter to eat slowly and to eat bulky foods first (so the feeling of fullness will hit before the high-kcalorie foods are consumed); and not allowing the dieter to purchase high-kcalorie foods unless they are for other family members, in which case they should be kept out of sight.(27)

To become aware of the cues in your environment that trigger eating, keep a food diary (Figure 6–7). This is a record of the time and circumstances of your eating. It allows you to judge whether you are eating because of hunger or in response to stress or other intervening factors. You should keep this diary for at least a week, and then try to change those variables in your environment that are prompting your eating behavior.

FIG. 6–7

Food diary

FOOD EATEN Quantity Type	TIME Circle time if food was part of meal	SOCIAL Alone? With whom?	WHERE EATEN Home Work Restaurant Recreation	MOOD WHEN EATING A—Anxious B—Bored C—Tired D—Depressed E—Angry
1 C. Coffee 2 TBs. half & Creamer half	2 pm	with Kate	espresso house	tired
croissant	"	"	"	"
butter - 1 TBs.	"	"	"	"
Jam 1 TBS.	"	"	"	"

Here are some general rules to follow when you diet:

1. Never skip a meal, especially breakfast. Eat at regular mealtimes and try to sit down at a table with your place set. Use a small plate and fork to make your meal look more substantial. Snacks are permitted, provided you have included them in your daily food allotments.

2. Eat slowly. It takes about 20 minutes after eating before you will begin to feel full.

3. Cook only enough food for a particular meal.

4. Low-kcalorie dishes can be made to look more appetizing if you add garnishes. Try planning low-kcalorie gourmet meals.

5. Don't give up your favorite dishes completely, but try to cut down on the number of times a week that you eat them and on the portion sizes.

6. Plan your meals ahead of time so you don't have to throw something together at the last minute.

7. Be aware of eating as a response to environmental cues or stress. A food diary is a useful tool to keep for a week or two. You may be surprised to discover how often you eat for reasons other than hunger.

8. If you are in the habit of heading to the refrigerator the minute you step foot into the house, force yourself to go into another room and allow yourself to enter the kitchen only when it is time to prepare meals.

9. Go grocery shopping after you have eaten. That way you will not be as tempted to buy everything in sight. Try to shop from a list.

10. Make sure you have ready-to-eat low-kcalorie foods available in the refrigerator. Wash fresh fruits and vegetables before you put them in the refrigerator so when you find yourself grabbing something, it is a carrot, not a piece of leftover banana cream pie.

11. When you attend social events, do not be pressured into overeating. If you know of an upcoming event (birthday, wedding) at which you would like to indulge in some high-kcalorie foods, begin the week before to cut back on some of your fat and carbohydrate allowances so that your diet will continue smoothly throughout the weekend.

12. If you go out to eat at a restaurant, try to keep to your diet. Ask to be allowed to put on your own salad dressing—or better yet, lemon juice; order broiled and baked rather than fried items. Have fruit compote before dinner and skip the dessert.

13. If you tend to overeat in the evening, try to arrange something to do that prevents you from hovering around the kitchen. Turn off the TV and join a softball league or take a long walk after dinner.

14. Set reasonable goals for yourself. A 500-kcalorie diet is doomed from the beginning.

15. Weigh yourself no more than once a week. Weight loss is rarely consistent. To avoid discouragement over uneven losses, it is best not to weigh yourself daily. Fluctuations in body water may cause you to give up your dieting entirely.

16. Reward yourself for adherence to the diet. You may want to punish yourself if you have gone off the diet on an eating binge, but do not make up the kcalories the next day. Instead, go back on the diet and try again.

17. If you find it impossible to diet alone, check in your local directory for groups like Weight Watchers, which provide balanced diets and group support sessions. If you join a weight-reducing group, be sure it is not promoting an unusual or fad diet.

UNDERWEIGHT

Considering the prevalence of obesity, it is difficult to believe some people have a hard time gaining weight. But the problem does exist. The causes of underweight (defined as weight less than 90 percent of ideal for height, age, and body build) are similar to those of overweight: the combination of genetic, metabolic, and psychological factors leading to possibly fewer fat cells, rapid metabolism, and/or lack of appetite. Although being slightly underweight may improve your life expectancy, being too thin can put you at risk of serious deficiency if you were to get sick. A young pregnant woman who is underweight is at higher risk of delivering a low-birth-weight infant.

A few practical suggestions can help underweight persons achieve weight gain:

1. Cut down on needless physical activity. Make sure you have enough rest.

2. Be sure to get enough daily exercise to ensure a good night's sleep. You won't use as many kcalories as you would from insomnia.

3. Eat nutritious snacks between meals, but not so much as to ruin your appetite. Recommended snacks include peanut butter, oatmeal cookies, ice cream, cheese, avocados. Drink whole milk instead of low-fat milk.

4. Try eating more rapidly than usual so that you can get a few extra bites in before your satiety mechanism goes into action.

Anorexia Nervosa

In February 1976, Frances O., a "well-behaved" teenager and straight-A student, weighed a stocky 134 pounds. By June 1976 she showed marked personality changes; she became easily upset and hostile, appeared constantly restless, and had lost much of her scalp hair. In the months between February and June, Frances had become obsessed with her weight and, through restricted eating and self-induced vomiting, dropped to a mere 72 pounds and was still losing.

Frances O. was suffering from an unusual and rather bizarre problem called anorexia nervosa, a state characterized by extreme emaciation resulting from self-starvation. Those who develop this syndrome exhibit a strong fear of becoming fat, a fear usually related to personality disorders. Almost all are white females aged 13 to 30 years. These women are usually well-off, high achievers, and described as having been model children.(46)

Women with anorexia nervosa tend to have distorted ideas about the size of their bodies. Though most are normal weight or slightly underweight prior to their illness, they believe they are too fat even after severe weight loss and see themselves as normal when they are in fact emaciated. They do not lose their appetites, but instead are constantly preoccupied with thoughts of food. Sometimes they go on eating binges, gorging on all kinds of fattening foods, only to force themselves to vomit or take diuretics and laxatives to bring the weight back down. These women may limit food intake to an incredibly small amount and develop odd eating habits. They may chop food into the tiniest fragments in order to slow eating and give the meal the appearance of being more substantial. Some eat only late at night so that they can go to sleep before the guilt sets in. Most know the kcalorie value of foods to a precise degree and are compulsive about keeping track of each gram entering their mouths. Women with this disorder enjoy cooking rich foods for others, but refuse to indulge themselves. Besides restricting food intake, anorexics become hyperactive, restless, and obsessed with exercise, even doing calisthenics when confined to a small room.

The pursuit of overthinness provides these people with a sense of control over their lives, a deviation from years of trying to please others. They show a total lack of self-confidence—never doing things they want, only responding to others' demands. Physical and emotional changes are evident. Menstrual periods cease. Since constipation is common, many take laxatives, and then suffer diarrhea. They become depressed, moody, and hostile, but will continue to deny being sick.

It would seem that anorexia nervosa is a symptom of the times, when there is so much emphasis on thinness. But although the incidence is on the rise, the first case was officially identified in 1682 by D. Richard Morton, a British physician. Dr. Morton described an 18-year-old patient who had ceased to have menstrual periods as "a skeleton, only clad in skin." The girl to whom he was referring died three months after treatment.(46) Even with a better understanding of this disease today, about 15 to 21 percent of those with anorexia nervosa die of starvation and ensuing complications.(46) Immediate medical and psychiatric measures are needed. Once the person is under medical supervision, individual and family therapy is begun to help the person develop a better self-awareness and to eliminate any factors in the home that may be involved. For permanent recovery, patients must develop positive feelings toward their bodies and a desire to be healthy. Without a realistic view of their bodies, they will relapse into their old patterns. There are now several national, nonprofit educational and self-help organizations dedicated to alleviating problems of eating disorders. Anorexia Nervosa and Associated Disorders, Inc. (ANAD) provides counsel, referral lists for professional assistance, educational materials, and research. Write: ANAD, Suite 2020, 550 Frontage Road, Northfield, IL 60093. Other groups are: National Anorexic Aid Society, Box 29461, Columbus, OH 43229, and American Anorexia Nervosa Association, 133 Cedar Lane, Teaneck, NJ 07666. If you are interested in learning more about anorexia nervosa, a good resource is H. Bruch's *The Golden Cage: The Enigma of Anorexia Nervosa.*(46)

REFERENCES

1. A.A. Rimm and P.L. White, "Obesity: Its Risks and Hazards." In *Obesity in America*, G.A. Bray, ed. (Public Health Service, National Institutes of Health, November 1979), pp. 103–24.

2. Dr. Maria Simonson, "Weight Clinic at Johns Hopkins," *The Washington Post*, March 1, 1977, p. A-10.

3. National Center for Health Statistics, *Weight by Height and Age of Adult 18–24 Years: United States, 1971–1974.* Vital and Health Statistics Advance Data No. 14, November 30, 1977.

4. E.A. Sims, "Definitions, Criteria, and Prevalence of Obesity." In *Obesity in America*, G.A. Bray, ed. (Public Health Service, National Institutes of Health, November 1979), pp. 20–36.

5. A.J. Stunkard, "Obesity and the Social Environment: Current Status, Future Prospects." In *Obesity in America*, G.A. Bray, ed. (Public Health Service, National Institutes of Health, November 1979), pp. 206–40.

6. R.B. Stuart and B. Davis, *Slim Chance in a Fat World* (Champaign, Ill.: Research Press, 1972).

7. "Obesity in America: An Overview." In *Obesity in America*, G.A. Bray, ed. (Public Health Service, National Institutes of Health, November 1979), pp. 1–19.

8. R.S. Goodhart and M.E. Shils, *Modern Nutrition in Health and Disease* (Philadelphia: Lea and Febiger, 1980).

9. R.E. Frisch, "Food Intake, Fatness, and Reproductive Ability." In *Anorexia Nervosa*, R.A. Vigersky, ed. (New York: Raven Press, 1977), pp. 149–61.

10. G.F. Cahill, Jr., T.T. Aoki, and A.A. Rossini, "Metabolism in Obesity and Anorexia Nervosa." In *Nutrition and the Brain*, Vol. 3, R.J. Wurtman and J.J. Wurtman, eds. (New York: Raven Press, 1979), pp. 1–70.

11. L.B. Salans, "Natural History of Obesity." In *Obesity in America*, G.A. Bray, ed. (Public Health Service, National Institutes of Health, November 1979), pp. 69–94.

12. P. Nestel and B. Goldrick, "Obesity: Changes in Lipid Metabolism and the Role of Insulin," *Clinics in Endocrinology and Metabolism* 5(1976):313–35.

13. American Diabetes Association and American Dietetic Association, *Application of Exchange Lists for Meal Planning*, 1977.

14. J.V. Durnin and J. Womersley, "Body Fat Assessed from Total Body Density and Its Estimation from Skinfold Thickness: Measurements on 481 Men and Women Aged from 16 to 72 Years," *British Journal of Nutrition* 32(1974):77–97.

15. S. Davidson et al., *Human Nutrition and Dietetics*, 3rd ed. (New York: Churchill Livingstone, 1979).

16. J. Mayer, *Overweight: Causes, Cost and Control* (Englewood Cliffs, N.J.: Prentice Hall, 1968).

17. *National Commission on Diabetes Report*, Vol. 3, Part 1. DHEW Publ. No. (NIH) 76–1021. (Washington, D.C.: U.S. Government Printing Office, 1975).

18. B.N. Chiang, L.V. Pearlman, and F.H. Epstein, "Overweight and Hypertension: A Review." *Circulation* 39(1969):403–21.

19. W.B. Kannel and T. Gordon, "Physiological and Medical Concomitants of Obesity: The Framingham Study." In *Obesity in America*, G.A. Bray, ed. (Public Health Service, National Institutes of Health, November 1979), pp. 125–63.

20. G.A. Bray, "Treatment of Obesity with Drugs and Invasive Procedures." In *Obesity in America*, G.A. Bray, ed. (Public Health Service, National Institutes of Health, November 1979), pp. 179–205.

21. A. Angel, "Pathophysiology of Obesity," *Canadian Medical Association Journal* 110(1974):540–48.

22. J.L. Kittle and J. Hirsch, "Effect of Early Nutrition on the Development of Rat Epididymal Fat Pads: Cellularity and Metabolism," *Journal of Clinical Investigation* 47(1968):2091.

23. G.B. Forbes, "Nutrition and Growth," *Journal of Pediatrics* 91(1977):40.

24. J.H. Himes, "Infant Feeding Practices and Obesity," *Journal of the American Dietetic Association* 75 (1979):122–25.

25. L.B. Salans, S.W. Cushman, and R.E. Weisman, "Studies of Human Adipose Tissue: Adipose Cell

Size and Number in Nonobese and Obese Patients," *Journal of Clinical Investigation* 52(1973):929–41.

26. J. Hirsch and B. Batchelor, "Adipose Tissue Cellularity in Human Obesity," *Clinics of Endocrinology and Metabolism* 5(1976):299–311.

27. T.J. Coates and E.C. Thoresen, "Treating Obesity in Children and Adolescents: A Review," *American Journal of Public Health* 68(February 1978):143–51.

28. S.M. Garn, S.M. Bailey, and I.T.T. Higgins, "Fatness Similarities in Adopted Pairs, A Letter to the Editor," *American Journal of Clinical Nutrition* 29 (1976):1067.

29. L.B. Salans and S.W. Cushman, "The Roles of Adiposity and Diet in the Carbohydrate and Lipid Metabolic Abnormalities of Obesity." In *Advances in Modern Nutrition, Obesity, Diabetes and Vascular Disease*, H.K. Katzen and R.J. Mahler, eds. (Washington, D.C.: Hemisphere, 1978), pp. 267–302.

30. S. Schacter, "Obesity and Eating: Internal and External Cues Differentially Affect the Eating Behavior of Obese and Normal Subjects," *Science* 161 (1968):751.

31. T. Van Itallie, "Obesity: The American Disease," *Food Technology* 33, no. 12 (1979):43–47.

32. R.I. Simon, "Obesity as a Depressive Equivalent," *Journal of the American Medical Association* 183 (1963):208–10.

33. A.J. Stunkard, "Environment and Obesity: Recent Advances in Our Understanding of Regulation of Food Intake in Man," *Federation Proceedings* 27 (1968):1367–73.

34. S. Abraham, M.D. Carroll, C.N. Dresser, and C.L. Johnson, *Dietary Intake Source Data: Vital and Health Statistics*. (Hyattsville, Md.: National Center for Health Statistics, DHEW Publ. No. (PHS) 79-1221).

35. C.M. Young, "Dietary Treatment of Obesity: Carbohydrate Content and Feeding Frequency." In *Treating the Obese*, W.L. Asher, ed. (New York: Medcom Press, 1974), pp. 51–72.

36. B.A. Bullen, R.B. Reed, and J. Mayer, "Physical Activity of Obese and Nonobese Adolescent Girls Appraised by Motion Picture Sampling," *American Journal of Clinical Nutrition* 14(1964):211–23.

37. T.B. Van Itallie, "Conservative Approaches to Treatment." In *Obesity in America*, G.A. Bray, ed. (Public Health Service, National Institutes of Health, November 1979), pp. 164–78.

38. "The Cambridge Diet," *Nutrition and the M.D.* VI (1980):2.

39. J. Mazel, *The Beverly Hills Diet*, (New York: Macmillan, 1981).

40. G.B. Mirkin and R.N. Shore, "The Beverly Hills Diet, Dangers of the Newest Weight Loss Fad," *Journal of the American Medical Association* 246 (1981):2235–2237.

41. L. Fenner, "Cellulite: Hard to Budge Pudge," *FDA Consumer*, May 1980, pp. 5–9.

42. *Community Nutrition Institute (CNI) Weekly*, April 13, 1980.

43. H. Gilder et al., "Components of Weight Loss in Obese Patients Subjected to Prolonged Starvation," *Journal of Applied Physiology* 23(1967):304–10.

44. *The Healthy Way to Weigh Less* (Council on Foods and Nutrition, American Medical Association, 1965).

45. H.A. Guthrie, *Introductory Nutrition*, 4th ed. (St. Louis: Mosby, 1979), pp. 119–20.

46. H. Bruch, *Eating Disorders: Obesity, Anorexia Nervosa, and the Person Within* (New York: Basic Books, 1973).

Vitamins
7

"Vitamins, if properly understood and applied," wrote biochemist Szent-Gyorgi in 1937, "will help us to reduce human suffering to an extent which the most fantastic mind would fail to imagine." It is not surprising he felt this way. From the early 1900s on, researchers were discovering vitamin after vitamin and curing deficiency diseases like beriberi and pellagra that had caused enormous suffering for centuries. Who wouldn't have been excited over the possibilities for vitamins?

Today, however, U.S. doctors rarely see vitamin-deficiency diseases except in certain groups like alcoholics. We do not hear people talking about taking supplements because they are worried about scurvy, beriberi, or rickets either. Instead, modern zealots promote vitamins as cures for so many unrelated disorders that it staggers the imagination. One current almanac lists 82 disorders alleviated by vitamin E, 102 by vitamin A, and 119 by vitamin C. To understand how vitamins achieved the dubious status of being curealls, we must examine them as a group and individually.

Vitamins are lumped together because they all contain carbon, do not provide energy, and are needed in small amounts in the diet to regulate biological reactions. Aside from these characteristics, they are totally unrelated. A substance can be a vitamin for one species yet not for another, depending on whether the animal's body can make the vitamin.

The vitamin era began in 1897 when Eijkman found that a diet of polished rice could cause beriberi because it was missing a certain factor vital to health. He discovered this factor in the rice polishings that had been removed during processing. Adding these polishings (later found to contain thiamin) back to the diet cured the disease.

Casimir Funk coined the term *vitamine* in 1912, from the roots *vita* (life) and *amine* (the chemical structure of the vitamin he was researching). When it was discovered that not all vitamins are amines, the *e* was dropped. Early researchers named vitamins alphabetically according to their time of discovery. Later they found that many substances originally classified as vitamins were not essential for humans and dropped them from the list. So there are many gaps in the alphabetical listing. Other vitamins thought at first to be one chemical turned out to be many, so the alphabetical name had to be broken down by numbers (B-1, B-2, and so on).

Based on solubility, vitamins fall into two groups: those dissolving in water and those dissolving in fat or oil. To date there are 13 recognized vitamins: four are fat-soluble and nine are water-soluble.

- *Fat-soluble:* A, D, E, K.
- *Water-soluble:* thiamin, riboflavin, niacin, vitamin B-6, folacin, vitamin B–12, pantothenic acid, vitamin C, biotin.
- Uncertain vitamin status: inositol, choline.

Vitamins in each of the two solubility categories share certain characteristics. Several vitamins exist in more than one chemical form, and these forms may vary in activity in the body.

FAT-SOLUBLE VITAMINS

You find fat-soluble vitamins in the fatty portions of food; these vitamins need fat for their absorption. Like fats, they are absorbed through the intestine with the help of bile. Any factor that impedes fat absorption also slows the absorption of the fat-soluble vitamins. For example, at one time manufacturers added mineral oil to dietetic salad dressings because the oil cannot be absorbed by the body. It coats the lining of the digestive tract, preventing foods from being absorbed. Dieters using these dressings absorbed fewer nutrients (and kcalories), but they also lost their fat-soluble vitamins. Since the body stores fat-soluble vitamins, humans do not have to consume them daily. Excessive doses, on the other hand, pose a danger of toxicity (see Issue: Megadoses).

Two of the fat-soluble vitamins (A and D) have *precursors* or provitamins. These substances, chemically related to the vitamin, must be converted to an active form before the body can use them. The conversion occurs in different locations (intestines, kidney, skin), depending on the precursor. Precursors cannot perform the vitamin function until converted to the vitamin and the conversion is less than 100 percent. Thus the amount of vitamin activity provided by a food is not equal to the actual amount of precursor in the food. For this reason some of the fat soluble vitamins are measured in units like "International Units" (I.U.) or "vitamin equivalents." Instead of indicating the amount of the precursor or vitamin contained in a food by weight, these units describe the amount of activity or vitamin action the food provides to the body. The I.U. is the older measure and the one used in most food composition tables. It is, however, being replaced gradually by "vitamin equivalents."

Vitamin A

Vitamin A has three different chemical forms, called retinaldehyde, retinol, and retinoic acid. People have recognized deficiency signs of vitamin A for centuries. Hippocrates prescribed raw liver for night blindness, a common symptom. In more recent times, during World War I, children in Denmark began to suffer from severe eye problems, and some became completely blind. An investigating doctor noted that the government was exporting all the butter to Britain, leaving the diets of Danish children devoid of milkfat. Once they added the butter and whole milk back to the diet, the incidence of these eye problems dropped.

Although researchers have studied vitamin A since its discovery in 1913, its metabolic roles are still baffling. Vitamin A is needed for bone growth, reproduction, the stability of cell membranes and healthy epithelial cells (those lining the skin and mucous membranes) and for the visual process. The only one of these roles that is clearly understood at the chemical level is that in the visual process.

The retina of the eye has two types of cells: rods and cones. The rod cells sense low light intensities required for vision in dim light. The cone cells are sensitive to high light intensities and colors. The photosensitive pigment of rods is called rhodopsin (or visual purple), and it is formed by the combination of a protein (opsin) and the retinaldehyde form of vitamin A. In dim light opsin combines with vitamin A to form rhodopsin. In bright light the opsin breaks apart from the vitamin, destroying the rhodopsin. When this occurs some of the vitamin A is recovered and recycled back into the system, although a little is lost and must be continuously replaced by vitamin A from the diet (Figure 7–1).

With a short-term vitamin A deficiency, rhodopsin synthesis is impaired and night blindness results. The person's vision does not adjust rapidly to dim light and objects cannot be seen even at relatively close distances. With longer-

FIG. 7–1

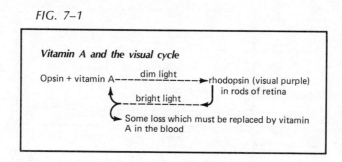

Vitamin A and the visual cycle

Opsin + vitamin A ----dim light----→ rhodopsin (visual purple) in rods of retina

----bright light----

Some loss which must be replaced by vitamin A in the blood

term deficiency, the corneas in the eyes become dry, thick, and wrinkled. If the deficiency continues, the person will become permanently blind, a condition called xerophthalmia. Xerophthalmia is one of the most important public health problems in the world today, with over 100,000 people, usually children, going blind yearly in countries such as Bangladesh, Brazil, El Salvador, Iraq, and Vietnam.

Vitamin A also maintains healthy epithelial cells. These cells form the outer layer of the skin, the lining of the gastrointestinal tract, and the respiratory tract. Although scientists are not sure how vitamin A functions in this role, a deficiency of the vitamin brings about well-recognized signs. With adequate vitamin A the epithelial tissue is smooth, moist, ciliated, and secretes mucus, the first line of defense against infections. With inadequate vitamin A, the epithelial tissue becomes irregular and deciliated. Instead of secreting mucus and remaining moist, the cells become dry and hard. This is called keratinization and the cells are said to be keratinized. The tissue breaks easily and is not able to ward off microorganisms, so infections develop (Figure 7–2).

Requirements for vitamin A are in direct proportion to weight. The average man needs more than the average woman and children's needs increase progressively as they grow. Excess intakes of vitamin A accumulate in the liver and lead to toxic symptoms of vomiting, nausea, and skin rashes. Children are especially susceptible. Toxic doses can be avoided if vitamin A is obtained solely from the diet and not from supplementary pills. (A unique exception is polar bear liver which contains incredibly high amounts of vitamin A. But how many people eat polar bear liver?)

Only animal products contain the active form or preformed vitamin A. Good sources include dairy products (milk, cream, butter) and liver. Skim milk and low-fat milk must be fortified with an amount of vitamin A equivalent to that in whole milk. Fortification of dry skim milk is optional. Margarine is fortified with enough of the vitamin to approximate that in butter. In plant foods, vitamin A is in the precursor form. Actually there are several related precursors which are collectively called carotene. Carotene is a yellow-orange pigment that is converted to active vitamin A in the intestinal wall (only about

FIG. 7–2

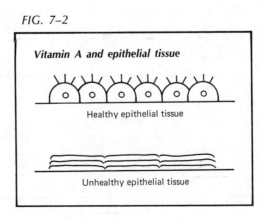

Vitamin A and epithelial tissue

Healthy epithelial tissue

Unhealthy epithelial tissue

one-third of ingested carotene is converted to the active form). Red, deep yellow, or orange vegetables generally are high in carotene, although these colors can also be caused by other pigments that have no potential vitamin A activity. In addition, dark green vegetables (dandelion greens, spinach, collard greens, mustard greens, broccoli, dark green lettuce, kale, beet greens, bok choy) may be good sources of carotene, even though the green chlorophyll-containing pigment masks the underlying yellow-orange color. Fruits, except for apricots, peaches, and cantaloupe, are generally low in carotene.

Vitamin D

The chemical name for this vitamin is calciferol, and it is also known as the sunshine vitamin because it can be obtained in two ways: from food and by the action of the ultraviolet rays in sunlight. The latter comes from the irradiation of a cholesterol-like substance in the skin that is converted to active vitamin D in the kidney. The amount of vitamin D formed in this way depends on the length and intensity of light exposure and the pigmentation of the skin. (Darker pigments are harder to penetrate.) The necessary ultraviolet light is also filtered out by fog, smoke, smog, and ordinary window glass. People living in cities, where exposure to sunlight is often minimal, should have a dietary source of the vitamin. Some nutritionists prefer to classify vitamin D as a hormone instead of a vitamin because it can be synthesized in the body, given exposure to sunlight. If you do not have much exposure to the sun, however, you should have a dietary source of the vitamin.

Food sources of vitamin D include eggs, vitamin D-fortified milk, butter, fatty fish, liver, and fish liver oils. Milk is a poor source unless it is fortified. Many foods are now fortified with vitamin D so that you can meet your daily requirement without relying on pills as a supplement.

Vitamin D promotes calcium and phosphate absorption in the intestinal tract and helps maintain blood calcium and phosphorus levels to permit the normal calcification of bone. A deficiency causes faulty bone mineralization. In children this condition is called rickets, in adults osteomalacia. With rickets, the newly synthesized bone matrix fails to calcify and harden, resulting in soft bones. Many infants and children in Europe and the United States suffered from rickets before the widespread use of vitamin D in milk. In recent years, rickets has occurred among some children of strict vegetarians who drink no milk. Deficiencies arise mainly among those individuals who are rarely exposed to direct sun and have no source of vitamin D in the diet. Although deficiencies are uncommon in adults, they can still be found in Muslim women whose practice of *purdah* restricts their exposure to sunlight and in the elderly on very limited diets and who seldom go outside. If women do not receive enough vitamin D during pregnancy and lactation to allow for adequate absorption of dietary calcium, it will be drawn from their bones, thus weakening their skeletal frames.

The RDA for vitamin D is highest for infants, children, and adolescents because of their growing bones. Pregnant and breastfeeding women have an increased requirement. Supplements may be needed by low-birth-weight infants and breastfed infants (commercial infant formulas contain vitamin D). Others (miners, night workers) who are deprived of sunlight because of smog, fog, or working conditions should plan their diets carefully to include adequate vitamin D.

Excess vitamin D can be toxic: it can cause vomiting, diarrhea, loss of weight, and kidney damage.

Vitamin E

This vitamin has several forms, known as tocopherols. The most active form is alpha-tocopherol. Vitamin E is the vitamin "in search of a deficiency disease." A deficiency of the vitamin in animals results in spontaneous abortions, wasting of muscle tissue, especially the heart, and leaky blood capillaries. Because it is in so many foods, deficiencies are rare in humans. The vitamin does not travel well across the placenta of the pregnant woman, so premature infants may not have adequate stores and become deficient if the vitamin is not provided in their diet. They become irritable, anemic, and show edema. The small reserves of the vitamin that adults have are hard to deplete. In adults, the only symptom of low vitamin E levels is a shorter survival time for the red blood cells. Persons with a fat malabsorption problem, like that which occurs in cystic fibrosis, may have a vitamin E deficiency.

Vitamin E is an antioxidant. That means it prevents oxygen from reacting with susceptible compounds like vitamin A and PUFAs. Various agents (radiation, chemicals) can cause hydrogens to break off at the carbons between two double bonds, the most vulnerable link in the carbon chain (Figure 7–3). When this happens, oxygen can come in and bond with the carbon between the double bonds, bringing about a series of reactions that may eventually break the carbon chain. PUFAs are major components of cell membranes, so when they are destroyed, the cell membrane becomes unstable. Once the cell membrane

FIG. 7–3

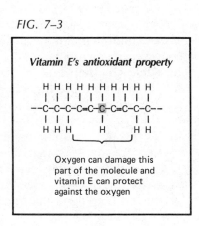

Vitamin E's antioxidant property

Oxygen can damage this part of the molecule and vitamin E can protect against the oxygen

has been damaged, the cell dies. Vitamin E protects the PUFA by acting as a decoy for the oxygen. It prevents the oxygen from bonding with the vulnerable carbon in the chain, thus protecting the double bonds in the PUFA.

Because the vitamin protects PUFA, your requirement will depend on how many of these fatty acids are in your diet. On an average, adult men require more than adult women. Children's needs increase as they get older. Pregnant and lactating women have slightly increased needs.

Luckily both vitamin E and polyunsaturated fats are present in the same foods, so increasing the amount ingested of one will automatically increase the other. The vitamin E in diets varies widely, depending on the amount and types of fat consumed. Principal sources include vegetable and seed oils (soybean, cottonseed, corn), shortening, margarine, egg yolk, butter, milk fat, grains, especially the germ, liver, nuts, and green leafy vegetables such as lettuce and cabbage.

Vitamin K

Vitamin K was named for the Danish word "koagulation" because it plays a role in the development of the protein prothrombin, a necessary factor for blood clotting.

Humans have two sources of the vitamin: food and intestinal bacteria. Good dietary sources are dark green vegetables (spinach, kale, cabbage leaves, peas), cauliflower, tomatoes, wheat bran, soybeans, and soybean oil. There is little in animal products, although egg yolks, milk, cheese, and organ meats contain some.

There is no RDA for vitamin K. Deficiencies are uncommon except in newborn infants, whose intestinal tracts are free of bacteria and who have low stores of vitamin K. It takes several days for the bacterial population in the intestines to become large enough to provide significant amounts of the vitamin. Adults have a problem only if they have some absorption defect or are on prolonged treatment with drugs that kill the intestinal bacteria. For example, since antibiotics destroy natural intestinal bacteria, dietary sources of the vitamin are important when you are taking these drugs. People using anticoagulants and those about to have surgery may receive vitamin K supplements. A synthetic form of vitamin K, menadione, may be toxic to newborn infants if taken in excess.

WATER-SOLUBLE VITAMINS

Most of the water-soluble vitamins are not stored in the body to the extent that fat-soluble vitamins are stored. Excesses are usually excreted in the urine or lost through perspiration, so daily consumption is recommended. Excessive doses generally are not toxic. Due to their solubility in water, however, large amounts of these vitamins can be lost during food processing, storage, and preparation if improper methods are used.

The B Vitamins

The B complex includes a group of vitamins with four common properties: All function as coenzymes for biochemical reactions in the body; are natural constituents of yeast and liver; are water-soluble; and promote the growth of bacteria. The complex includes thiamin, riboflavin, niacin, vitamin B-6, vitamin B-12, folacin, pantothenic acid, and biotin.

Researchers discovered the B vitamins by their absence rather than their presence in food. Usually, if there is a deficiency of one of these vitamins there will be deficiencies of the others, since they tend to occur in the same foods. The only reason they are sometimes called the "B complex" is because of their similar functions; their structures are completely different. As coenzymes, they serve in these reactions:

- Reactions that release energy from fats and carbohydrates: thiamin, niacin, riboflavin, pantothenic acid, biotin
- Reactions that break down and rebuild amino acids: pyridoxine
- Reactions necessary for proper formation of red blood cells: folic acid, cobalamin, pyridoxine

Remember that vitamins help release energy from carbohydrates, fats, and proteins and do not provide any energy themselves. Granted, if your diet contains enough fuel nutrients but too little of the vitamins needed to act as coenzymes in energy release, you will lack energy. On the other hand, if your diet contains enough vitamins yet is lacking in carbohydrates, fats, and proteins, no extra vitamins will add to your energy level.

Like all nutrients, the B vitamins function together, so that any excess intake of one may create a greater need for the others. If you are in the habit of routinely taking vitamins, it would be wiser to buy a multivitamin B complex capsule rather than a capsule containing only one or two specific B vitamins.

Thiamin (B-1). Nutritionists have long known thiamin to be the factor that prevents *beriberi,* a disease prevalent in areas where polished rice is the staple food. The incidence of beriberi jumped once it became popular to refine rice. The word itself means "I cannot," so named because its victims suffer paralysis. During the late nineteenth century the disease was rampant in the Japanese navy, where sailors would receive white milled rice as the mainstay of their diets over a period of many months at sea.

Thiamin is required to release energy from carbohydrates and trap it in

ATP. Thiamin helps transmit nerve impulses, possibly by acting in the formation or release of acetylcholine, one of the substances needed for impulses to be passed from one nerve cell to another. Thiamin is also required for breaking down alcohol. Individual requirements for the vitamin depend on carbohydrate intake and are calculated on the number of kcalories consumed. More thiamin is needed whenever there is an increased need for kcalories: during growth spurts, pregnancy and lactation, and athletic training, and during periods of illness.

Severe thiamin deficiency produces mental confusion and muscular cramps. Low intake can lead to decreased coordination, with lessened ability to work. In the United States, the major groups at risk of deficiency are alcoholics and those following certain food fads where milled rice is the primary food eaten. Alcoholics may experience a neurological condition called *Wernicke-Korsakoff syndrome,* which produces stumbling, loss of memory, and reduced mental ability. Some doctors recommend putting thiamin in alcoholic beverages or providing thiamin-enriched snacks at bars. Other support immunizing alcoholics with periodic thiamin shots.

Pork is the richest common food source of thiamin, although whole grains and enriched or fortified cereals are also high. Other good sources are liver, poultry, fish, eggs, potatoes, dried beans and peas, nuts, dark green vegetables, brewer's yeast, and wheat germ.

Riboflavin (B-2).   Riboflavin was first called "lactoflavin" because it was found in milk. Researchers have not identified a riboflavin deficiency disease, but low intakes lead to cracked skin around the mouth, inflamed lips, sore tongue, and sensitivity to light.

Riboflavin, as a coenzyme, helps release energy from carbohydrates, fats, and proteins. It is essential for growth and healthy skin. Riboflavin requirements depend on body size, metabolic rate, and rate of growth, so that more is needed in periods of growth, pregnancy, and lactation. Few individuals in the United States except alcoholics and the very poor show deficiencies of this vitamin.

Riboflavin is well distributed in animal and vegetable foods, and is especially high in milk. Meat (particularly organ meats), poultry or eggs, enriched breads and cereals, green leafy vegetables, beans, and yeast are all good sources. As a rule of thumb, foods high in calcium will usually be good sources of riboflavin.

Niacin (B-3).   Niacin is a chemical relative of nicotine, the toxic substance found in cigarette smoke, but its effects are far from harmful. It exists in two forms: nicotinic acid and nicotinamide (also called niacinamide). All living cells need niacin to release energy from carbohydrates, proteins, and fats. Niacin is also needed for making proteins and nucleic acids. *Pellagra* results if there is too little of this vitamin. Many Americans in the southeastern United States suffered from this disease in the early part of the twentieth century. In 1914, a U.S. Public Health team headed by Goldberger discovered that, contrary to the widely held belief, the disease was not caused by a germ, but was the result of a vitamin deficiency. The disease is found in areas where corn is a major dietary staple and is caused by a diet built around the three Ms of a pellagra-causing diet: meal (corn), meat (salt pork), and molasses. None of these foods is a good source of niacin, although many other meats are.

Individuals deficient in the vitamin experience weakness and indigestion, and lack energy and appetite. Later these symptoms develop into what are known as the three Ds of pellagra: dermatitis (inflammation of skin exposed to the sun), diarrhea (from inflammation of the lining of the intestinal tract), and dementia (mental confusion from degeneration of the brain cells and tracks of the spinal cord). Today in the United States deficiencies are limited to chronic alcoholics and persons with intestinal disturbances.

Niacin is synthesized in the body from the amino acid tryptophan. You should remember this indirect source of the vitamin when evaluating your diet. Sixty milligrams of tryptophan are equivalent to 1 milligram of niacin. If a quart of milk contains only 1 milligram of niacin but 480 milligrams of tryptophan, there is enough tryptophan to make 8 milligrams of niacin equivalents. The total niacin equivalents then equal 9 milligrams. Your need for niacin increases as you consume more kcalories, so if you are pregnant, breastfeeding, sick, or stressed, you will need more niacin.

The richest food sources are liver, meat, poultry, peanut butter, and legumes. Strict vegetarians must rely on nuts and legumes for niacin. The niacin in cereals and vegetables such as corn is usually bound to other compounds which lessens the body's ability to use it. Sources of tryptophan include milk, eggs, meat, legumes, and nuts.

Vitamin B-6.   This vitamin has three forms, pyridoxine, pyridoxal, and pyridoxamine. Its primary role is helping change one amino acid into another. It is also required for the production of antibodies and red blood cells, and for the functioning of the nervous system. Vitamin B-6 helps convert the essential fatty acid linoleic to another important fatty acid, arachidonic, and is required for the conversion of the amino acid tryptophan into niacin.

Vitamin B-6 is found in so many foods that a deficiency was once thought an oddity because researchers had seen it only in laboratory animals fed special diets. Ironically, B-6 deficiencies occur almost entirely in wealthy, developed countries. The first recorded cases were in infants fed formulas in which the vitamin had been destroyed during processing. One group at risk of deficiency is tuberculosis patients, because an important antituberculosis drug (isoniazid) increases the body's need for B-6. A deficiency affects the central nervous system, causing convulsions and behavioral abnormalities. Other symptoms include poor growth, anemia, and decreased antibodies. Need for the vitamin increases with increased protein intake. There also is a greater requirement during pregnancy, with the use of oral contraceptives, and with advancing age.

Good food sources of vitamin B-6 include muscle meats, liver, dark green leafy vegetables, avocado, whole grain cereals, egg yolks, potatoes, dried beans and peas, fish, and dairy products.

Folacin (Folic Acid).   Folacin is required for cells to regenerate and is involved in the synthesis of such important compounds as the nucleic acids DNA and RNA. The requirement for folacin is directly related to the rate at which the body is forming cells and the activity of these cells. The need increases when the metabolic rate increases, as in pregnancy, lactation, growth of malignant tumors, infections, hyperthyroidism, and with certain anemias. Both alcohol and oral contraceptives increase the requirement for folacin.

A deficiency of folacin slows growth and interferes with cell regeneration. Cells that are short-lived, such as red blood cells, are the first to succumb. For this reason, a folacin deficiency produces megaloblastic anemia which is characterized by red blood cells that are too large and too few in number. The oxygen-carrying ability of the blood is reduced. Folacin works together with vitamin B-12 and if taken in excess can mask a B-12 deficiency. This is why the Food and Drug Administration restricts folacin supplementation to small amounts in vitamin pills. Persons can become folacin-deficient if they consume too little, have a malabsorption problem, or certain diseases such as leukemia, Hodgkin's disease, or cancer.

The term folacin comes from the Latin word "folium" meaning leaf, because it is found in high amounts in green leafy vegetables. Other rich sources include liver, kidney and muscle meats, legumes and beans, asparagus, broccoli, orange juice, brewer's yeast, torula yeast, and the germ and bran of wheat (milling and processing of grain products destroys much of the vitamin). Good sources include lean beef, nuts, sweet potatoes, cantaloupe, melons, potatoes, corn, lima beans, parsnips, green peas, and pumpkins.

Pantothenic Acid.   During World War II, prisoners of war developed "burning feet syndrome," a feeling of tingling and great tenderness in the feet. A pantothenic acid deficiency was partly to blame. Pantothenic acid is so widespread in foods (its name comes from the Greek "pantos" meaning everywhere) that there is little to no evidence of a spontaneous dietary deficiency in humans, except in such rare situations as a prisoner of war camp.

Like other B-vitamins, pantothenic acid helps release energy from carbohydrates, fats, and protein. It also aids in the formation of cholesterol, hemoglobin, and certain hormones. The richest food sources include organ meats, fish, and whole grain cereals.

Vitamin B-12.   This vitamin, sometimes called cobalamin, is so named because it contains cobalt. In order to be absorbed by the body, it must first bind to a protein called the intrinsic factor, which is secreted by cells in the stomach lining. Anything interfering with normal stomach secretions will hinder B-12 absorption. Once the intrinsic factor and the vitamin (plus calcium) have been bound, the vitamin can pass through the intestinal wall into the bloodstream. Some people with a defective gene do not synthesize the intrinsic factor. Even though there is enough of the vitamin in their diets, they cannot absorb it and must be given B-12 injections. How well the body absorbs B-12 is also influenced by the body's level of B-6 and iron. Low levels may repress absorption. Absorption probably decreases with age and increases with pregnancy.

B-12 is required for growth, maintenance of healthy nervous tissues, and normal red blood cell formation. The exact manner in which it performs these functions is not entirely clear, but it does serve as a coenzyme in a number of reactions involving breakdown products of carbohydrate, fat, and protein. A deficiency, usually from an absorption problem or stomach injury, leads to *pernicious anemia,* a condition in which red blood cells are abnormally large, too few in number, and incompletely developed. Other symptoms of pernicious anemia include weakness, indigestion, abdominal pain, constipation, diarrhea, a sore and glossy tongue, and damaged nerve fibers. The elderly are most at risk of developing pernicious anemia, although the reason is not completely understood.

B-12 is made only by microorganisms. Since most of these microorganisms exist in the intestines of animals, animal products are the main food source of the vitamin. Plant products containing B-12 include those contaminated by organic fertilizers, fermented soybean foods, and sea vegetables. Few of these foods are consumed in this country, but they are popular in Asia. None is considered a reliable source. In this country, rich dietary sources of B-12 include clams, oysters, and organ meats such as lamb and beef liver, kidney, and heart. Moderately large amounts are found in seafood and eggs. The normal liver can store enough B-12 to meet daily requirements for over two years, but strict vegetarians may develop a deficiency over time if they are not careful about their food choices.

Biotin (H).   Biotin is a sulfur-containing vitamin that functions in the metabolism of fats and carbohydrates. Deficiencies are unknown, because intestinal bacteria produce the vitamin. Biotin, however, can be bound by avidin, a protein in raw eggs, and become unabsorbable. This is how researchers create biotin deficiencies in lab animals. Almost all foods contain biotin, but liver, kidneys, milk, egg yolk, and yeast are particularly rich sources.

Vitamin C (Ascorbic Acid)

Vitamin C's best-known role is in the formation of collagen, the protein binding cells together. Vitamin C also aids in the absorption of iron and in healing of wounds. Like vitamin E, it is an antioxidant, protecting substances from oxidation.

Scurvy is the vitamin C deficiency disease. Known since ancient times, it was described on papyrus rolls from 1500 B.C., and in the writings of Hippocrates in 400 B.C. Because vitamin C is found mainly in fresh fruits and vegetables, scurvy became one of the leading causes of death for explorers undertaking long sea voyages. British navy doctors prescribed the use of lemons and limes aboard ships to avoid this disease, which is why British sailors were called "limeys." With scurvy, the poorly formed collagen leads to abnormal bones, joint pains, bleeding gums, and tiny hemorrhages beneath the skin surface. Few Americans, except infants fed exclusively on unsupplemented cow's milk, are at risk of scurvy. In adults, the poor or alcoholics may show symptoms. Infections, burns, and injuries decrease the amount of vitamin C in tissues and body fluids.

The adult RDA for vitamin C is 60 milligrams. Pregnancy and lactation increase the requirement. Needs can easily be met by including good vitamin C sources in the diet, such as fresh, canned, and frozen citrus fruits, as well as other fruits, potatoes, green peppers, broccoli, and raw or lightly cooked greens or cabbage. In some fruits and vegetables the vitamin accumulates with ripening, examples of which are asparagus, green pepper, and apples. The opposite, however, has been reported for others, such as bananas and cantaloupes. The only significant animal source is liver.

COMPOUNDS OF UNCERTAIN STATUS AND NONVITAMINS

Choline and Inositol

Scientists are not quite sure whether to call certain compounds like choline and inositol vitamins. Even though they function like vitamins, they are made by the body. There is, however, some disagreement as to whether the amount would be adequate if there were none in the diet for a long period. If future researchers find a human dietary need for them, they will be reclassified as vitamins.

Both choline and inositol may be found in food and in the body as part of a fatty substance called lecithin. Choline functions in a number of important reactions in the body and, since it is part of the coating of nerves, helps transmit impulses. The body makes choline from the amino acids glycine and methionine, with the help of vitamins B-12 and folacin. Concern about choline adequacy has arisen only for infants and young children with severe protein deficiency. Researchers have not found any deficiency disease or toxic symptoms in humans. Good food sources of choline are egg yolk, liver, brewer's yeast, and wheat germ. Inositol functions in the growth of liver and bone marrow cells, and humans can make it from glucose. It is in all plant and animal tissues, but the best food sources are fruits, meat, milk, nuts, vegetables, and whole grain cereals.

Nonvitamins

If you have passed a health food store recently, you may have seen an ad in the window declaring, "We Now Have B-15." You may have been relieved to know that now you can buy B-15, or maybe you wondered where it has been all this time. For B-15 you can substitute terms such as bioflavonoids, PABA, vitamin T, but you still have the same situation: These are all substances with no known nutritional value that are promoted and sold as vitamins. Some of these so-called vitamins simply bleed your wallet; others have dangerous side effects. Their absence from the diet does not cause illness or disease.

A good example of widely promoted "vitamins" are the *bioflavonoids,* a group composed of substances (sometimes called vitamin P) that include citrin, hesperidin, rutin, flavones, and flavonals. Bioflavonoids were first found in the white segments of citrus fruits. Promoters claim that these substances can cure ulcers, inner ear disorders, and asthma, and prevent miscarriages, bleeding gums, eczema, hemorrhage, rheumatism, rheumatic fever, and muscular dystrophy. They also supposedly protect the body from X-rays.

Not to be outdone by the bioflavonoids is *pangamic acid* or B-15. Other names for it include Aangamik and Caldiamate. Scientists do not know the composition of B-15 because no two manufacturers use the same ingredients. Even so, regardless of the chemicals used, B-15 has no vitaminlike activity, and there is no evidence that it is safe. Both Canada and the United States have banned its sale as a food or drug. There are claims that it cures high blood pressure, asthma, rheumatism, rheumatic heart disease, alcoholism, athero-sclerosis, and cancer; lowers cholesterol levels; improves circulation; and delays aging. None of the claims, however, is substantiated by sound research.

B-15 promoters recommend its use along with *laetrile* for cancer therapy. Laetrile, also known as B-17, amygdalin, or nitrilosides, is a substance present in apricot pits. It is not a vitamin, can be harmful, and is worthless as a cancer remedy.

Para-aminobenzoic acid (PABA) is a water-soluble substance often found with folacin. The body makes its own PABA, so there is no dietary requirement. Promoters of PABA supplements claim it can restore the natural color to graying or white hair, and that it soothes burns, delays aging, and can be used to treat depigmented skin and certain parasitic diseases like Rocky Mountain Spotted Fever.

Other nonvitamins include vitamin T (sesame seed factor), promoted as a cure for anemia, hemophilia, and fading memory; vitamin U, the supposed answer to peptic ulcers; and B-13 (orotic acid), a treatment for multiple sclerosis, cancer, and high blood pressure. One of the oddest is vitamin F, or unsaturated fatty acids. Somehow fats are now being billed as vitamins and promoted as cures for ulcers, eczema, psoriasis, and dermatitis, and as preventing heart disease.

Preserving Vitamins

When storing, preparing, and cooking vegetables, the main concern is to spare as many nutrients as possible.

The first way to do this is to avoid buying wilted or old produce. Next, be careful how vegetables are stored. Dark green leafy vegetables should be put in plastic bags or stored in tight-fitting containers and refrigerated. Vegetables in pods should be left whole until ready to use. Tuber or root vegetables (potatoes, onions, squash) should be kept in a cool, well-aired place. Tomatoes can be ripened in the sun for up to a week (if left in the refrigerator, they become soft, watery, and begin to decay).

Wash vegetables and fruits, preferably unpeeled, quickly and without soaking. Do not let them stand in the light or air. If vegetables must be soaked, this should be done before paring or peeling them. When washing leafy greens, dry them immediately by shaking off the excess water and blotting gently. When you eat a raw fruit or vegetable, don't hack away half of it to remove the peel. Vitamins are usually concentrated just under the skin of fruits and vegetables, so if the skin is edible, wash it and eat the whole thing. If you have to peel the skin, remove as thin a layer as possible. Do not throw away the outer leaves of vegetables because these contain more vitamin A, calcium, and iron than the inner leaves. Be careful not to bruise produce, because bruising exposes the cellular contents to air, reducing vitamins A and C. Vegetables such as spinach eaten raw will provide more of the water-soluble vitamins and fiber. Cooking vegetables such as carrots softens the cell walls, allowing release of more of the fat-soluble vitamins (particularly vitamin A) during digestion.

If you are going to cook vegetables, keep them whole or in large pieces to preserve as many water-soluble nutrients as possible. When boiling, place them in a pan with very little water and use a tight-fitting lid, and minimal cooking time. Steaming, sautéeing, or waterless cooking are also recommended. Pressure cooking is fine if the cooking time is short and little water is used. To steam vegetables, put a steamer in a pot with about an inch of water, cover with a tight-fitting lid, and place over medium heat. Avoid opening the lid, as the steam will escape. Five to seven minutes of cooking is enough for most vegetables. Save the water for soups, casseroles, or cooking grains and beans. Waterless cooking uses natural juices from the vegetables and the water left on the vegetables after washing. Use a pot that distributes heat evenly. Preheat the pot and put at most about two tablespoons of water in to provide steam until the vegetables release their juices. After the water boils, add the vegetables, cover, and turn heat to low. Cooking time will be slightly longer than steaming.

Stir-frying vegetables in oil or butter cuts down on vitamin C losses, but adds kcalories from the absorbed oil. To keep vegetables crisp, cook just a short time. Deep-fat frying reduces the level of many heat-sensitive vitamins. Boiling and baking make starch more available in tuber and root vegetables and grains. Keep the skins on to retain most of the vitamins. When cooking vegetables, do not use baking soda. Although it gives the vegetables a bright green color, it destroys thiamin and vitamin C and breaks down the cellulose, causing changes in texture. Cooked vegetables will lose some nutrients during refrigeration; up to one-half may be lost after two to three days. Reheating causes more losses.

Canning fruits and vegetables reduces the level of heat-sensitive vitamins, but enough remain to make a significant contribution to the diet. Few nutrients are lost from canned fruits and vegetables during storage provided they are kept in a cool, dry place and storage time is not lengthy.

If blanched first, frozen fruits and vegetables retain vitamins well if they are kept at very low temperatures. You can minimize loss by keeping a constant freezer temperature below 0°F (−18°C). Wrap foods tightly in plastic or place them in tightly-covered, vaporproof containers. Do not thaw frozen vegetables before cooking.

Frozen fruit juices keep most of their vitamin C for up to one year, but you should not thaw frozen juice by running hot water over the can since this will reduce the level of heat-sensitive vitamins. Frozen citrus juice concentrates retain 95 percent or more of their vitamin C when reconstituted and refrigerated in a covered container. After 8 days about 85 percent of the vitamin is still present.(1)

Do not wash rice before cooking because the B vitamins are added to the outside of the grain. Cooking cereals in too much water, draining off the excess and rinsing afterward wastes nutrients. When baking breads, be careful not to use too much baking powder; quick breads, made with baking powders composed of sodium bicarbonate, contain less thiamin than yeast breads since thiamin is more readily destroyed in the presence of this alkali. The list below shows the major ways nutrients are lost from plant products.(2)

- Spoilage of unprocessed plant foods
- Excessive refining, trimming, cutting, chopping, slicing, washing, soaking
- Excessive use of water in cooking
- Excessive use of heat in cooking
- Discarded cooking water
- Use of alkaline processes in cooking or baking
- Refrigeration of cooked foods longer than one day
- Reheating

SUMMARY

Vitamins are organic compounds, required in the diet in small amounts to regulate biological reactions. Based on solubility, vitamins are classified as fat-soluble (A, D, E, K) or water-soluble (thiamin, riboflavin, niacin, B-6, folacin, B-12, pantothenic acid, C, and biotin).

Fat-soluble vitamins are present in the fatty portions of food and follow fat in absorption. Because fat-soluble vitamins can be stored, humans do not need to consume them daily. Excessive intakes can be toxic, particularly in the case of vitamins A and D. Some of the fat-soluble vitamins have precursor forms that must be converted to the active vitamin before they can be used by the body. Daily consumption of the water-soluble vitamins is recommended because most are not stored to any great extent. Since they are in the water portion of foods, these vitamins can easily be lost due to improper food processing, storage, and preparation procedures.

None of the vitamins provides energy; they only help to release energy from the three fuel nutrients—carbohydrates, fats, and proteins. As such, they act as coenzymes for biological reactions but are not part of body tissues.

Some compounds have vitaminlike activity but are not classified as vitamins because they can be made by the body. Others have no vitaminlike activity but are often promoted as "vitamins" and as cures for numerous illnesses and diseases.

Issue

Nutrients as Drugs: Megavitamin Therapy

The first herbalists were never quite sure whether, after eating a plant, they would feel euphoria or nausea—or drop dead. Trial and error was the only way they could learn the medicinal value of plants. By choosing those leaves, fruits, flowers, seeds, and fungi with beneficial properties, these foragers laid the foundation for modern medicines. They knew that drugs and food were closely related. Only recently have modern researchers begun to rediscover just how intimate this relationship is.(3)

Nutrients can be considered drugs when they are used for treating nonnutrition-related diseases. For instance, vitamin C is sometimes used to acidify the urine of persons with bladder infections.(4) Recently, promoters of nutrient pills and tonics have linked massive doses of vitamins with the prevention and treatment of practically every known disease. This treatment is called *megavitamin therapy*.

Megavitamin proponents argue that vitamins are not drugs because they are natural to the body, but that they must be balanced properly for optimal health. Drugs are foreign to the body and used to attack a specific agent; they often cause harm to the body. They further insist that humans today have increased nutrient needs because of supermarket diets and the added stresses of pollution, drugs, worry, illness, alcohol, and overwork. Thus, they claim that people need massive vitamin doses as preventive medicine or vitamin insurance.

Scientists opposed to megavitamin therapy see a different situation. Vitamins in amounts required by the body's physiological processes are called physiological doses. These levels can be obtained from a varied diet that does not rely heavily on refined foods. When taken in amounts that greatly exceed these levels, the dosage is pharmacological and the vitamins become drugs. At such levels the vitamin's activity may be greatly altered. For instance, water-soluble vitamins act as coenzymes, hooking up with enzymes to promote reactions in the body. Excess vitamins do not improve the reactions because there is only a limited amount of the various enzymes with which to combine. In rare cases megadoses may be useful if there is a defect in the enzyme machinery and flooding of the system is required.

Opponents of the megavitamin concept further argue that vitamins are not isolated in nature, but are found along with other nutrients in food, so ingesting large amounts in pills may lead to problems. In large doses certain vitamins are toxic; some may interact harmfully with other substances. Since nutrients are needed in proper proportions, taking large doses of one may throw off the balance of others. Excessive amounts of some vitamins may mask deficiencies of others. And if a person takes large doses for a long period of time, he or she may become dependent on the large doses. Every pharmacist knows that in a given amount a medication is effective, but in increasing amounts toxic effects are likely to occur.(5) So the heart of the controversy is this: What is the most effective dose for vitamins? Megavitamin supporters say people should aim for optimal (some even say "super") health; opponents challenge them to define optimal health before trying to medicate for it.

More is at stake in the megavitamin controversy than just a person's right to self-medicate. What are the claimed benefits of large doses? And what are the potential side effects? Let's take a closer look.

MEGADOSES: RISKS AND BENEFITS

Fat-Soluble Vitamins

Misuse of the fat-soluble vitamins poses a great health risk because excessive amounts are stored in the liver, muscle, kidneys, and fat tissues of the body. Vitamins A and D can accumulate in the body and become toxic. Vitamins E and K, although fat-soluble, to date have not been known to cause toxic symptoms. However, a synthetic substance with vitamin K activity can cause vomiting if taken orally and may be harmful to infants if large doses are injected.

Vitamin A. Some symptoms of a vitamin A deficiency, such as abnormal drying and cracking of the skin that allow for development of infected areas, resemble acne. As a result, vitamin A has been touted as a cure for acne and oral doses are often prescribed for its treatment. The problem with this is that the doses prescribed are often very high and to make matters worse the overzealous patient may decide to double or triple the dose. In situations like this where toxic levels are easily reached, treatment of acne with oral doses of vitamin A is definitely not recommended except under continuous supervision by a physician. Researchers are studying the use of vitamin A analogs or retinoids for acne and they appear to hold great promise for certain types of acne. These retinoids are forms of the vitamin which perform many of its functions but are less toxic in high doses. However, they too should be used only under careful medical supervision.

The topical application of one form of vitamin A (retinoic acid) is proving effective in treatment of some types of acne.(6) This topical treatment to the skin does not carry the risk of toxicity found with high oral doses of vitamin A, but skin irritations are often a side effect.

Another claim for vitamin A is that it can prevent cancer. Rats deprived of vitamin A have a higher rate of colon cancer than rats with adequate amounts. Several epidemiological studies have shown that the risk of lung cancer is lower when intake of vitamin A is high.(7,8) Some scientists say vitamin A may prevent cancer by bolstering the body's defenses in the early stages of disease; others think it protects against certain chemicals like those found in cigarette smoke. Since large doses of vitamin A are toxic, researchers are looking at the less toxic retinoids for cancer treatment. The retinoids can be targeted in large doses to specific organs that may develop cancer. Although these retinoids are not totally safe, they have been effective in preventing certain cancers in experimental animals and certainly offer some possibilities for use with humans.(9)

A variety of other claims surround vitamin A, none supported by data: it is said to improve vision for those working under artificial light; calm hyperactive children; cure warts, dry and wrinkled skin, stress ulcers, respiratory infections, and eye disorders (other than those caused by vitamin A deficiency); delay heart disease; and retard aging.

Large doses of vitamin A over long periods of time can lead to symptoms like those of a deficiency. A person taking at least 25,000 IU for 30 days or longer shows fatigue, lethargy, brittle nails, sparse hair, dry and scaly skin, abdominal pain, liver damage, and calcium loss from the bones. People may experience pressure on the brain that mimics a brain tumor (severe headaches, nausea, vomiting). One teenager was hospitalized and prepared for brain surgery for what turned out to be a vitamin A overdose.(10) Figure 7–4 shows the symptoms of too little and too much vitamin A.

It is so easy to obtain vitamin A in large doses without prescription that vitamin A toxicity is on the rise. Researchers have reported several cases of acute toxicity in infants due to single, massive doses. Chronic vitamin A toxicity in adults occurs most often in people taking large doses to treat skin problems, and those who continue high intakes without medical supervision. Consumption of large amounts of carotene, the precursor of vitamin A, will not bring serious side effects, although the skin may take on a jaundicelike orange tinge until consumption is reduced.

FIG. 7–4

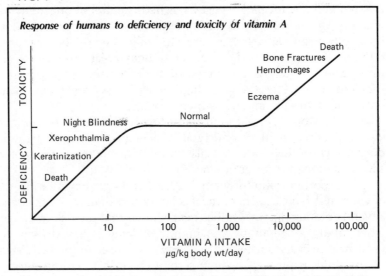

Response of humans to deficiency and toxicity of vitamin A

Source: Adapted from J.C. Bauerfeind, *The Safe Use of Vitamin A, A Report of the International Vitamin A Consultative Group* (Washington, D.C.: The Nutrition Foundation, 1980), p. 7.

Vitamin D. Megavitamin enthusiasts have spared vitamin D many of the outlandish claims given to the other vitamins. Even so, it is claimed to lower blood cholesterol, prevent or cure osteoporosis in the elderly, and strengthen bones. The dosage required for these feats is 3,000 to 4,000 IU, a level that can lead to serious problems. Tolerance for high doses of vitamin D varies with individuals, so it is difficult to set a minimal dose above which toxicity occurs. Most cases of vitamin D toxicity in children occur with doses of from 25,000 to 60,000 IU per day for one to four months.(11) Vitamin D megadoses can cause excess calcium in the blood, weakness, lethargy, loss of appetite, and constipation.

Vitamin E. If all the claims for vitamin E were true, Ponce de Leon would have had better luck finding the elixir of youth inside a jar of wheat germ or safflower oil. Vitamin E proponents base most of their claims on deficiency signs seen in animals. Laboratory animals deprived of the vitamin show reproductive, muscular, and circulatory problems.

When the early findings on vitamin E deficiency in laboratory animals were reported, researchers hoped they could use the vitamin for curing human disorders with similar symptoms. Unfortunately, careful studies that attempted to relate vitamin E deficiency in animals to human symptoms have failed to find such a link. The vitamin E deficiency induced in experimental animals over a long period of time simply does not occur in humans eating ordinary food, and ethics prevent human studies from proceeding to the point where deficiencies are so profound. But despite the lack of data, many supporters of vitamin E are still using the findings of animal studies to justify their claims. The claims for vitamin E are so extensive that it is best to break them down by categories: reproduction, heart disease, muscular disorders, aging, pollution, cosmetic uses, and others.

1. *Reproduction.* Researchers interested in the effects of vitamin E on reproduction have collected data for over 35 years. They have found some beneficial effects, but the weight of the evidence shows that vitamin E is not very effective in this area. Most nutritionists agree there is no value in using vitamin E to prevent male impotence or sterility or to alter the outcome of pregnancy.

2. *Heart disease.* The first announcement that vitamin E could combat heart disease appeared in *Time* magazine on June 10, 1946.(12) Based on clinical trials and personal experiences with patients, two Canadian physicians proclaimed that large doses of vitamin E could cure rheumatic fever, eliminate hypertension, and stop anginal pain from heart disease. In 1947 the Shute brothers reported on 84 patients they had treated with vitamin E. According to these researchers, all the patients had symptoms of angina pectoris, and the majority had a positive response to the treatment. Other researchers have not been able to duplicate these results.(13) By 1950, 13 studies, involving 32 researchers and more than 450 patients, had been published in medical journals. None of the researchers found any value in using vitamin E with heart disease patients. The results of a more recent study are shown in Table 7–1.

3. *Muscular disorders.* Vitamin E deficient animals suffer from a muscle-wasting disease that can be cured once they receive the vitamin. Human muscular dystrophy causes similar symptoms, but the muscles of humans with dystrophy show no deficiency of vitamin E. Giving the vitamin does not prevent or cure the disorder.

4. *Aging.* Dr. Al Tappel of the University of California at Davis believes vitamin E may retard aging. According to Tappel, cells age because they are damaged by cosmic rays breaking the bonds of polyunsaturated fats in their membranes. The total damage to the cells, concludes Tappel, is what causes you to age and vitamin E may offer some protection against this damage.(14) This theory certainly deserves more investigation but it is highly unlikely that vitamin E will stop or even significantly slow the aging process.

TABLE 7–1 **Effect of Vitamin E on Angina Symptoms**

Effect	Subjects Given 3200 mg/day	Subjects Given Placebo
Much Improved	1	0
Improved	4	3
Slightly improved	0	2
No change	13	12
Slightly worse	0	1
Total	18	18

Source: T.W. Anderson and D.B.W. Reid, "A double-blind trial of vitamin E in angina pectoris," *American Journal of Clinical Nutrition* 27 (1974): 1174–1178.

5. *Pollution.* Some rat experiments show that vitamin E might protect lung tissue from the harmful effects of smog. Laboratory rats fed different amounts of vitamin E and then exposed to artificial smog showed more damage at low vitamin E levels than at higher levels. Tappel is also involved in this research, and in one of his experiments rats were exposed to ozone, an air pollutant from automobiles.(15) The amount of ozone in the air the rats inhaled was comparable to the worst possible smog conditions in Los Angeles. After one week, 10 percent of the rats receiving no vitamin E died, whereas none of the rats fed an amount of vitamin E equivalent to human RDA levels died. The implications of these findings for humans must await further investigation.

6. *Cosmetic claims.* Vitamin E is reported to heal skin blemishes, soften dry skin, erase wrinkles, and give new life to aging skin. Despite advertising claims, however, vitamin E does nothing to toilet soaps or skin care cosmetics but increase the price. At one time vitamin E was a popular ingredient in deodorants. The theory was that its antioxidant properties would prevent bacteria from using oxygen to break down underarm secretion into the substances that cause body odor. Not only was this theory wrong, but one popular vitamin E deodorant was recalled in 1973 because it caused severe rashes.(10)

7. *Other claims.* One claim for vitamin E that does have some basis is as a treatment for fibrocystic breast disease, a condition in which women experience sore breasts due to noncancerous tumors. The grabbag of claims for vitamin E that have no supporting evidence includes promoting it as a cure for ulcers, warts, mental retardation, diabetes, and cancer, and as bringing relief from burns and menstrual cramps.

Vitamin E is the least toxic of the fat-soluble vitamins, but researchers have not yet assessed the risks from taking large doses (100 to 800 IU) over several years. They have reported isolated cases of fatigue, dermatitis, diarrhea, hemorrhage, and muscle damage with very high intakes, and some persons taking 800 IU daily have complained of flu-like symptoms.(16,17) Excess vitamin E may interfere with function of the other fat-soluble vitamins. There are no reports of toxic effects from the use of vitamin E for short periods (two to three months). Most people have an adequate intake of vitamin E. The only persons who may require supplementation are premature infants and those with a fat malabsorption problem. The benefits and risks of megadoses remain a grey area.

Water-Soluble Vitamins

"Our sewers run with the richest urine in the world," goes a popular nutrition joke. It is true that massive amounts of the water-soluble vitamins pass out of the body in the urine. This makes them less likely to be toxic, although it does not guarantee there will be no harmful side effects from megadoses.

Niacin.　One of the symptoms of the niacin deficiency disease pellagra is mental confusion. Observing this, researchers got the idea of using massive amounts of niacin as a cure for schizophrenia. The use of niacin megadoses and vitamins C, B-6, and E to treat mental disorders is called *orthomolecular psychiatry.*

Since megadoses are given to mental patients along with conventional treatment, it is hard to assess the effectiveness of the vitamin supplements alone. In 1973, however, the American Psychiatric Association Task Force on Vitamin Therapy in Psychiatry convened a group of experts who reviewed the accounts of megavitamin "cures" and found that they were not supported by sound research findings; most, in fact, were uncontrolled observations.

Niacin is also claimed to lower serum lipid levels, thereby reducing the risk of heart disease. This, of course, does not prove that the atherosclerotic plaques causing heart disease can be reduced with megadoses of niacin. Niacin supplements do not reduce deaths from heart disease. Ironically, some persons taking high doses show heart abnormalities, gastrointestinal problems, and abnormal blood tests.[18] Other symptoms include an initial flushing and itching of the skin, later worsening into severe skin problems, liver damage, elevated blood glucose, and peptic ulcers.[13]

Other claims for niacin that are not supported by research are its ability to promote recovery in alcoholism, improve circulation, and reduce stiffness in old age.

Thiamin.   Thiamin is claimed to stimulate mental responsiveness and cure skin disorders, multiple sclerosis, infections, cancer, and impotence, and relieve symptoms of alcoholism. No data exist for any of these claims except for the relief of symptoms of alcoholism when the symptoms are caused by a thiamin deficiency.

Pantothenic Acid.   A severe deficiency of pantothenic acid in black rats causes their hair to turn gray. When the vitamin is given, the natural color of the hair returns. Despite the claims, humans with graying hair will not benefit by taking massive pantothenic acid supplements. Among the other unproved claims for pantothenic acid are its ability to speed up wound healing and cure liver cirrhosis, Addison's disease, and cancer, as well as to combat cancer-producing agents.

Other B Vitamins.   Claims made for megadoses of other B vitamins are that riboflavin reduces susceptibility to infections; that folacin increases resistance to pain; and that vitamin B-12 hastens recovery from mental depression and alcoholism, prevents kidney stones, and controls nausea in pregnant women. No evidence exists to support any of these claims.

Vitamin C.   About a decade ago, Linus Pauling, twice a Nobel laureate (though not in nutrition), published a book called *Vitamin C and the Common Cold* in which he asserted that large doses of vitamin C reduced the incidence of the common cold. He claimed that regular ingestion of 1000 milligrams (1 gram) of vitamin C daily produced a 45 percent reduction in the incidence of colds and a 60 percent reduction in total respiratory illness. Nutritionists have conducted a great deal of research since then to see if Pauling was right. Thousands of subjects and numerous studies later, they still do not have the answer. Trying to

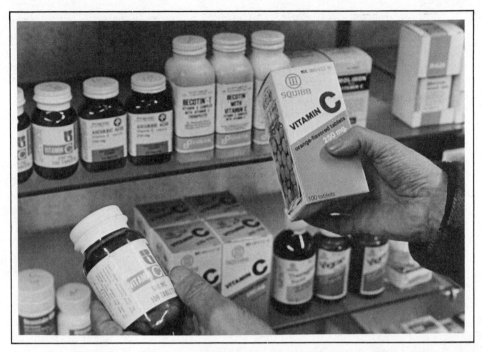

People who use supplements should be careful to note the dosage they are buying because certain vitamins and minerals are toxic in large amounts. Others, such as vitamin C, can give the same positive effects at lower dosages as at higher ones.

measure the beneficial effects of vitamin C on the natural course of a cold is difficult because colds are usually self-limited, of short duration, and caused by different strains of viruses, so that large numbers of subjects must be studied to observe a meaningful effect. Also, many of the studies showing beneficial effects are uncontrolled, and the conclusions are based on subjective and clinical impressions. In some studies vitamin C was given with other active agents, making it impossible to evaluate any effect of the vitamin alone.

A few researchers have conducted well-controlled double-blind studies using large numbers of subjects. Anderson and co-workers conducted three of these studies in Toronto. During the winter of 1971–72,(19) they tested the claim that taking 1 gram of vitamin C per day (increased to 4 grams at the onset of symptoms) reduces the frequency and duration of the cold. Of 818 adult subjects, 411 were on a placebo and 407 were on 1 gram of vitamin C. Subjects could not tell the difference between the placebo and the vitamin C tablet. Table 7–2 summarizes the findings. The researchers found no difference in the total number of colds or "winter illness" among the vitamin C group. The length of time confined to the house, however, was reduced by 30 percent, and significantly more subjects in the vitamin C group remained free of illness of any

TABLE 7–2 First Toronto Double-Blind Study, Vitamin C and Colds

Summary of Findings	Vitamin C	Placebo	Statistical Significance of Difference
Total number of colds	561	609	Not significant
Number of days symptoms were present	5.25	6.02	Not significant
Average number of days confined to the house	1.30	1.87	Significant
Number of subjects free from illness during the study	105(26%)	76(18%)	Significant

Source: T.W. Anderson, G. Suranyi, and G.H. Beaton, "The effect on winter illness of large doses of vitamin C," Canadian Medical Journal III (1974): 31–36.

kind. These differences were much less dramatic than Pauling's claims. Yet the fact that subjects in the vitamin C group were confined to the house for a shorter time shows they experienced less severe symptoms.

Anderson's group conducted a second study(20) between December 1972 and February 1973 on 2349 adult volunteers to assess the effect of different levels of vitamin C on winter illness in adults. They concluded that 250 milligrams daily was as effective as 2 grams of vitamin C per day. In the winter of 1973–74, the same researchers wanted to see what even lower doses of vitamin C would do.(21) This time the vitamin C group was given 500 milligrams of the vitamin once a week, with the dosage increased to 1500 milligrams on the first day of illness; then 1000 milligrams per day for the next four days of the illness. Again the vitamin C group had the same number of colds but experienced milder symptoms. The lower levels of vitamin C used in this study (500 milligrams per week) were as effective as the higher daily levels used in the previous study. Anderson explained that although the vitamin cannot kill the cold virus, it may act like an antihistamine helping the person cope with the infection. Other studies show similar results: Subjects taking vitamin C experience as many episodes of illness as those taking the placebo, but the severity of the illness in the vitamin C groups is reduced. In regard to the usefulness of taking massive doses of vitamin C, smaller doses (500 milligrams per week or about 75 milligrams per day) are as effective as massive ones.

Many other claims are made for vitamin C. One to six grams are recommended for treating a hangover, viral diseases, bacterial infections, cancer, vertebral disc lesions, fractures and burns, wounds, and heart disease; and for increasing mental alertness and achieving the "normal concentration" of vitamin C in the blood of cigarette smokers. Pauling suggests a minimum of 200 to 400 milligrams vitamin C per day in order to maintain "optimal health." Proof is still lacking for these claims.

Some researchers feel excess vitamin C will simply be excreted; others believe high doses may build up unnatural reserves with unforeseeable results. General risks do exist, though specific side effects will depend on an individual's tolerance level. Rebound scurvy occurs in some persons who have taken large doses of vitamin C over a long period of time and who then discontinue the megadoses "cold turkey." What happens is that the body's machinery for breaking down vitamin C is accelerated with large doses. If the person does not taper off slowly, the body continues to break down the vitamin at a fast rate, resulting in a temporary case of scurvy (swollen, bleeding gums and loosened teeth). There is little hazard to adults, but such effects are potentially dangerous to the newborn. Vitamin C megadoses may interfere with certain drugs. Diabetics taking large doses may receive inaccurate readings on blood sugar tests, and persons suspected of intestinal bleeding will show false negatives on tests for blood in their stools. Large doses of vitamin C may also cause gastrointestinal upset and diarrhea. They may also increase the risk of kidney stones. At one point research findings indicated that vitamin C megadoses could cause a B-12 deficiency, but recent evidence does not support this idea.(22)

Until the claims made for vitamin C can be proved, it is not wise to consume large amounts. If you insist upon taking high doses to ward off colds, try reducing your intake to about 75 milligrams per day (500 milligrams per week). If you are pregnant, you should avoid unnecessary drugs of any type, including megadoses of vitamin C. The amount prescribed in prenatal supplements is ample, but not excessive, in meeting the needs of pregnant women.

Megadoses: Where Do We Stand Now?

Does all this mean you should just write off using megadoses? Not necessarily. Knowledge of the body's biochemical machinery and enzyme systems is still limited. As scientists learn more, they may find new ways to use vitamins to promote health. In the future doctors may use vitamins to treat a variety of disorders, but it is not likely that they will be the answer to all problems.

VITAMIN AND MINERAL SUPPLEMENTS

A 4-year-old in Kansas once took an entire bottle of children's vitamins all at once. Instead of becoming the superkid on the block, he spent the following two days in intensive care with iron poisoning.(10)

Vitamins and minerals do not bear out the commonly held belief that if some is good, more is better. If you are going to buy a multivitamin-mineral supplement, your best choice would be one that contains nutrients in amounts close to RDA levels. Table 7–3 shows a good balance of vitamins and minerals as recommended by a special FDA panel. The minerals fall short of the RDA because researchers are uncertain how well they are absorbed in both supple-

TABLE 7–3 Panel Recommendations on Vitamin and Mineral Dosages to Prevent and/or Treat Deficiencies

Vitamins	Minerals
Vitamin C (ascorbic acid) 50–100 mg/day prevention 300–500 mg/day treatment **Niacin (niacinamide or niacinamide ascorbate)** 10–20 mg/day prevention 25–50 mg/day treatment **Vitamin B-6 (pyridoxine)** 1.5–2.5 mg/day prevention 7.5–25 mg/day treatment **Vitamin B-2 (riboflavin)** 1–2 mg/day prevention 5–25 mg/day treatment **Vitamin B-1 (thiamin)** 1–2 mg/day prevention 5–25 mg/day treatment **Vitamin A** 1,250–2,500 IU/day prevention 5,000–10,000 IU/day treatment **Vitamin B-12** 3–10 micrograms/day prevention Not to be used to treat deficiency **Folic acid** 0.1–1.4 mg/day prevention 1.0 mg/day for pregnant and lactating women Not to be used to treat deficiency **Vitamin D** 400 IU/day prevention, infants and growing children under 18 years of age 200 IU/day prevention, adults Not to be used to treat deficiency	**Calcium** For prevention only Adults, children 1–10, and 12 and over—400–800 mg/day Children 10–12, and pregnant and lactating women—600–1,200 mg/day Adults over 51—500–1,000 mg/day Infants 6 months to under 1 year—300–600 mg/day Infants under 6 months—200–400 mg/day **Iron** For prevention only Menstruating and lactating women—10–30 mg/day Pregnant women—30–60 mg/day Children 6 months to under 5 years—10–15 mg/day In combination products other than for use in pregnancy: adults and children over 5—10–20 mg/day **Zinc** For prevention only Adults, and children 1 year and over—10–25 mg/day Pregnant and lactating women—25 mg/day

Source: Annabel Hecht, "Vitamins over the counter: take only when needed," *FDA Consumer* 13 (1979): 17–19.

ments and foods and because tablets would be hard to swallow if larger amounts were given.

Natural versus Synthetic Vitamins

Many people believe natural vitamins are better than synthetic and that the natural ones contain no synthetic ingredients. Both beliefs are wrong. First, manufacturers can make all the vitamins. When the molecular structure of the synthetic vitamin is the same as the natural, the body cannot tell the difference between the two. Most laboratory-made vitamins do have structures identical to those of the natural ones, although some formulations of vitamins E and K may differ slightly from the natural items.

Second, natural vitamins are not always natural. In processing tablets and capsules, vitamin manufacturers must hold the tablet together with such substances as ethyl cellulose, Polysorbate 80 and gum acadia.(10) A recent investigation also found that some of the products advertised as "natural" actually had synthetic vitamins added to the natural sources. Try to take a vitamin C tablet made from only rose hips and you will find yourself trying to swallow a horse pill. There is one difference between natural and synthetic vitamins: the natural ones cost about twice as much.

Who Should Take Supplements?

You are not going to compensate for a poor diet by taking vitamin and mineral supplements. Many nutrients in food are not included in supplements. Certain groups in the population, however, are at higher risk of deficiencies than others, and for them a supplement is generally recommended. They include:

- Women during pregnancy and lactation
- Infants from birth until they can eat a variety of table foods (commercial formulas have the entire array of vitamins added, so no further supplement is needed)
- Individuals on weight reduction diets of less than 1000 kcalories per day
- Persons with certain malabsorption diseases
- Strict vegetarians who eat no animal products
- Those convalescing from surgery or illness
- Women during the reproductive years who have an unusually heavy menstrual flow and who may need iron supplements
- Some of the elderly who may have poor diets due to loneliness, ill-fitting dentures, poor absorption, and budgetary problems

The elderly do not need special types of vitamins. Claims for such preparations are as false and misleading as claims of "high" or "super" potency.

Issue: Oral Contraceptive Agents (OCA)

OCA (also known as birth control pills or the Pill) are combinations of the synthetic forms of two sex hormones, estrogen and progesterone. Because these drugs are hormones, they influence many of the body's biochemical processes, including the metabolism of nutrients. The degree to which OCA affect nutritional status depends on previous hormonal balance, diet, and age as well as the composition of the drug and the length of time taken. Changes in nutrient needs during OCA use mimic those of pregnancy.

Protein metabolism is slightly changed in OCA users, but since Americans consume ample amounts of protein, there should be little cause for concern unless meals are skipped. Women taking OCA may have higher blood sugar levels than nonusers. This problem worsens with age, with excess kcalorie intake, and with weight gain. For this reason there is particular concern about the use of these drugs by diabetics or women with a family history of diabetes. Lipids and cholesterol tend to be higher in the blood of OCA users than nonusers. These elevated levels do not necessarily increase the risk of heart disease, although there may be greater change of this with prolonged OCA use. Women are generally less susceptible to heart disease than men.

The requirements for some vitamins and minerals are affected by OCA. Some evidence indicates that folacin absorption is decreased. This could increase the risk of developing a type of anemia caused by low folacin levels in the body. Under the influence of the OCA, the rate of tryptophan conversion to niacin is increased. Since this process uses vitamin B-6 as a coenzyme, the requirements for this vitamin may be increased. With discontinuation of the OCA, B-6 status returns to normal. Since vitamins B-6 and riboflavin are interrelated, the increased need for one may increase the need for the other.

Menstrual blood losses are smaller in OCA users, so their need for iron often is not as high as among non-OCA users. Copper, a component of an enzyme necessary for iron metabolism, is increased in the blood of many OCA users, but whether this has any adverse consequences is yet to be determined. In contrast, vitamin C blood levels are reduced, so women using OCA may have increased needs for this vitamin. Vitamin A levels are reduced in the liver but raised in the blood. Since liver stores are better indicators of vitamin A status, it is possible that, over time, a vitamin A deficiency may result. Reports of effects on vitamin E run from an increase, through no change, to a decrease in blood levels. The effect seems to depend on nutritional status.

Recommendations for OCA Users. Due to the changes in blood lipids, it is important for women on OCA to have their serum triglycerides and cholesterol checked at least once a year. If blood levels rise, it may be wise to discontinue use.

There is a disagreement among nutritionists as to whether vitamin B-6 and folacin supplements are needed by OCA users. Many believe that the lower blood levels of OCA users do not necessarily indicate a true deficiency. Even so, the diets of these women should provide rich sources of these vitamins. OCA users should be careful to avoid excess kcalories and should reduce if overweight. Sugar, fat, and alcohol intakes should be moderated. Suggested low-fat sources of protein include legumes, fish, poultry, eggs (in moderation), and skim milk. Polyunsaturated oils should be used when frying foods, but fried foods should generally be avoided. Since OCA use does influence nutrient status, women who plan to become pregnant are advised to discontinue use for a few months prior to conception. This will allow time to replenish the stores of those nutrients that may have been diminished due to the OCA use.

REFERENCES

1. F.E. Andrews and J. Driscoll, "Stability of Ascorbic Acid in Orange Juice Exposed to Light and Air During Storage," *Journal of the American Dietetics Association* 71(1977):140–42.

2. J.W. Erdman, "Effect of Preparation and Service Food on Nutrient Value," *Food Technology* (1979):31–48.

3. C.E. Butterworth, "Interactions of Nutrients with Oral Contraceptives and Other Drugs," *Journal of the American Dietetic Association* 62(1973):510–14.

4. "Diet-Drug Interactions," *Dairy Council Digest*, March–April 1977, pp. 7–12.

5. G.B. Forbes, "Food Fads: Safe Feeding of Children," *Pediatrics in Review* 1(1980):207–10.

6. P.M. Elias and M.L. Williams, "Retinoids, Cancer, and the Skin," *Archives of Dermatology* 117 (1981):160–80.

7. E. Bjelke, "Dietary Vitamin A and Human Lung Cancer," *International Journal of Cancer* 15(1975):561–65.

8. C. Mettlin, S. Graham, and M. Swanson, "Vitamin A and Lung Cancer," *Journal National Cancer Institute* 62(1979):1435–1438.

9. M. Sporn and D. Newton, "Chemoprevention of Cancer With Retinoids," *Federation Proceedings* 38 (1979):2528–2534.

10. "Myth of Vitamins," *FDA Consumer*, February 1978.

11. J.C. Bauerfeind, *The Safe Use of Vitamin A. A Report of the International Vitamin A Consultative Group* (Washington, D.C.: The Nutrition Foundation) 1980, p. 37.

12. R.E. Hodges, "Vitamin E: Uses and Misuses," In *Selections from Nutrition and the M.D.*, G. McKee, ed. (Van Nuys, CA.: PM, Inc., 1978), pp. 7–8.

13. V. Herbert, "Facts and Fictions about Megavitamin Therapy," *Journal of the Florida Medical Association,* April 1979, pp. 475–81.

14. A.L. Tappel, "Where Old Age Begins," *Nutrition Today*, December 1967, pp. 2–7.

15. B.L. Fletcher and A.L. Tappel, "Protective Effects of Dietary α-tocopherol in Rats Exposed to Toxic Levels of Ozone and Nitrogen Dioxide," *Environmental Research* 6(1973):166–75.

16. P.M. Farrell, "Excessive Vitamin E Consumption," *Nutrition and the M.D.*, April 1977, pp. 1–2.

17. J.G. Bieri, "Vitamin E in Human Nutrition." In *Selections from Nutrition and the M.D.*, G. McKee, ed. (Van Nuys, CA.: PM, Inc., 1978), pp. 16–18.

18. R.B. Alfin-Slater, "Vitamin Supplementation: An Appraisal of Values—and Dangers," *Professional Nutritionist*, winter 1980, pp. 8–11.

19. T.W. Anderson, D.B.W. Reid, and G.H. Beaton, "Vitamin C and the Common Cold: A Double-Blind Trial," *Canadian Medical Association Journal* 111 (1974):31–36.

20. T.W. Anderson, G. Suranyi, and G.H. Beaton, "The Effect on Winter Illness of Large Doses of Vitamin C," *Canadian Medical Association Journal* 111 (1974):31–36.

21. T.W. Anderson, G.H. Beaton, P.N. Corey, L. Spero, and B. Pharm, "Winter Illness and Vitamin C: The Effect of Relatively Low Doses," *Canadian Medical Association Journal* 112(1975):823.

22. S. Ekvall, I-Wen Chen, and R. Bozian, "The Effect of Supplemental Ascorbic Acid on Serum Vitamin B-12 Levels in Myelomeningocele Patients," *American Journal of Clinical Nutrition* 34(1981):1356–1361.

Minerals and Water Balance

8

In nutrition, the term *minerals* refers to elements such as iron that cannot be broken down into simpler compounds. They are inorganic (no carbon) substances present in rock or soil rather than originating from living matter. The carbon, hydrogen, oxygen, and nitrogen of the other nutrients account for about 96 percent of the body's weight. The remaining 4 percent, about 5 pounds of total weight, is minerals.

Like vitamins, minerals are micronutrients because the body needs them only in small amounts. Within the category of minerals, however, the elements are divided into two groups:

- Minerals present in the body in relatively large amounts (greater than 5 grams or 1 teaspoon) that are required at levels of 100 milligrams daily or more. (The 100 milligrams is still very small compared to the requirements for carbohydrates, fats, and proteins.)

- Minerals present in the body in relatively small amounts comprising less than 0.005 percent of body weight and required in trace amounts. For this reason they are called *trace minerals.*

Of the 60 known minerals, about 17 are essential to humans and another 4 may prove to be essential (Table 8–1). Minerals are released from food during digestion, absorbed intact through the walls of the small intestine into the blood, and carried to the tissues. Of increasing importance to researchers is the concept of *bioavailability.* As regards minerals, this is the amount of an element that the body can absorb and use; it is influenced by the chemical form of the element and the other nutrients consumed at the same time. For instance, vitamin C helps in the absorption of iron. Not only do minerals interact with other nutrients, they interact with each other: calcium and phosphorus work together

TABLE 8–1 **Minerals Essential to Human Nutrition**

Minerals Present in the Body in Relatively Large Amounts	Trace Minerals	Uncertain Status
Calcium	Iron	Cobalt
Phosphorus	Zinc	Silicon
Potassium	Selenium	Vanadium
Sulfur	Manganese	Nickel
Sodium	Copper	Tin
Chlorine	Iodine	Arsenic
Magnesium	Molybdenum	Cadmium
	Chromium	
	Fluorine	

in forming bones and teeth; iron, copper, and cobalt are important in hemoglobin synthesis and red blood cell formation; sodium, potassium, calcium, phosphorus, and chlorine act to keep body fluids properly distributed among the circulatory system, the cells of tissues, and the spaces between the cells. The level of minerals in the body is dependent on the amount absorbed, the amount excreted or lost in perspiration, and the function of the mineral. The body contains a lot of calcium, for example, because of the role calcium plays in the structure of bones and teeth.

Although the body needs minerals in small amounts, the current American diet may not be supplying enough of certain minerals to meet the RDA, especially those of women and the elderly. Particular minerals in question are calcium, magnesium, zinc, copper, and chromium.

MINERALS PRESENT IN RELATIVELY LARGE AMOUNTS

As a group, these minerals share some general functions. They act as cofactors in biological reactions, a role they share with vitamins. They also help maintain the acid-base balance of the body. Some of these minerals (chlorine, phosphorus, and sulfur) are acid forming and are present mainly in protein-rich foods like poultry, fish, meat, and cereals. Others (potassium, sodium, calcium, and magnesium) form alkali or base and occur more in fruits and vegetables. You may think of citrus fruits as acid, but actually the ash they form after they are oxidized in the body is alkaline, not acid. A mixed diet contains equal amounts of acid and alkaline minerals that work together to keep the body's acid-base balance at an optimal level.

Certain minerals (especially sodium and potassium) occur in large amounts in body fluids and serve to maintain water balance. These two, along with other minerals (calcium, sodium, potassium, and magnesium) are needed for nerve impulse transmission and muscle contraction. Unlike vitamins, minerals can become part of biological compounds and body tissues, like the calcium and phosphorus in bones and teeth. The list below summarizes the general functions of the minerals present in relatively large amounts in the body:

- Regulate biological reactions
- Maintain the acid-base balance of the body
- Maintain the water balance of the body
- Assist in nerve impulse transmission
- Regulate muscle contraction
- Serve as constituents of body tissues

Calcium

Calcium is present in the body in larger amounts than any other mineral; it accounts for about 2 to 3 pounds of body weight. About 99 percent of body calcium is in bones and teeth, where it is part of the hard crystals that give strength and resilience to these structures. Since it is involved in bone formation, calcium is needed for normal growth.

Functions. Bone acts as a reservoir for calcium. If the levels in the tissues or blood fall, the body draws calcium from the bones to restore these levels. If there is too much calcium in the blood, less is drawn from the bones and absorbed from the intestines. Calcium turnover in hard tissues varies; teeth give up their calcium much less rapidly than bone. The amount of calcium in the blood, then, is determined not so much by diet as it is by the hormones that cause calcium to be pulled from or deposited in the bones.

It is crucial that the calcium in tissues and blood be kept at a constant level because it is needed to maintain the cement substances holding cells together, to transmit nerve impulses, to regulate muscle contractions (including heartbeat), and to control the flow of many substances into and out of cells. Without it, the brain could not trigger nerves to send impulses and the cells would not be as able to regulate what enters them. Calcium is a cofactor in blood-clotting reactions as well as in other biological activities, such as the absorption of vitamin B-12.

Although an individual may consume enough calcium in the diet, many factors can enhance or impede its absorption. The amount absorbed varies with the individual and with the stage of life. Here are the factors that increase calcium absorption:

- *Adequate vitamin D in the body.* Vitamin D is necessary for adequate calcium absorption across cell membranes of the intestinal tract.
- *Acid conditions in the digestive tract.* Acid conditions make calcium more soluble. Some elderly people secrete less hydrochloric acid in the stomach, which leads to less acidic conditions. Such individuals may have trouble absorbing sufficient calcium.

- *Presence of the milk sugar lactose in the digestive tract.* Lactose and calcium form a soluble compound that is better absorbed than either alone. Since milk contains both lactose and calcium, it is an excellent source of the mineral.

- *Lack of stress.* Emotional upheavals can lower the efficiency of calcium absorption.

- *Ingestion in small amounts throughout the day.* Calcium is more efficiently absorbed if small intakes are consumed throughout the day rather than a large amount being consumed all at once.

- *Physiological need for calcium.* Persons with greater needs, such as adolescents and pregnant women, are more efficient at absorbing calcium. Infants and children absorb up to 60 percent of ingested calcium; pregnant women about 50 percent; other adults about 30 percent; and those with deficiencies close to 60 percent.

Despite all the factors that increase calcium absorption, there are just as many that decrease it:

- *Oxalic acid.* This substance, found in rhubarb, spinach, chard, and beet greens, forms a complex with calcium that makes it insoluble and difficult to absorb.

- *Phytic acid.* Present in the outer husks of cereal grains, phytic acid can also form an insoluble complex with calcium.

- *Rapid movement through the intestines.* The liberal use of laxatives and diets high in bulk speed foods through the intestines, resulting in reduced calcium absorption.

- *High-fat diet.* Fats can form insoluble complexes with calcium, which is then excreted in the feces.

- *Lack of exercise.* The body requires some type of physical exercise or mechanical stress to maintain a healthy balance between the calcium absorbed and that lost from the body. Both calcium and phosphorus losses from bone are triggered by bed rest or immobilization. Astronauts experiencing zero gravity show a loss of bone mass, though the how and why of this are unknown.

Other nutrients, including protein, phosphorus, and fluorine affect the body's use of calcium. Research during the last ten years indicates that high protein intakes lead to high levels of calcium being excreted in the urine. High levels of dietary protein may cause calcium to be withdrawn from the bone, though it is not clear why this occurs. When phosphorus intake increases along with protein, the increase in calcium excretion is not as great as when protein alone increases.(1)

Requirements. In experimental animals, diets high in phosphorus depress calcium absorption. There is disagreement as to whether phosphorus has the same effect on human calcium absorption but many experts feel that absorption is best when the ratio of dietary calcium to phosphorus is one. Others think that the calcium to phosphorus ratio has little effect if calcium intake is optimal. Americans consume higher quantities of phosphorus than calcium because phosphorus is much more abundant, being present in large amounts in processed meats and cheeses and soft drinks. Meat, poultry, and fish have 15 to 20 times more phosphorus than calcium; organ meats have 25 to 50 times more.

The RDA for calcium for adult men and women is 800 milligrams daily. Adolescents and pregnant and lactating women have a higher allowance of 1200 milligrams. The extra amount for pregnant women is to protect the mother's bones, since they will give up their calcium to the fetus if the mother's diet does not provide enough of the mineral. Children, because of their rapid growth, need more calcium per unit of weight than adults. The level of calcium in the body often changes with age. More calcium is withdrawn from the bone and excreted in women, particularly white women, after menopause. Less is absorbed from the diet by both sexes after age 60.

Abnormalities. Calcium deficiency only becomes apparent once bone reserves are severely depleted, and this can take months to years on a poor diet. Two bone abnormalities related to calcium metabolism are osteoporosis and osteomalacia.

Osteoporosis affects 14 million Americans, mostly women between 40 to 60 years of age. Affected persons show a loss in total amount of bone. The remaining bone is of normal composition, but it is weaker and fractures easily. The condition is probably due to many factors including imbalances in hormone secretions; anything that interferes with or decreases calcium absorption; and long-term calcium deficiency, with inadequate intakes of vitamin D. High intakes of protein or phosphorus throughout life may also play a part, as may reduced physical activity. One of the first symptoms of osteoporosis may be certain forms of periodontal disease. Periodontal disease affects the supporting structures of teeth, making them loose. At this stage, the condition may be reversible with a change in diet. Once significant amounts of bone are lost, it is difficult, if not impossible, to reverse the situation.

Persons with osteomalacia have demineralization of bone, that is, the loss of calcium and phosphorus crystals, so that the remaining bone is of abnormal composition. Both conditions weaken the body's structural support. Rickets is usually defined as a vitamin D deficiency disease, but low intakes of calcium and phosphorus or an imbalance in their ratio can also cause this disease. Abnormal hormonal secretions can cause transient changes in blood calcium levels. Low blood levels result in muscle spasms, while high levels cause abnormal muscle contractions. But although hormones control blood levels of calcium, over a long period of time the levels of calcium in the body are a function of diet.

Sources. Unless you are a very picky eater, your diet will likely provide enough calcium. Milk and dairy products are the richest sources. There is little in butter or margarine because calcium is not fat-soluble. Other sources include baked goods containing added dried milk solids, broccoli, okra, dried beans and peas, dark green leafy vegetables (collard greens, mustard, Swiss chard, bok choy, and kale), shellfish, eggs, canned sardines, and salmon (both with bones). Certain greens (spinach, chard, sorrel, parsley, beet greens), rhubarb, and cocoa contain oxalic acid, which binds calcium so that its bioavailability in these foods is not as high as in dairy products. Grains and legumes contain phytic acid, which can also hinder absorption. Strict vegetarians should use calcium-enriched soybean milk to ensure an adequate intake.

Phosphorus

Next to calcium, the mineral present in the body in largest amounts is phosphorus. About 85 percent of the body's phosphorus is in bones and teeth. Phosphorus is needed in order for the body to lay down calcium in these tissues and so is important for growth. It is also part of all body cells and probably has more functions than any other mineral.

Functions.   Phosphorus is needed for energy to be released from the fuel nutrients. This mineral helps transfer energy from food to cells for use in body processes. Many enzymes and B vitamins are active only with a phosphate group (phosphorus, with oxygen attached). Phosphorus assists in the absorption and transport of many nutrients; it helps maintain the body's acid-base balance by its buffering action in the blood; and it is part of the structure of cell membranes and many body compounds, like the nucleic acids DNA and RNA.

Requirements and Sources.   Except for infants, the RDA for phosphorus are the same as those for calcium. Phosphorus is so widespread in foods that deficiencies are rare. Individuals who consume large amounts of antacids containing aluminum hydroxide may become deficient, since these interfere with phosphorus absorption. Symptoms include severe muscle weakness, loss of appetite, pain in bones, and loss of minerals from the bones.

Rich food sources of phosphorus are also rich protein sources, such as milk, dairy products, meat, fish, poultry, and eggs. Whole grain cereals, nuts, and legumes are also good sources. The storage form of phosphorus in seeds is phytic acid, the substance that binds many minerals and hinders their absorption. Phytic acid is broken down by yeast, so leavened bread will not contain as much as nonleavened breads. Usually if the diet is adequate in protein, it is also adequate in phosphorus.

In the United States, people generally need to be more concerned about getting enough calcium than enough phosphorus. Soft drinks are often overlooked as sources of phosphorus, but frequent consumption can disrupt the body's calcium-phosphorus balance. Phosphorus is also high in processed foods and rich sources, like meat, are all commonly consumed foods.

Magnesium

Most of the body's magnesium is in bones, with much of the remainder in muscle. Magnesium, is essential for providing body cells with a readily available supply of chemical energy. Cardiac and skeletal muscles and nerves depend on a proper balance of calcium and magnesium to function. Magnesium is essential for relaxation of muscles after they have contracted. Some evidence shows that the function of insulin and other hormones may be involved with binding or releasing magnesium within the cells. The amount of magnesium the body absorbs is influenced by the total intake of magnesium, fiber, calcium, phosphorus, and lactose.

Requirements and Sources. The RDA for magnesium is 350 milligrams daily for men, 300 milligrams for women, with an additional 150 milligrams for pregnant and lactating women. Deficiencies are unlikely except for those who suffer recurrent vomiting or diarrhea, alcoholics, postsurgical patients, those using diuretics, and those suffering from protein malnutrition. Symptoms include convulsions and extreme muscle contractions. Good food sources of magnesium include nuts; legumes; cereals (especially oats and wheat germ); dark green vegetables; seafoods; chocolate and cocoa; poultry; sunflower, caraway, and pumpkin seeds; and whole grains.

Sodium

Sodium is one of the two minerals that make up sodium chloride or table salt. The level and distribution of body fluids depend on sodium and potassium ions. Ions are charged forms of minerals that occur when they are placed in water. Proper distribution of fluid depends on the cells' ability to keep sodium on the outside of the membranes and potassium on the inside. Nerve impulses are transmitted when there is a temporary exchange of these sodium and potassium ions.

It is important that blood levels of sodium be within a certain range. If they increase, the thirst center is activated and the person drinks to equalize the sodium-to-water ratio. If the blood level of sodium drops—as a result of vomiting, diarrhea, sweating, or blood loss—both water and sodium must be replaced. If only the water is replaced, fluid migrates into the cells and causes water intoxication. Symptoms include muscle weakness, apathy, nausea, and loss of appetite.

Requirements and Sources. There is no RDA for sodium, but an estimated safe and adequate intake ranges from 1.1 to 3.3 grams daily for adults. Intakes vary greatly. Asians, with their liberal use of soy sauce and monosodium glutamate (MSG), consume about 30 to 40 grams of salt (12 to 16 grams of sodium) per day, while daily consumption in the United States is closer to 6 to 18 grams. Deficiencies of sodium are rare. Sodium enters body fluids freely, with the kidneys filtering any excess from the blood into the urine. The kidneys conserve salt during a deficiency and return it to the blood. A person cannot gain permanent weight by eating salt and drinking water, because both will eventually be excreted.

Too much sodium likely leads to high blood pressure in some people. With excess sodium, there is an increase in blood volume that puts pressure on the arteries. The heart has to work harder to pump blood. Persons with certain conditions such as high blood pressure and kidney, liver, and heart disease are usually advised to limit salt intake.

Animal products are higher in sodium than foods from plants. Diets high in grains may be low in both sodium and chloride. Processed foods such as cured ham, bacon, pickles, potato chips, canned vegetables, and cold cuts contain large amounts of the mineral, as do table salt, soy sauce, and MSG. Some water supplies have high sodium contents. It is not necessary to salt food, since many foods naturally contain sodium. People who are used to heavily salted foods can, with time, adjust to the taste of foods that have only minimal salt added. For those, especially athletes, who have lost water and salt through sweat, replacement of sodium losses can be met by increasing the amount of salt added to meals.

Chloride

Chloride is the other half of table salt. Depending on the dose and form, it can be poisonous when taken alone; combined with sodium, it is an essential mineral. Chloride is part of the hydrochloric acid that is necessary for maintaining acid conditions in the stomach. Chloride helps maintain the body's acid-base balance. A sudden loss of chloride from the stomach, such as in vomiting, disrupts this balance. There are no RDA for chloride, but the estimated safe and adequate daily intake for adults ranges from 1.7 to 5.1 grams. The most common food sources are animal products and table salt.

Potassium

Potassium is the main positive ion inside cells, where it helps maintain water balance and thus healthy functioning. Nerve and muscle cells are rich in potassium because it is the sodium and potassium ions that exchange places during nerve transmission and muscle contraction. This includes keeping the heart beating regularly. Diets low in potassium, such as the liquid protein diet, can cause heart abnormalities. Potassium also plays a role in protein and carbohydrate metabolism.

Requirements and Sources.   There is no RDA for potassium, but the estimated safe and adequate daily intake for adults ranges from 1.9 to 5.6 grams. Deficiencies usually occur when large volumes of water are lost through prolonged diarrhea, use of diuretics, or heavy sweating every day. Because of potassium's role in muscle contractions, deficiencies cause muscle weakness and eventually paralysis. Potassium is dangerous when taken in large amounts, as in the potassium chloride or potassium salt supplements sold in health food stores. Excessively high intakes can raise blood levels, a potentially fatal condition.(2) Supplements should be taken only when prescribed by a doctor. To replace losses from heavy sweating, a better choice would be rich sources such as orange juice, bananas, tomatoes, carrots, citrus juices, dried fruits, and potatoes.

Sulfur

Sulfur is present in all tissues, but all its functions are not yet known. Certain amino acids contain sulfur in their side chains, which link together to form bridges between the chains as they fold over themselves or one another. This gives proteins their shape and, for some like hair, skin, and nails, their rigidity. Sulfur is also part of the vitamins thiamin and biotin. There is no RDA for sulfur and no recognized deficiency. Intake is adequate if protein intake is adequate.

TRACE MINERALS

The body needs trace minerals in such tiny amounts that it is hard to believe researchers discovered they were essential. To many nutritionists, trace mineral research is the next frontier. Scientists need to determine the amounts necessary for health and decide whether certain minerals, always thought to be poisonous to humans, are actually essential in tiny amounts. Researchers have identified nine trace minerals that are necessary for humans and have placed seven more on the uncertain list. There is evidence that these latter seven are required by several animal species, but human requirement has not been proven. These trace minerals are as follows:

NECESSARY	UNCERTAIN STATUS
iron	silicon
zinc	vanadium
selenium	nickel
manganese	tin
copper	cobalt
iodine	arsenic
molybdenum	cadmium
chromium	
fluorine	

Like those minerals present in relatively large amounts in the body, trace minerals act as cofactors in body reactions, are required for growth of tissue, and become part of body compounds. For instance, iodine and zinc are part of the hormones thyroxin and insulin, respectively, while iron is crucial to the hemoglobin molecule.

With a few exceptions, deficiencies of trace minerals result from inadequate intake or poor absorption over a long period of time. Nutritionists in the United States are concerned, however, that the trend toward greater use of processed and refined foods could be decreasing overall intake of trace minerals. Taking multivitamin supplements is not the solution. Minerals do not function in isolation, so it is important to consume them in proper proportion to one another. High intakes of one will disturb the balance of the others, and often manufacturers market supplements that contain large amounts of the cheaper minerals and small amounts of the more expensive ones, with little regard to their interactions.

Trace minerals can be toxic. Many of them, necessary for health in small quantities, are health hazards when ingested in large amounts. Often a trace mineral is acquired from the environment, not the diet. Miners who breathe air high in selenium and manganese experience toxicity symptoms. Apart from such occupational hazards, the general public is exposed to substantial amounts and combinations of minerals through sources such as air, water, and paint. Some of these, like lead, are extremely dangerous.

The amount of the trace minerals in food depends on the mineral content of the soil where the food was grown. Since minerals *leach* into water, the mineral content of water also reflects soil levels. Today Americans are at less risk of mineral deficiencies from poor soil than in the past because interstate commerce has shuffled the food supply. People in Michigan eat oranges from Florida; apples from Washington are found in produce sections of Arizona supermarkets; and grains from the wheat belt are sold as baked goods on the East Coast.

Iron

Iron is present in every cell, though it makes up only 0.004 percent of weight. Most of it is in the blood as part of hemoglobin in red blood cells, but muscle tissues and enzymes also contain a sizable proportion.

Functions.   The body has over 25 trillion red blood cells, each living for about 120 days. As these cells die, the body takes the iron in their hemoglobin and incorporates it into the new red blood cells being made in the bone marrow. As part of hemoglobin, iron carries and releases oxygen to the cells. It is also a part of myoglobin, a compound similar to hemoglobin but located mainly in the muscle, where it aids in providing oxygen during sustained muscle contraction. Iron plays a role in collagen synthesis, production of antibodies, removal of fats from the blood, conversion of carotene to vitamin A, detoxification of drugs in the liver, and conversion of the fuel nutrients to energy.

In general, humans absorb only about 10 percent of the iron they ingest. Many factors affect ability to absorb iron. Factors that enhance absorption include these:

- *The chemical form of the iron.* The iron in mixed diets is either in the heme or the non-heme chemical form. Heme is a very complex, large compound containing one atom of iron. Iron exists in this form in hemoglobin and myoglobin so it is found mainly in meat, fish, and poultry. The non-heme form of iron has a much simpler chemical structure. It is the major form of iron in foods of plant origin but is also found in animal-origin foods. Heme iron is much more readily absorbed (about 23 percent on the average) than is non-heme iron (3 percent to 8 percent on the average). In addition, iron can exist in either the oxidized or reduced state. It is more easily absorbed in the reduced state.

- *A physiological need for iron.* During periods of life such as growth or pregnancy, when there is a greater need for iron, the body is more efficient at absorbing the nutrient.

- *Acid stomach conditions.* The hydrochloric acid secreted into the stomach makes iron more soluble and so more easily absorbed. *(Presence of vitamin C in the intestines)* Vitamin C keeps iron in the reduced form that is better absorbed. For this reason, iron supplements often include vitamin C.

- *High altitude.* Because there is less oxygen in the air at high altitudes, the blood must have higher levels of hemoglobin to deliver enough oxygen to the cells. This increases the need for iron and thus its absorption.

Factors that lessen absorption are these:

- *A diet high in fiber.* Fiber moves food through the intestines quickly, reducing absorption time.

- *Phytic acid present in cereals and grains.* Phytic acid binds with iron and forms a large complex that is poorly absorbed.

- *Animal tissue intake.* The addition of animal tissue (meat, fish, or poultry) to the diet increases non-heme iron absorption by twofold to fourfold. Eggs, milk, and cheese, however, do not have this effect.(3)

The body tightly controls absorption of iron because, once absorbed, little is excreted. Iron losses occur with cell loss (about 1 milligram per day), so varying amounts are found in hair, nails, sloughed-off cells from skin and the intestinal tract, menstrual fluid, and other blood losses such as from chronically bleeding hemorrhoids, peptic ulcers, nosebleeds, and blood donation. Once absorbed, iron moves in one of three directions: It becomes a part of cells, it is incorporated into hemoglobin, or it is stored in the liver, bone marrow, spleen, and muscles.

The RDA for iron for men and older women are 10 milligrams daily. For women of childbearing age who must replace menstrual losses and for the teenage male who has the demands of growth, the RDA are 18 milligrams per day. A 30 to 60 milligram iron supplement is recommended for pregnant women. Actual iron needs by body cells are much less than this, but the RDA must allow for the fact that only a small percentage of dietary iron is absorbed— 3 to 23 percent—depending on whether it is the none-heme or heme form and other dietary factors.

Deficiency and Excess.   Although the body conserves as much iron as possible, low intakes will lead to *iron-deficiency anemia*, one of several nutritional anemias. Anemia means that the red blood cells are few in number or are of poor quality. When the anemia is caused by lack of iron in the diet, the red blood cells are small, light in color, contain little hemoglobin, and can carry much less oxygen than normal red blood cells. Low iron levels can result from slow blood loss or from dramatic loss, as in hemorrhage. In these cases red blood cells will look normal, but there will be too few to meet the body's oxygen needs.

One indication of whether a person is getting enough iron can be obtained by measuring hemoglobin. Normal hemoglobin values for men are 14 to 15 grams hemoglobin per 100 milliliters of blood; for women, 13 to 14 grams hemoglobin per 100 milliliters of blood. Values below this can indicate a problem. The tissues of an anemic individual must function with less oxygen and so have less energy. Thus, fatigue is one of the first symptoms, followed by decreased work performance and increased risk of infection.

Iron-deficiency anemia is one of the few nutrient deficiencies that affects a large number of Americans especially during four periods of life: (1) during infancy, when iron stores are exhausted at 6 months of age and the baby is fed only milk, a poor iron source; (2) during the rapid growth of childhood and adolescence, when blood volume and iron stores are expanding; (3) during the female reproductive period to replace menstrual losses; and (4) during pregnancy to meet the needs of the expanding blood volume and tissues of the mother and the needs of the fetus, as well as to cover blood losses in childbirth. Infants born to iron-deficient mothers are at greater risk of becoming anemic during the first months of life. There are several ways to obtain iron if you are in one of the high-risk groups for anemia. Physicians of ancient times would dip a sword in water and have patients drink the liquid to absorb the strength of the sword's iron.(4) Today it is easier to just plan the diet to include iron-rich food sources. For many women in childbearing years, a supplement may be desirable.

Even though the body strictly controls how much iron it absorbs, excesses have occurred in humans. Researchers first noticed this among the African Bantu tribe, whose members consume large amounts of beer fermented in iron kettles. The iron leaches into the beer, giving it a high iron content. In the United States, excessive intakes have occurred from unrestricted use of therapeutic iron supplements or from large intakes of cheap wines, which are known to be high in iron. This is the kind and amount of wine usually consumed by the chronic alcoholic. Chewable multiple vitamin tablets containing iron are dangerous for preschoolers, who eat them like candy, because iron is absorbed faster when the tablets are chewed rather than swallowed. Too much iron in the body allows harmful organisms to multiply, increasing the chances of infection.

Sources. Good dietary sources of iron include liver and other organ meats, red meat, blackstrap molasses, whole grain or enriched and fortified breads and cereals, cocoa, oysters, clams, and dried beans. Some fruits and vegetables, such as the dark green ones, are high in fiber, which reduces iron absorption. Drying concentrates the iron in fruits, so a cup of raisins contains more iron than a cup of fresh grapes. The iron content of vegetables reflects soil conditions. The iron in eggs is poorly absorbed and may interfere with iron absorption from other foods. The iron in meat, fish, and poultry is better absorbed than that in plants. You can increase iron absorption from plant foods by including small amounts of meat in a meal. You can also eat a vitamin C source with meals to help iron absorption. Cooking in unenameled iron pots adds iron to food because the mineral leaches from the pot into the food, particularly if the food is acid (simmering spaghetti sauces, for instance).

Iodine

About 70 to 80 percent of the body's iodine is in the thyroid gland. There it is used to synthesize thyroid hormones that regulate growth and development in children and controls basal metabolic rate or the rate at which the body uses energy for fuel.

Requirements and Deficiencies. The RDA for iodine are 100 to 140 micrograms per day, and in large amounts it is toxic. If there is an iodine deficiency, the thyroid gland enlarges to capture what little iodine is available in the blood. This enlargement, called goiter, appears as a swelling in the neck. Simple goiter is painless, though unsightly. Those with the condition may become sluggish and gain weight. With increased swelling, the goiter blocks normal breathing. Children born to mothers with low iodine intakes during adolescence and pregnancy may suffer from cretinism—these children show dwarfism and mental retardation.

Most iodine deficiencies occur in areas where the soil lacks iodine. In the United States, soils rich in iodine are coastal or located in southern states; the Plains States are poor, and foods grown in such areas have little iodine. Goiter is rare in this country because of interstate commerce and the use of iodized salt and other sources of the mineral.

Currently there is more concern about the United States diet having too much rather than too little of the mineral because of inadvertent iodine sources such as dough conditioners used in commercial breadmaking and substances used as teat dips for milk cows which pass into milk.(4)

Rich food sources of iodine include seafoods such as lobsters, shrimp, oysters, and salt-water fish, and iodized salt. Sea salt contains some trace minerals, but iodine is lost during the drying process. The amount in meat, poultry, eggs, dairy products, and cereals depends on the soil content as well as any iodine-containing substances which inadvertently enter the products. Some foods, mainly those of the cabbage family (rutabagas, turnips, cabbages), contain substances called goitrogens which prevent the body from using iodine.

Zinc

Zinc is present in every tissue, but the highest concentrations are in the eyes, the male reproductive organs, the liver, muscle, and bone. It is a cofactor for many enzymes essential for such processes as the release of carbon dioxide from tissues to lungs, where it is exhaled, and for the synthesis of protein and collagen, the cellular cement substances. It is part of insulin and is important for growth, wound healing, and tissue repair.

Requirements and Deficiencies. The RDA for zinc are 10 milligrams for children 1 to 10 years old. It increases to 15 milligrams for everyone over 11 years. Usually if people eat enough protein, they get enough zinc.

Researchers first identified zinc deficiency in Egyptian adolescent males who suffered from retarded growth and poor sexual development. These young men were eating diets high in cereals containing phytic acid and fiber, which bind zinc. Many ate clay, a practice called *pica* and common in groups with mineral deficiencies. Intestinal parasites and high temperatures that caused sweating increased the zinc losses from their bodies. Other signs of zinc deficiency are abnormal hair and nails, deformed bones, poor healing, and loss of taste.

There is growing concern that the American diet may be deficient in zinc. In 1972 Denver scientists discovered several children from middle- and upper-class families whose sense of taste was poor. Later this was attributed to zinc deficiency. Individuals most at risk are children and teenagers undergoing rapid growth, pregnant women, especially pregnant teenagers, and the nursing infant. Others such as alcoholics, those with liver cirrhosis, protein malnutrition, and chronic infections, or those suffering severe trauma, may be susceptible. Certain genetic disorders can also cause lower levels of zinc in the body.

Sources. The richest food sources of zinc are herring, oysters, clams, poultry, oatmeal, corn, whole grain cereals, meats, liver, milk, fish, eggs, nuts, legumes, and peanut butter. Zinc in grains is not as well absorbed as that from meat because the phytic acid, oxalic acid, and fiber that grains contain reduce the bioavailability of the mineral. Vegetarians who eat mainly grains may have difficulty absorbing sufficient zinc.

Copper

Copper is a part of the enzymes necessary to stimulate iron absorption. It is also involved in iron storage, release, and incorporation into the hemoglobin of red blood cells. It is a component of compounds required for energy release and helps form collagen and maintain the sheath around nerves.

There is no RDA for copper, but estimated safe and adequate intakes should range from 2 to 3 milligrams per day for adults. Deficiencies in humans are rare except in the malnourished or those with certain genetic disorders. Recently another group has been recognized as being at risk: premature infants born with low copper reserves who are fed only cow's milk for the first two to three months of life.

Most unprocessed foods contain copper. The richest sources include oysters, nuts, liver, kidney, corn oil margarine, legumes, shellfish, chocolate, and cocoa. The amount in water depends on the metal piping and water hardness.

Fluoride

The highest concentrations of fluoride are in bone and the enamel of teeth. An essential role for fluoride has not been established, but where fluoride is lacking in the water supply, dental decay is high. Dental caries or cavities are decreased by 50 to 70 percent with water fluoridation, topical applications, or toothpastes, since fluoride makes tooth enamel more resistant to decay.

People living in areas like parts of Colorado and the Texas Panhandle, where fluoride is naturally high in drinking water, show tooth mottling (that is, brown discoloration of the teeth). With prolonged consumption of high levels, skeletal deformities can develop. Fluoride toxicity is rare and usually caused by an accidental overdose. Artificially fluoridated water does not pose a danger of toxicity because levels are kept within a narrow range.

The main sources of fluoride in the diet are drinking water and foods and beverages prepared from fluoridated water, such as tea.

Other Trace Minerals

Chromium works with insulin to help the cells take up glucose and break it down for energy. It also protects against the toxic effects of lead. There is some concern that the American diet may be low in chromium. A deficiency produces a condition similar to diabetes. Good sources include brewer's yeast and whole grain cereals.

Molybdenum is part of many essential enzymes. No deficiency has been identified in humans, so the requirement for the mineral is probably low enough that it can be met by a normal diet. A greater problem than deficiency is toxicity. High concentrations in a province of the Soviet Union caused adverse effects on the inhabitants. A safe and adequate range of intake is established to be 0.15 to 0.5 milligrams per day. Good food sources include meat, grains, and legumes.

Manganese is a component or cofactor of many enzymes and plays a role in brain function. It helps maintain normal tendon and bone structures. A deficiency in humans is unknown, so the amount required has not been determined. Toxic symptoms have been seen only in workers exposed to high concentrations of manganese dust in the air, and not from any dietary excess. A safe and adequate intake is in the range of 2.5 to 5 milligrams daily. Manganese is abundant in many foods, especially bran, coffee, tea, nuts, peas, and beans.

Selenium is part of enzymes and its action is similar to that of an anti-oxidant. In many cases this anti-oxidant action "spares" vitamin E. In the liver it protects against cirrhosis. It also counteracts the toxic effects of heavy metals such as cadmium and mercury. There are no RDA for selenium, but an intake of 50 to 200 micrograms a day is considered safe and adequate. Selenium is usually present in protein foods, such as seafoods, kidney, liver, and other meats. There is little in fruits and vegetables. Few toxicity cases have been seen in humans, but this may change now that selenium is being added to vitamin-mineral supplements.

Trace Minerals of Uncertain Status

A number of trace minerals are essential for other animal species but have not been proved to be essential for humans. No human requirement or range of intake has been established for them, and some are known only to be toxic.

Cobalt is supplied to the body as part of vitamin B-12. There is no known deficiency or requirement for this mineral except as part of B-12, which is needed to form red blood cells.

Silicon is the most prevalent element on earth next to oxygen. It used to be considered a contaminant, since silicon dust inhalation caused a respiratory disorder called silicosis. Silicon has since been shown to be a component of collagen, and it may play a role in the formation of bone, cartilage, and connective tissue by providing strength and resilience. *Vanadium* may play some role in maintaining healthy bones and teeth, though its specific function is unknown. *Nickel* and *tin* have no known functions, but future research may show them to be essential for humans. Research may also reveal some essential function for *arsenic* and *cadmium* but presently there is more concern about their toxic effects. Cadmium interferes with the functioning of iron, copper, and calcium. Environmental exposure causes anemia, kidney damage, and loss of bone material.

Two other trace minerals exist which to date have not been shown essential for humans but are well known for their toxic effects. These are *lead* and *mercury*. Lead is present in food, air, water, and as a base in some paints. The main victims of lead poisoning are children from 1 to 6 years of age who eat paint flakes in old buildings. Mercury poisoning is an increasing concern as industrial pollution of waters becomes more widespread. Fish consume the mineral as methylmercury and pass it on to humans. The worst incidence of mercury poisoning occurred in Minamata, Japan, in the 1960s and resulted in a number of cases of nerve disease and death.

It is not necessary to eliminate fish from the diet to avoid mercury. The FDA has set a concentration level above which the fish cannot be sold. At present, the American diet contains foods with mercury levels much lower than

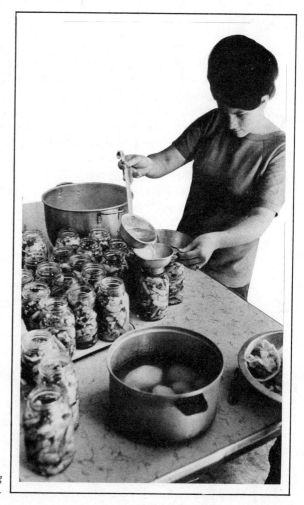

Proper methods of preserving food help to conserve nutrients.

the guideline. And researchers have not only found no change in mercury concentration in the oceans in recent years, but the mercury content of today's fish is the same as that of fish in the nineteenth century. *Selenium*, a mineral that accumulates along with mercury, is protective and helps negate mercury toxicity.

SUMMARY

Minerals are inorganic substances needed by the body in small amounts. They function either as part of tissues and biochemical compounds or as regulators of body functions. Mineral deficiencies usually result from malabsorption problems. The amount of these nutrients in food is a function of the soil where the plant was grown or the animal raised, so that poor soil may result in low intake.

Humans can survive without food for 30 days, but they will die in 5 to 6 days without water. Ironically, if asked to name the different nutrients, most people would forget to even mention water. Most of the human body is composed of water. It accounts for about 50 to 70 percent of body weight, and makes up 70 percent of muscle, 30 percent of fatty tissue, and 10 percent of bone. In general, water is present in larger amounts in active tissues like muscle than in metabolically sluggish tissue like fat. Total body water is higher in muscular than obese adults, since the obese have a higher ratio of fat to muscle. With age, muscle mass decreases because of reduced exercise and hormonal changes and is accompanied by a decrease in body water.

Animal life evolved in a watery environment that provided living organisms with all the necessities for survival. Once these organisms crawled out of the primeval sea, they had to adapt to new and hostile surroundings. To survive on land they were forced to carry the salty, watery environment of their tissues within their own structures. Within the body, the water pools into different compartments. Most stays in the cells and is called intracellular fluid. All the remaining water is outside, or extracellular, and is divided into three groups: (1) the intercellular fluid filling the spaces surrounding the cells; (2) the intravascular fluid flowing through the blood vessels, arteries, veins, and capillaries; and (3) the transcellular fluids present in special tissues (Figure 8–1).

Electrolyte Balance

Water moves freely across membranes; increases or decreases in the level of one compartment affect the levels in other compartments. Body water is in fact a solution filled with minerals which, when placed in water, break up into charged particles called ions or electrolytes. The positively charged ions (+) are sodium, potassium, calcium, and magnesium; the negatively charged ones (−) are chloride, bicarbonate, phosphate, and sulfate. These particles are distributed within different water compartments in a certain way (Table 8–2). The positive and negative charges must be carefully regulated for cells to function. When the body loses ions, it loses not only the mineral itself, but also the charge.

Potassium, phosphate, calcium, and magnesium are present mainly in the fluid within the cells (intracellular fluid). The major ions in the fluid bathing the cells are sodium and chloride. This fluid is ideal for exchanges of nutrients and wastes between the cell and its surrounding environment. The cell sits like a bather in an inner tube bouncing around the body's own internal ocean.

Two other ions are important in body fluids. These are hydrogen ions (H+) and hydroxyl ions (OH−). Positive mineral ions match up with the OH−; negative mineral ions with the H+. By having the proper concentration of positive and negative ions, the body can maintain its acid-base balance. Tissues

FIG. 8-1

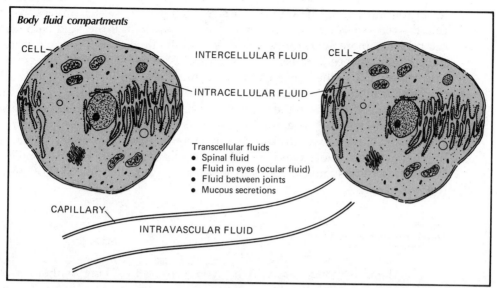

Body fluid compartments

CELL

INTERCELLULAR FLUID

CELL

INTRACELLULAR FLUID

Transcellular fluids
- Spinal fluid
- Fluid in eyes (ocular fluid)
- Fluid between joints
- Mucous secretions

CAPILLARY

INTRAVASCULAR FLUID

have more acid or base depending on the best environment for their enzymes. Buffers can pick up extra positive or negative charges to keep a solution neutral.

To control the amount of water and to keep the distribution of ions constant, ions must constantly be pumped across membranes. If the proper distribution of ions is not maintained on the inside and outside of the cell membrane, the cell dies. Ions attract water and drag it along when they move from one compartment to another. If ions increase in concentration on one side of the membrane, water flows in that direction, diluting the ion solution so that proper concentration is maintained and balance restored.

TABLE 8-2 Primary Salts Present in Body Fluids*

Large Amounts	Moderate Amounts	Small Amounts
Extracellular Fluid		
Sodium	Bicarbonate	Phosphate
Chloride	Oxygen	Sulfur
	Glucose	Potassium
	Fatty acids	Calcium
	Carbon dioxide	Magnesium
	Other wastes	
Intracellular Fluid		
Potassium	Magnesium	Sodium
Phosphate	Sulfur	Chloride
	Protein	
	Calcium	

*Salts are minerals with a neutral charge; once they dissolve in fluids they become positively or negatively charged and are called ions.

The cell must also keep a certain amount of pressure between itself and its surrounding fluid. If sodium, passively followed by water, moves into the cell, the cell swells unless it can pump out the sodium. If the fluid bathing the cell becomes more concentrated in ions than the fluid within the cell, water is pulled from the cell, causing it to shrink. Not only must the pressure be maintained across the cell membrane, it must also be maintained across the capillary membrane. Protein molecules in the blood vessels are too large to move across the membrane into the intercellular spaces. These molecules are charged and act like ions. By remaining in the blood vessels, they help maintain the pressure on either side of the capillary membrane. With a protein deficiency, the number of protein molecules in the blood vessels drops, so much of the pressure is lost. Water leaks into the area surrounding the cells, and puffiness of the skin (edema) results.

Functions in the Body

There is good reason why you cannot live long without water, considering the vital functions it performs in the body. These important functions are listed below.

- Give cells shape
- Provide a neutral medium for chemical processes
- Participate in chemical processes
- Transport nutrients to cells and wastes from cells
- Regulate body temperature
- Distribute heat evenly throughout the body
- Lubricate joints
- Protect eyes and spinal cord

Water is a structural component of cells, giving them shape. As part of body fluids, it provides a neutral medium for all chemical processes and often participates in the reactions. For instance, when a sugar containing two glucose molecules splits apart, water is also split. Water, by dissolving amino acids, glucose, minerals, and other substances, can transport them to the cells and remove cellular waste products. Water holds heat and so can regulate body temperature and distribute heat evenly throughout the body. Enzymes work best at a temperature of 98.6° F. Wide fluctuations in body temperature threaten their ability to function and can lead to death. For water to evaporate from the skin, it must vaporize. When this occurs, energy is lost in the form of heat. Thus, through evaporation of water, the body rids itself of excess heat. As a component of mucus, water acts as a lubricant. Because they are hard to compress, water molecules are ideal for protecting joints. Fluid also protects the eyes and the spinal cord.

Trace minerals, dissolved in water, are easily absorbed. The amounts in a given volume of water are affected by the source of the water, water treatment practices, and type of piping. Some minerals, such as calcium and magnesium, are responsible for water hardness. To soften it, these are exchanged for sodium. Public health officials often add two other minerals to water: chlorine to stop growth of algae and harmful bacteria, and fluoride to help prevent dental caries.

Requirements

The body is able to keep its water level within a fairly strict range. It does this by juggling intake and output. Humans need about 2.5 liters (about 2.4 quarts) a day, or 1 milliliter of water for every kcalorie. Body water comes from the diet and from internal metabolic processes. The most obvious sources are beverages: water, tea, milk, and juice. Next is solid food. Fruits and vegetables can be high in water, whereas nuts and grains tend to be low; fats and oils do not contain water. The third source is the metabolic water derived from the breakdown of foods during biological oxidation:

$$\text{Glucose} + \text{oxygen} \longrightarrow \text{water} + \text{carbon dioxide} + \text{energy}$$

(For a discussion of the effects of caffeine-containing beverages, see Issue: Caffeine Consumption.)

Much of the body's water is recycled, but about 3 pints are lost daily through urine, feces, and perspiration. Larger amounts, depending on type of physical activity, temperature, humidity, and wind velocity, can be lost through sweating. Smaller amounts, called insensible losses, are lost through the lungs and skin. These losses are determined by metabolic rate. Water intake and output are shown in Table 8–3. Abnormally large losses of water occur with diarrhea, vomiting, and faulty kidney function.

TABLE 8–3 Water Intake and Output

Daily Intake Averages 2000–2500 milliliters (ml)	Daily Output Averages 2000–2500 milliliters (ml)
Sources of Intake	*Sources of Output*
Fluids (water, beverages, soup): 500 ml to several liters averages 1000 ml	Urine: 400 ml to several liters averages 1000 ml
Water in solid foods: 600 to 1200 ml	Feces: 80 to 200 ml
Metabolic water: 300 to 400 ml	Water vapor from lungs: 300 to 600 ml
	Sweat: 0 to several liters averages 200 ml
	Insensible loss: 300 to 500 ml daily

Source: Adapted from G.M. Briggs and D.H. Calloway, *Bogert's Nutrition and Physical Fitness* (Philadelphia: W.B. Saunders, 1979), p. 240.

Excessive Loss

With large water loss, there is a large sodium loss. This triggers the thirst center in the brain, which tells the person to drink. The kidneys control the excretion of water and ions by conserving these nutrients when body levels fall and excreting excesses when body levels rise too high. Since sodium is crucial to water and ion balance, the kidney can conserve almost all of it during periods of depletion by reabsorbing the ion instead of excreting it in the urine and sweat. The kidneys can excrete large amounts of sodium, but they use up much water in the process. This is why humans cannot survive by drinking salt water. The salt water is so concentrated that it forces the kidney to use more water to flush out the excess salt than the body gets from ingesting the water. The result is dehydration.

When the balance of water and salts is disrupted, sickness results. *Heat stroke* is usually caused by high temperatures, high humidity, poor body ventilation, and several hours of water deprivation before intense physical activity. It is an extremely dangerous condition and can cause high body temperature (106–110° F), coma, and even death. Early symptoms include absence of sweat and urine and convulsions. *Stokers' disease* is named after coal stokers who worked in steamship boiler rooms and sweated profusely. They would routinely drink water to replace the fluids but not compensate for the salt losses. Cells would take in the water and expand because there was too little salt to maintain balance. With small water and salt losses, sodium can be replaced by a more liberal salting of food. Salt tablets should be taken with careful supervision if at least 4 quarts (8 pounds) of water have been lost.

When water is limited, a person should restrict intake of protein and salt and moderate kcalorie intake. When salt is scarce, a person should avoid sweating and excessive physical exercise. Over time, however, the body has the capacity to adapt to amazingly low salt intakes. And certain people have higher water needs than others. This includes individuals who have suffered prolonged vomiting or diarrhea, those taking diuretics or consuming high-protein diets, and those living in hot climates.

Excessive intakes of water can cause water intoxication. This condition is rare and affects mostly patients with malfunctioning kidneys. Symptoms include headaches, nausea, poor coordination, and high blood pressure.

SUMMARY

A proper distribution of water within the body is important because water performs essential functions, including being a component of body fluids, a medium for chemical reactions, a substrate for chemical reactions, and a regulator of body temperature. Minerals (as ions) serve many functions within the fluid compartments of the body. The distribution of water and ions within each of the body's compartments must be held within a certain range. Sources of water include food, beverages, and outputs from the combustion of food within the body (metabolic water). Loss of excessive water and ions disrupts balance with adverse effects on health.

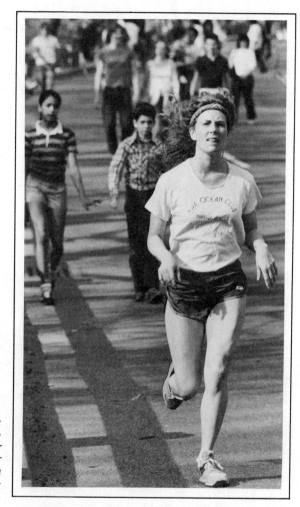

Although most people are not professional athletes, many have learned to set aside a part of their day for a brief workout. It is better to exercise at least five times a week than to restrict vigorous activity to the weekend.

Issue

Nutrition and the Athlete

I took some of the best long-distance runners in America and I dehydrated them with diuretics. After they ran for 55 minutes, they all passed out.

David Costill, Ph.D.
Director, Human Performance Lab,
Ball State University(5)

Boxer Leon Spinks takes a meal of raw eggs and two bottles of beer; tennis pro Billie Jean King, once a self-proclaimed "junk food addict," now rarely indulges in sweets; Olympic marathon winner Frank Shorter drinks de-fizzed colas during races. Do the successes of these three athletes come from their diets or in spite of them?

Athletes have the same basic nutritional needs as nonathletes except for an increased energy requirement. Their need to maintain an efficient body weight and to meet the increased energy demands of training and competi-tion determine the amount of food they require. Though both athletes and nonathletes require a nutritionally balanced diet, de-ficiencies are of particular con-cern to athletes because their performance is impaired. This section explains how training and performance, whether of Olym-pic contenders or suburban vol-leyball players, can affect and be affected by nutrition.

NUTRIENT NEEDS OF ATHLETES

A prudent distribution of nutrients for anyone is about 15 percent of kcalories from protein, 30 to 35 percent from fat, and 50 to 55 percent from carbohydrate. As energy needs increase, this distribution should remain the same, with only the number of grams of each nutrient increasing.

Protein.   Athletes need protein to maintain tissues, to develop muscle during conditioning, to allow for growth if the athlete is not yet physically mature, and to replace the nitrogen lost in sweat. The protein RDA for adults is 0.8 grams per kilogram of body weight. Athletes have the same RDA unless they are enlarging muscles or prone to repeated trauma (football or hockey players). These individuals require slightly more protein for increases in lean body mass, enzymes, myoglobin, and hemoglobin. Such persons may need 1 gram per kilogram of body weight per day, while growing athletes may have protein needs as high as 1.5 grams per kilogram of body weight per day.(6) Some nutritionists believe that 20, instead of 15, percent of the diet of young athletes should be high-quality protein. With an intake of 3000 kcalories, this would be about 600 kcalories from protein or about 150 grams.(7) Athletes with these higher protein needs can meet their requirement without liquid or powdered supplements through the normal increase in food necessary to meet their higher energy needs. Once in condition, the athlete's protein needs differ little from those of the nonathlete. Heavy sweating does increase protein needs somewhat, but 0.8 to 1.0 grams per kilogram of body weight will easily cover that extra need, because physical activity does not destroy cellular protein.(8)

Increasing protein intake will not improve performance and may actually hinder it. High-protein diets increase the need for water, since more fluid is needed to rid the body of the nitrogen by-products in the urine. Such diets create more work for the liver and kidneys; can lead to ketosis, dehydration, loss of appetite, and diarrhea; and deprive the body of the more efficient fuel, carbohydrate. Even though there is no need for the traditional steak diet, it may give some athletes a psychological lift.

Fat.   Athletes have the same need for dietary fat as nonathletes. It is a misconception that they should avoid all fats, fried foods, and oily dressings. As is true for everyone, those wishing to lose a few pounds might try cutting back on fat intake. On the other hand, there is no need for athletes to increase fat intake dramatically to cover extra energy needs.

Carbohydrates.   Carbohydrates are the most efficient energy source for athletes and nonathletes alike. Although athletes have a greater energy requirement and can consume more sugary foods without gaining weight than can sedentary people, they should be careful to indulge in these foods only after they have met all other nutrient needs. In order to use the energy from the fuel nutrients the body needs certain vitamins and minerals, so consuming many foods of low nutrient density reduces the chances of meeting all needs. As marathon runner George Sheehan put it: "How can one play and think and find truth when stuffed with jelly doughnuts?"

Kcalorie Needs.   The average man needs about 2700 to 3000 kcalories per day. The typical male athlete requires 3000 to 6000 kcalories per day. An athlete's kcalorie requirement depends on body size, age, weight, height, type of competition, and level of training. Kcalorie needs increase as the number of muscle contractions increase, so swimmers and runners have higher needs than gymnasts, who sustain their muscle contractions.(9)

In general, an athlete's appetite increases in proportion to increased training. Table 8–4 shows how to determine kcalorie needs for athletic events. When energy needs are from 5000 to 6000 kcalories per day, the athlete may find it easier to eat five or six meals instead of three.(8) An athlete's ability to perform is determined first by the level of training, and second by body fat. The work of exercise increases with increased fat. Highly trained male athletes have about 5 to 8 percent body fat; females, about 9 to 10 percent. Women whose body fat drops below this level often experience amenorrhea, or cessation of menstruation.(9) But even the body of the leanest marathon runner contains at least 4 percent fat. In certain sports (sumo wrestling, weight lifting, and channel swimming) it is an advantage for athletes to have more fat; in most sports, however, leanness (less than 15 percent body fat) is better.(6,9)

Many athletes find themselves weighing too much or too little for their best performance. The methods by which they choose to lose or gain weight will affect their overall health and ultimate ability to perform.

Weight Control.   Athletes get overfat if they consume too much food, just like anyone else. This extra weight means a greater workload for the heart and can hinder agility and coordination. A one- to two-pound loss per week is a sound goal. Fad diets promising faster losses can cause fatigue, mild dehydra-

TABLE 8–4 Caloric Requirements for Participation in Athletic Events

Sport	Reference Athlete		Daily Requirement for Maintenance and Light Work (kcal)	Kcalories Expended per Minute of Activity	Minutes of Activity per Event	Kcalories Expended per Event	Requirement for Maintenance and Light Work and Event Participation (kcal)
	Height (ft./in.)	Weight (lb)					
Men							
Football	6 2	195	2700	10.2	10.0	102	2800
Wrestling	6 3	218	3000	14.2	8.0	114	3100
Gymnastics (apparatus)	5 10	153	2100	6.5	6.0	39	2100
Hockey	6 3	195	2700	11.5	15.0	173	2900
Long-distance running (5 miles)	5 9	155	2100	14.4	25.0	360	2600
Swimming	6 1	174	2400	11.0	20.0	220	2600
Tennis	5 10	160	2200	7.1	45.0	320	2500
Baseball	6 1	200	2700	4.7	60.0	282	3000
Basketball	6 3	175	2400	8.6	40.0	344	2800
Women							
Swimming	5 4	137	1800	11.0	25.0	275	2100
Tennis	5 5	115	1600	7.1	60.0	420	2000
Gymnastics (apparatus)	5 7	120	1600	5.0	4.5	23	1625
Basketball	5 10	160	2200	8.6	32.0	275	2500
Running (1 mile)	5 7	120	1600	10.6	5.5	58	1700

Source: D.M. Huse and R. A. Nelson, "Basic, Balanced Diet Meets Requirements of Athletes," *The Physician and Sportsmedicine* 5 (1977): 52–56.

tion, decreased muscular strength and work performance, and problems with controlling body temperature. Semi- or total starvation diets dehydrate the body. Weight loss is accompanied by loss of protein, glycogen, minerals, enzymes, and other important body constituents. Such diets reduce body reserves needed for athletic demands. Some athletes have experienced abnormal heartbeats on such regimens. In the young athlete, normal growth can be slowed.

Young wrestlers and boxers are often told to lose weight by "drying out" for the early weigh-in. This forced dehydration can reduce the urine volume to a point where kidney damage can occur. The weight loss is from water loss, not fat. Dehydration, semi-, and total starvation have been condemned by the American Medical Association and the American College of Sports Medicine. The best way to lose weight is to eat less at each meal (cut down on fats and sugars first). Skipping meals will impair performance during training and during the event itself.

The best way for athletes to gain weight is to eat larger than normal portions of food. They should also eat snacks that are high in both kcalories and nutrients. If an athlete increases food intake dramatically to achieve a fast weight gain, the gain will often be fat, not muscle. Effective muscle gains depend on increased exercise combined with a nutritious diet.

Vitamins. Athletes undergoing rigorous training do not require extra vitamins. Contrary to another popular belief, vitamin needs do not increase in cold weather. Nutritionists do not recommend supplements because water-soluble vitamins in excess of needs are excreted, while excess fat-soluble vitamins can be toxic (see Chapter 7). Some athletes take extra vitamin C to improve endurance and performance, and to reduce the duration of injuries. There is no evidence to back up the effectiveness of this particular practice unless there was a prior deficiency.(9) Athletes may need extra B vitamins (thiamin, riboflavin, and niacin) to meet increased energy requirements, but they can meet these needs by eating extra food. Excess B vitamins do not improve endurance, time of recovery, or strength.

Water and Minerals. Water is the nutrient most often depleted and most easily restored. All athletes engaged in prolonged activity or in settings conducive to dehydration should ingest fluids. One way to determine which athletes are susceptible to dehydration is to measure their weights before and after practice. Athletes do not experience harmful side effects from fluid losses up to 2 percent of body weight.(10) Anyone who loses greater than 4 to 5 percent body weight in sweat should be encouraged to drink during exercise.(9) Since marathoners may lose 8 to 13 pounds (16 to 26 cups) of water during an event, they should drink several glasses of fluid before a race and at regular intervals during the race. Sir Edmund Hillary, the first person to climb Mt. Everest, attributed his success to adequate water during the last few days of the ascent.

The minerals most affected by heavy exercise are iron, sodium, and potassium. Iron deficiency is common in athletic women, particularly during enstruation, and intake should be increased according to need. Well-trained endurance athletes may experience "athlete's anemia," a borderline low hemoglobin level. Part of the reason for the condition may be the large loss of iron in sweat.(6) Since this type of anemia does not improve with supplementation, some physiologists think it may be a normal adaptation to training. Unless there is a definite iron deficiency, the athlete should avoid iron supplements, which can cause nausea, stomach upset, and constipation. In some genetically disposed persons, the iron can accumulate to harmful levels.(9) Athletes should include iron-rich foods in the diet, however.

Sweat loss is mostly water, but some electrolytes like sodium and potassium are also lost and must be replaced through the diet.

SPECIAL DIETARY CONSIDERATIONS

Carbohydrate Loading

During rest, the major source of the body's energy is fatty acids from stored fat, though some comes from carbohydrate in the form of glucose. During exercise, the proportion of energy coming from fat or carbohydrate varies with the intensity of exercise and the athlete's level of conditioning. When there is plenty of oxygen available to contracting muscle, fatty acids remain the chief energy source. When oxygen availability does not keep pace with the intensity of the exercise, the muscles rely more on glucose.

During prolonged heavy exercise, the blood cannot carry oxygen to tissues fast enough to meet the oxygen needs for breaking down fats. Instead, it switches to carbohydrates (glycogen) for energy, since they can be broken down to provide energy without oxygen. Thus, an athlete's ability to sustain prolonged exercise is directly related to initial glycogen stores. The higher the liver and muscle stores of glycogen, the longer the athlete can avoid fatigue. This has led to the practice of carbohydrate loading.

Carbohydrate loading, a practice developed by the Swedish scientist P.O. Astrand, is a way to increase glycogen stores in the muscles of athletes in order to delay glycogen depletion and fatigue during competition. Carbohydrate loading can double the glycogen content of muscle through a procedure that involves depleting the body's glycogen reserves and then eating a series of diets that cause the body to store more glycogen than normal.

Here is how it works. One week before an event, the athlete exercises to exhaustion, depleting muscle glycogen stores (a marathon runner can do this by a long-distance run). The athlete then consumes a high fat, high-protein, low-carbohydrate diet for three days to keep the glycogen content of the exercising muscles low. For the best effect, researchers recommend the athlete refrain from exercising during this time. Three days before the competition, the athlete eats large amounts of carbohydrates, particularly starchy foods, not sweets like sugar, candy, soft drinks, or honey, and normal amounts of protein and fats.

This not only replenishes but actually increases glycogen stores. During this three-day period, minimal to no exercise is also recommended. Such a regimen is useful only for activities lasting 60 minutes or longer (cross country skiing, cycling) and for high altitude sports such as mountain climbing, where little oxygen is available for burning fats.

The technique is fairly easy, so why don't all endurance athletes use it? As you may have guessed, there are as many risks and disadvantages as there are gains. First of all, the program requires days, not hours, yet the endurance gained is not much more than that from a simple high-carbohydrate diet. The diet is potentially dangerous to cardiac rehabilitation type runners and older athletes and may have long-range cardiac effects on any healthy athlete. (Glycogen is deposited in all muscles, including the heart, and there are large changes in blood fats.) During the low-carbohydrate phase, the athlete eats large amounts of protein and fat, a diet that can produce fatigue, irritability, and nausea. During the high-carbohydrate phase, water is stored along with glycogen in the muscle, giving a feeling of heaviness and stiffness that can hinder performance. Weight gain from water retention can reduce the athlete's maximum ability to use oxygen. The change from low to high carbohydrates may cause nausea and cramping. Muscle damage can occur. The better trained the athlete, the less likely endurance will improve with carbohydrate loading, since well-trained athletes use glycogen slowly and rely for a longer time on fats.(9)

The risks of carbohydrate loading often outweigh the benefits. You should not try this regimen without expert supervision or for more than two or three times per year. Any unusual symptoms (chest pains) should be reported to a doctor at once. This practice should not be used by early adolescent or pre-adolescent athletes, and can be dangerous to those with diabetes or high fat levels in their blood.

Competition Meals and Dehydration

Pregame Meal. An athlete should eat the pregame meal about three hours before the event to allow for proper digestion and absorption. The stomach should be relatively empty before beginning strenuous exercise, because food in the stomach at the time of performance competes with the working muscles for the blood supply. An empty stomach also is desirable for contact sports in case surgery and anesthesia are required.

Gastric emptying is slowed by emotional excitement. Athletes may get indigestion if they eat foods high in protein or fat in the tense period before an event. Rather, they should eat bread, pasta, rice, and other grain products, instead of meat. They should not eat heavily salted foods because water retention may result. Other foods to avoid include concentrated sources of sugar, glucose tablets, undiluted honey (all these can cause cramps or temporary hypoglycemia), and gas-forming foods such as sauerkraut, cabbage, and beans, which can cause distention and discomfort.

A light carbohydrate meal (about 500 kcalories) such as skim milk, a sandwich, cookies, and a banana is adequate. Two to three glasses of a beverage should be included, but preferably not whole milk (too much fat) or caffeinated drinks, which act as diuretics and can increase nervous tension before the contest. (Some researchers point out that caffeine consumption equivalent to 2 cups of coffee one hour before exercise stimulates the release of fats into the blood, which may help spare glycogen from being used as energy. This would be helpful to endurance athletes. More research is needed to determine whether this possible advantage outweighs the unwanted side effects of caffeine.)(6)

Recommended beverages include slightly diluted fruit juices, skim milk, broth and bouillon. Iced drinks delay digestion and can cause cramping. Athletes should avoid alcohol, which can affect fine coordination and reaction time and can cause cramping. Table 8–5 gives guidelines for choosing pregame meals.

Some athletes find liquid meals reduce mouth dryness and the indigestion, nausea, vomiting, and muscle cramping caused by nervous tension.(11) Fluid meals are easier to digest because they skip the liquefaction step in digestion. It is not necessary to purchase special liquid meals since the homemade variety is cheaper and can be as or more nutritious (Table 8–5).

Fluid and Nutrient Replacement During the Event.   Water is the only nutrient of greater importance to athletes than nonathletes, especially during prolonged training in a hot, humid environment. Athletes need more water, and sometimes more salt, than usual to replenish sweat losses. It was once thought that athletes should not drink during exercise because of cramps. They could only suck on ice cubes or rinse out their mouths. It is now known that restricting

TABLE 8–5 Guidelines for Pregame Meals	
Composition of a Solid Food Meal	Composition of a Liquid Meal (one cup = 200 kcal)
1 serving of roasted or broiled meat or poultry	nonfat dry milk (¼ cup)
1 serving of mashed potatoes, 1 baked potato, ½ cup macaroni, noodles, or the like	skim milk (3 cups)
1 serving of vegetables	water (½ cup)
1 cup skim milk	sugar (¼ cup)
	flavoring, vanilla (1 teaspoon)
1 teaspoon fat spread or 2 teaspoons jelly or other sweets	
½ cup or a serving of fruit	
sugar cookies or plain cake (angelfood, sponge, white cake)	
extra beverages, 1 to 2 cups	

Sources: (solid food): E. Darden, *Nutrition and Athletic Performance* (Pasadena: The Athletic Press, 1977).; *(liquid meal):* American Alliance for Health, Physical Education, and Recreation, *Nutrition for Athletes* (Washington, D.C.: AAHPER, 1971).

water intake during performance can cause dehydration, leading to loss of appetite and a limited capacity for work, depending on how much body water is lost. A loss of 3 percent body water leads to impaired performance, a 5 percent loss causes heat exhaustion, a 7 percent loss causes hallucinations, and a 10 percent loss can lead to heat stroke.

Athletes cannot adapt to water intakes lower than their daily losses and should replace losses by periodic fluid intake. During activity, the largest amount of water is lost through the skin. It is almost impossible to drink enough fluid to replace this water as it is lost, but partial replacement by frequent drinking can prevent overheating. Potential dehydration is best monitored by close watch of body weight. Drinking to satisfy thirst does not ensure replacement of fluids, since tension, anxiety, and the large sweat losses distort the thirst sensation. During prolonged competition in warm weather, athletes should drink about two-thirds of what they have lost.(11) About two hours before an event, endurance athletes should drink about 600 milliliters (18 ounces) of fluid. Ten to fifteen minutes before performance, 400 to 600 milliliters (12 to 18 ounces) of cool water is recommended. Small amounts of water (100 to 200 milliliters or 3 to 7 ounces) every 10 to 15 minutes are better than larger amounts every hour.(8) The stomach can empty only about 1 liter of fluid per hour, so larger amounts should not be consumed.

The manner of replacing fluid and mineral losses during exercise is still controversial. Whatever fluid is chosen should be palatable and dilute enough to be emptied readily from the stomach.(9) Fluids that contain too much sugar or minerals will draw fluid into the stomach from other parts of thge body, increase dehydration, and possibly cause stomach upset or diarrhea. Drinks like plain water, orange juice, grapefruit juice, cola or ginger ale mixed with three parts water, or tomato, V-8 or other vegetable juices mixed with one part water will not cause any of these reactions. It may require 24 to 36 hours to replace fluid losses completely.

In the mid 1960s electrolyte solutions (Gatorade, Sportade, Electrolyte Replacement with Glucose or ERG, Bike Half Time Punch) were introduced. They differed in electrolyte concentration, but all contained sodium, potassium, and carbohydrate. No evidence exists to show their superiority over water, saline solutions or glucose syrup drinks in improving performance. Most have less potassium than milk, beer, or orange juice. These commercial solutions are generally more concentrated than recommended and should be diluted. The electrolytes lost during an event do not have to be replaced hour by hour, but can be ingested after the competition is over. All the nutrients lost during a competition, except water, can be replenished in a normal diet. Sodium and potassium losses can be replaced by putting extra salt on food, adding broth or boullion to the meal, and consuming potassium-rich foods like oranges and bananas. Taking salt tablets to maintain sodium levels is unnecessary until 4 quarts (8 pounds) of water is lost, since sweat is less salty than blood. Athletes should not take salt tablets except on the advice of the team physician. These are harmful if consumed with too little water. They also draw water from the body tissues into the intestines, sometimes producing nausea. Excessive salt intakes increase the requirement for water, which can impair an athlete's efficiency during training.

Some events, like marathons, require a great deal of energy expenditure. During these endurance events athletes can help avoid fatigue by eating a small cube of sugar every hour. Too much sugar, however, can draw fluid into the gastrointestinal tract, causing cramps, nausea, gas, and diarrhea. No more than 3 rounded tablespoons should be taken in a given hour. For short events, such as dashes, there is no benefit from sugar cubes, honey, or candy before or during competition.

Issue

The Weekend Athlete

Most of us are not athletes now nor will we ever be. Exercise, however, should be included in everyone's daily activities. If you are like many Americans, you probably spend more time making excuses than exercising. Some of the most common excuses follow: (12)

1. The key to staying fit is not exercise, but controlling how much you eat.

2. Too much exercise can enlarge the heart, which is harmful once you stop exercising.

3. People who exercise work up big appetites and then eat too much, making the exercise useless.

4. These fads about physical fitness come and go, and I'm not impressed by them.

5. In the things I have to do every day, I get enough exercise without doing any exercises.

6. I'm so busy that I don't have enough energy left when I get around to thinking about exercising.

7. Too many people, like joggers and weight lifters, become fanatical about physical fitness, which is not healthful.

8. The trouble with participating in a sport is that I can only get to it now and then and too much physical exertion at one time like that is bad.

9. Middle-aged and older people don't really need exercise other than occasional walking.

Ever heard these before? Maybe from your parents, or friends, or even in your own mind? You might be hearing them less often now, since Americans are showing a trend toward more exercise. Currently, more than 90 million Americans participate in some form of physical activity, about 54 percent of all those over 18 years. This is in contrast to a 1961 survey, which showed only

24 percent exercising.(12) Most of these people are weekend athletes; that is, they participate in an activity once or twice each week, for perhaps 15 minutes to 2 hours each time. Competition athletes, by contrast, are in training 3 or more days per week for a minimum of 10 to 12 hours per week, not including competition.(13)

Each different kind of exercise has its own special benefits. General body movement, such as slow walking or calisthenics, can aid in weight control but does not help in cardiovascular conditioning. Appendix E gives the number of kcalories expended for various activities. Aerobic exercise, on the other hand, is exercise that increases the strength and endurance of the heart, lungs, and circulatory system. It promotes improved use and consumption of oxygen in the body. Both can lower percentage of body fat. Exercise develops muscular strength, endurance, and tone; promotes greater flexibility, balance, coordination, and agility; and gives an improved sense of well-being.(14) Aerobic exercise, in addition, increases muscle efficiency in handling oxygen, improves work capacity, and can lower blood pressure and pulse rate. It can also decrease risk of CVD. With exercise, the heart beats stronger and steadier, requiring fewer strokes to pump the same amount of blood. Breathing becomes deeper, and circulation improves. Aerobic exercise increases the efficiency and supply of oxygen to the muscles. As endurance increases, the body recovers more quickly from vigorous activity. The individual can exercise longer before tiring because the size and number of vessels carrying blood to the tissues increase.

Before starting an exercise program, you should take into account family and medical history, age, physical fitness, blood pressure, smoking habits, and weight. See a doctor, especially if you are over 35 or have any risk factors for cardiovascular disease such as hypertension and elevated blood lipids. In planning a program, be sure to choose an activity you can continue, one that is convenient for your life style and not too expensive. The type of exercise you choose will affect your success at integrating it into your daily schedule. It is not surprising that the single most popular exercise for adults in the United States is walking.(12)

Sporadic exercise is not too useful, because it tends to stimulate the appetite. Regular daily exercise, even a short 15-minute program, will improve muscle tone and circulation without the rapid jump in appetite. The appetite-controlling mechanism does not work well if the person does not maintain a minimal level of activity. The goal should be 15 to 60 minutes of continuous aerobic activity 3 to 5 days each week. For nonathletic adults, low- to moderate-intensity activities should be chosen but performed for a longer period of time.(14) The exercise should be continuous and of sufficient duration and intensity to condition muscles and the cardiovascular system without being too strenuous. Aerobic activities include jogging, brisk walking, swimming, skating, cross-country skiing, cycling, jumping rope, aerobic dancing, rowing, and jumping on a trampoline. Handball, tennis, squash, and volleyball are not aerobic the way most people play them.(14) Golf and bowling are not aerobic for anyone. Jogging, though a good exercise for many people, can increase the risk of foot, leg, and knee injuries in others. Walking is aerobic if done at a quick pace (about 3.5 to 4 miles per hour for 30 minutes) and is recommended for all age groups.

The way to determine if you are getting any cardiovascular conditioning from your exercise program is to measure your pulse rate immediately upon beginning an exercise, at peak period, and at the end of the exercise. If you are performing at 85 percent of your maximal heart rate, you are getting cardiovascular benefits. (You can figure your maximal heart rate by subtracting your age in years from 220).(14) Try to maintain this rate for at least 15 to 20 minutes during each session.

Starting a physical conditioning program has helped many people improve their eating habits. One study found that people beginning active exercise programs increased their consumption of green vegetables, fruit and fruit juices, dairy products other than eggs, whole wheat products, yogurt, and vitamins and minerals.(12) There is no need to add special foods to the diet once you begin an exercise program, because by meeting the RDA, you can obtain adequate amounts of the nutrients. As you become more fit, though, you may find yourself cutting back on empty-kcalorie foods and trying to eat more nutrient-dense ones.

Issue

Caffeine Consumption

Sometime around 500 B.C. in ancient Abyssinia, a hungry goatherd probably started munching on the fruit of an evergreen bush. Not long after, the world became hooked on coffee.(15) From the Middle East, coffee spread to the West in the seventeenth century.

"This little bean is the source of happiness and wit," said the British physician William Harvey in 1657. Almost 200 years later, a German chemist discovered just what it was about that little bean that made it so appealing: caffeine.(16)

Other caffeine-containing drinks beside coffee have been known for centuries. There is the tea leaf in China, the kola nut in West Africa, the ilex plant for making *maté* in Brazil, and the cassina or Christmas berry tree in North America.(17) A chocolate drink made from cacao beans was served by Montezuma in 1519 to Spanish explorers. It caught on in Europe once it was sweetened with sugar.(18) In more recent years, John S. Pemberton, a druggist in Atlanta, Georgia, produced a cola drink from kola nut extract and a pinch of caffeine in a three-legged pot in his backyard. His first year sales totaled $50, but rapidly ballooned into the $5 billion industry now known as Coca-Cola.(18)

Caffeine is chemically related to a group of substances called *methylxanthines*. Other members of this group are theophylline and theobromine, found most often in tea and cocoa.

Caffeine Content of Foods and Drugs. Caffeine is naturally present in coffee, tea, chocolate, and kola nuts. It is added to colas, pepper drinks, some other soft drinks (Sunkist orange drink), and certain medications. Table 8–6 presents the caffeine, theobromine, and theophylline content of selected foods and drugs. The amount of caffeine in coffee and tea depends on the strength of the brew. The methylxanthine content of natural sources is also determined by the variety of plant, the location and climate where grown, and cultural practices like fermentation.(17)

Medications may contain caffeine; the obvious ones are "wake up" tablets. Caffeine, however, may also be present in lower doses in menstrual, pain-killing, and cold compounds. Beverages account for most of the caffeine consumed in this country. Smaller amounts enter the diet through foods like coffee-flavored ice cream, chocolate bars, and chocolate-flavored foods.

Caffeine Consumption. Exposure to caffeine can begin before birth because caffeine crosses the placenta. It also passes into breast milk.(18) A survey of caffeine consumption in the United States(19) found that almost one in five infants under 2 years consume some caffeine. Higher intakes occurred where mothers gave cola drinks to infants suffering from stomach and intestinal distress. The mean intake of a 6- to 11-month-old infant was 4.2 milligrams, but on some days these infants averaged 77 milligrams, an amount found in 1 cup of coffee or 19 ounces of a cola. Average caffeine consumption increases steadily but sporadically until the

TABLE 8–6   Methylxanthine Contents of Foods and Drugs

Product	Caffeine (mg)	Theobromine (mg)	Theophylline (mg)
Coffee (5 oz)			
Regular brewed			
Percolated	110	3	tr
Dripolator	150	3.5	1
Instant	66	1.5	tr
Decaf brewed	4.5	tr	tr
Instant decaf	2	tr	tr
Soft drinks (12 oz)			
Dr. Pepper	61	tr	tr
Mr. Pibb	57	tr	tr
Mountain Dew	49	tr	tr
Tab	45	tr	tr
Coca-Cola	42	tr	tr
RC Cola	36	tr	tr
Pepsi-Cola	35	tr	tr
Diet Pepsi	34	tr	tr
Pepsi Light	34	tr	tr
Instant or brewed tea			
(5 min. brew)	45	9	6
Cocoa (5 oz)	13	173	tr
Milk chocolate (1 oz)	6	42	tr
Drugs			
Vivarin Tablets	200	—	—
Nodoz	100	—	—
Excedrin	63	—	—
Vanquish	33	—	—
Empirin Compound	32	—	—
Anacin	32	—	—
Dristan	16.2	—	—

Tr = less than 1 mg per serving.

Nutrition Action, August 1980, p. 6.

late teens. Coffee intake increases during the early adult years, and once started, the number of cups increases.(18) Of adults in the United States (age 18 and over), 82 percent consume an average of 186 milligrams of caffeine per day, or about the amount contained in a little over 2 cups of coffee. According to industry figures, almost one-fourth of those who drink coffee consume 9 or more cups per day; only 10 percent consume it decaffeinated.(18) The mean intake of caffeine from all sources by pregnant women who consume such products is estimated to be 193 milligrams per day. Coffee consumption begins to decline after the age of 50.(18)

Absorption and Metabolism. Caffeine is rapidly absorbed, metabolized, and excreted in the urine. Within a few minutes after drinking a cup of coffee, the caffeine enters all the organs and tissues of the body and is distributed in proportion to the tissue water content.(18) Its peak ''pick-me-up'' effect occurs within one hour, and its effect diminishes to half within three hours. It takes about 18 to 24 hours to be completely excreted. Caffeine does not accumulate or build up in body tissues.

Biological Effects. Caffeine produces a variety of biological effects. It stimulates the central nervous system, dilates blood vessels, increases the heartbeat, promotes secretion of stomach acid, and increases the production of urine.(15) Three to four cups of brewed coffee can increase basal metabolic rate from 10 to 25 percent. The stimulant prevents lapses of attention and improves the performance of physical tasks, especially those related to speed. It does not improve intellectual performance.

Medicinal Properties. Caffeine is used for its stimulant properties in many dietary beverages and in a number of over-the-counter and prescription drugs. The amount required to have a pharmacological effect is 200 milligrams. Its diuretic effects are useful in a number of medicines. Doctors often use it to stimulate the heart and to stimulate the respiratory system of premature infants.

Harmful Effects. Heavy coffee drinking may produce symptoms of *caffeinism* (insomnia, nervousness, irritability, anxiety, stomach irritation, diarrhea, and disturbances in heart rate and rhythms).(15,16) There have been several reports of persons drinking 8 to 15 cups of coffee a day seeking medical and psychological help for dizziness, agitation, headaches, and sleep difficulties. The classic case was one involving a prison inmate, being treated without success for anxiety, who could not understand how his habit of consuming 50 cups or more of coffee a day could be involved.(20) Caffeinism has been reported among irritable and nervous children who rarely drink coffee but consume large amounts of cola, hot chocolate, and chocolate bars.(20) High levels of caffeine are definitely toxic and can cause convulsions and vomiting, with complete recovery in six hours.(17) Ten grams (70 to 100 cups of coffee) can be fatal.(15)

Caffeine is a mildly addicting drug, but its stimulating effects are not reduced with long-term consumption. It continues to make the person feel alert and

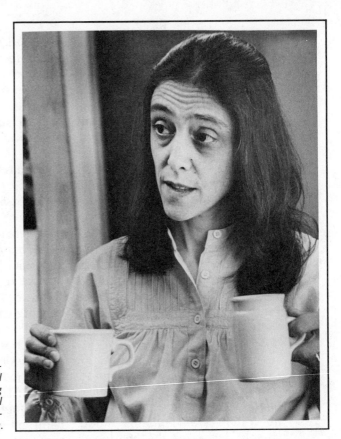

Many people, though unaware of all the physiological effects of caffeine, are willing to admit to a psychological dependence on this mildly-addictive drug.

active even with daily consumption, although some tolerance to its effects on the kidneys and circulation may develop. People who normally drink large amounts of caffeine-containing drinks may experience headaches or depression following abrupt withdrawal. There is also some psychological dependence ("Don't speak to me until I have my morning coffee!")(16)

Links between caffeine and heart disease have long been suspected. There is no evidence that coffee and tea drinking cause CVD, but excessive coffee drinking can cause arrhythmia (abnormal heartbeats) in a small percentage of the population.(17) The relationship of caffeine to the development of peptic ulcers has been debated, since caffeine does stimulate the production of stomach acid. Evidence fails to support this theory. There does seem to be some other ingredient in coffee besides caffeine that exerts similar effects on stomach acid and that may be responsible for stomach disturbances. People with sensitive stomachs may be better off eliminating coffee.

At one time General Foods used trichloroethylene (TCC) in the process for extracting caffeine from Sanka and Brim coffees. Studies showed that TCC produces liver cancer in mice. General Foods claimed that a person would have to drink 50 million cups of decaffeinated coffee a day to match the amount fed the animals, but voluntarily switched to a different chemical, methylene chloride.(20) Quite recently, a study(21) conducted at Harvard University showed a strong association between coffee drinking and the development of pancreatic cancer. There was no association, however, with this type of cancer and tea drinking so the culprit in coffee was apparently not caffeine. Some experts believe there were faults in this study such that the results should not be taken seriously unless they can be confirmed in further research.(22)

Methylxanthines may lead to fibrocystic breast disease, a benign condition that can necessitate surgery and sometimes precedes cancer. The symptoms of this disease are reduced in some women who give up products containing caffeine, theobromine, or theophylline.(23) Recently, evidence has emerged that caffeine may affect the developing fetus. The concern arose because many pregnant women have a high caffeine intake and caffeine crosses the placenta easily. Data from rat studies show complete or partial absence of toes in 20 percent of the young born to rats fed an amount of caffeine equivalent to 12 to 24 cups of strong coffee a day. At levels of 2 cups of coffee a day, pups showed slowed bone development.(15) One problem with these studies is that rats metabolize caffeine differently from humans. A recent study with 12,205 pregnant women found no relationship between coffee consumption and the birth weight or occurrence of malformation of babies.(24)

It is ironic that "cola" or "pepper" drinks, common beverages for children, must contain a certain amount of caffeine to meet standard regulations. These regulations were originally intended to assure consumers they were getting all the ingredients they expected in these drinks. With the recent evidence linking caffeine to birth defects in animals, the FDA has changed this so that noncaffeinated cola and pepper drinks will be available.

ALTERNATIVES TO CAFFEINE-CONTAINING PRODUCTS

1. If drinking coffee makes you jittery or anxious, you can cut down on the caffeine by switching to instant coffees blended with grain or chicory or to decaffeinated coffee (although decaffeinated coffee still contains some caffeine).

2. Tea may be easier on your stomach than coffee, but it still contains caffeine plus the other methylxanthines.

3. Children feel the stimulating effects of caffeine more than adults, so chocolate-containing foods and caffeinated sodas should be limited.

4. You can switch to special caf-feine-free products like Pero or Postum, both grain-based, or try herbal teas.

5. In cooking and baking, carob, also called St. John's bread, is a good substitute for chocolate. It is lower in fat and kcalories than chocolate, though it is usually sold at a higher price. It does not contain any caffeine.

Resources: Recommended Books for Athletes

- Best Foods, *Beyond Diet...Exercise Your Way to Fitness and Heart Health* (Englewood Cliffs, New Jersey: CPC International).

- N. Clark, *The Athlete's Kitchen: A Nutrition Guide and Cookbook* (Boston: CBI Publishing, 1981).

- E. Darden, *Nutrition for Athletes* (Winter Park, FL: Anna Publishing, 1978).

- F.I. Katch and W.D. McArdle, *Nutrition, Weight Control, and Exercise* (Boston: Houghton Mifflin, 1977).

- J. Parizlova, *Nutrition, Physical Fitness and Health* (Baltimore: University Park Press, 1978).

- N.J. Smith, *Food for Sport* (Palo Alto, CA: Bull Publishing, 1976).

- D.R. Young, *Physical Performance, Fitness, and Diet* (Springfield, IL: Charles C Thomas, 1977).

REFERENCES

1. M. Hegsted, S. Schutte, M. Zemel, and H. Linkswiler, "Urinary Calcium and Calcium Balance in Young Men as Affected by Level of Protein and Phosphorus Intake," *Journal of Nutrition* 111 (1981):553–62.

2. M. Stephenson, "The Confusing World of Health Foods," *FDA Consumer*, July–August 1978, p. 32.

3. T.A. Morck and J.D. Cook, "Factors Affecting the Bioavailability of Dietary Iron," *Cereal Foods World* 26(1981):667–72.

4. "Do You Need Iron Supplements?" *Consumer Reports*, September 1978, p. 502.

5. G. Mirkin and M. Hoffman, *The Sportsmedicine Book* (Boston: Little, Brown, 1978), p. 51.

6. E.R. Buskirk, "Diet and Athletic Performance," *Postgraduate Medicine* 61(1977):229–36.

7. M.H. Williams, "Nutritional Faddism and Athletes," *Nutrition and the M.D.*, December 1979, pp. 1–2.

8. Nutrition and Physical Fitness: A Statement by the American Dietetic Association," *Journal of the American Dietetic Association* 76(1980):437–43.

9. S.H. Vitousek, "Is More Better?" *Nutrition Today*, November–December 1979, pp. 10–17.

10. "Nutrition and the Athlete," *Nutrition and the M.D.*, April 1977, p. 3.

11. American Alliance for Health, Physical Education, and Recreation, *Nutrition for Athletes* (Washington, D.C.: AAHPER, 1971).

12. L. Harris and Associates, *The Perrier Study: Fitness in America* (New York: Great Waters of France, January 1979)

13. J. Garrie, "The Prudent Diet for the Competitive vs. the Weekend Athlete," *Nutrition and the M.D.*, January 1976, p. 2.

14. "Nutrition and Physical Fitness: A Statement by the American Dietetic Association," *Journal of the American Dietetic Association* 76 (1980:437–43.

15. C. Lecos, "Caution Light on Caffeine," *FDA Consumer*, October 1980, pp. 6–9.

16. *Consumer Reports*, October 1979, p. 571.

17. D.M. Graham, "Caffeine: Its Identity, Dietary Sources, Intake and Biological Effects," *Nutrition Reviews* 36 (1978):97–102.

18. Food and Drug Administration, *Report on Caffeine*, September 1980.

19. Committee on GRAS, *List Survey, Phase III: Estimating Distribution of Daily Intakes of Caffeine* (Washington, D.C.: National Academy of Sciences, 1977).

20. "Coffee: Three Updates," *Nutrition and the M.D.* 2 (August 1976):3–4.

21. B. MacMahon, S. Yen, D. Trichopoulos, K. Warren, and G. Nardi, "Coffee and Cancer of the Pancreas," *New England Journal of Medicine* 304 (1981):630–33.

22. I. Higgins, P. Stolley, and E.L. Wynder, "Correspondence: Coffee and Cancer of the Pancreas," *New England Journal of Medicine* 304 (1981):1605.

23. "For Others, Methylxanthine Withdrawal May Work," Medical News, *Journal of the American Medical Association* 244 (1980):1078.

24. S. Linn, S.C. Schoenbaum, R. Monson, B. Rosner, P.G. Stubblefield, and K. J. Ryan, "No Association Between Coffee Consumption and Adverse Outcomes of Pregnancy," *New England Journal of Medicine* 306 (1982):141–45.

The U.S. Diet: Safe and Nutritious?

9

In the early nineteenth century, English food sellers would often adulterate their goods. Practices such as putting leaves of other plants in tea, sawdust in spices, cheap oils in expensive ones, mineral oil in saffron, and chalk in watered-down milk were common. A merchant who attempted to defraud customers in these ways might find himself put in stocks in the center of town, with honey smeared on his face to attract flies and ants. Some people, no doubt, look at today's processed and fabricated foods and think that this practice should be revived. Many are part of the back-to-basics movement and view the past as the ideal way of living, preferring homemade foods to their processed counterparts. People who prefer to bake their own bread and prepare all their dishes from scratch probably have delicious meals, but for those who insist that the U.S. food supply must return to that of the turn of the century, a brief review of food safety and the nutritional status of Americans during the last century and today may prove enlightening.

FOOD REGULATION IN THE UNITED STATES

Legislation

Dr. Harvey Wiley, chief of the Department of Agriculture's Bureau of Chemistry in the early 1900s, was convinced food manufacturers were poisoning the American public. Prior to the Civil War, most food colors were made from fairly harmless vegetable dyes, but by the nineteenth century the use of minerals for coloring had become widespread. Copper sulfate, red lead, lead chromate, and vermilion are some of the toxic pigments manufacturers routinely used. Coal tar dyes, also highly toxic, became popular after 1856.

To draw attention to the problem, in 1902 Dr. Wiley organized what came to be known as Dr. Wiley's Poison Squad. Over a five-year time span, his 12 USDA volunteers consumed many kinds of commonly used food additives to see how the human body would react. Wiley chose young men because, as a rule, they would be more resistant to any harmful effects from the additives than children or older persons. If they became ill or showed signs of injury, other people could be more seriously injured. During this same period, Congressman Mann became interested in the addition of possible harmful chemicals to the food supply and in 1906 introduced into the *Congressional Record* a table of dangerous color additives, preservatives, and adulterants that were in widespread use (Table 9–1). Because of efforts such as these, Congress passed the Pure Food and Drug Act of 1906. This law held a food to be adulterated, and therefore illegal, if it contained any poisonous or deleterious substances.

Around the same time that Harvey Wiley was testing food on young men, a journalist named Upton Sinclair arrived in Chicago to chronicle the life of the meatpacking plant worker. His book *The Jungle,* intended as a statement of the injustices suffered by working people in America, unintentionally became an indictment of the filth and contamination found in the meat industry. Stories of workers falling into lard vats and going out of the world as pure beef lard shocked President Theodore Roosevelt into ordering a thorough investigation of stockyard conditions. As a result, the first comprehensive meat inspection law was passed in 1906. As Sinclair was later to admit, "I aimed at the public's heart and by accident I hit it in the stomach."(1)

The Pure Food and Drug Act of 1906 had many loopholes and was revised in 1938 as the Federal Food, Drug, and Cosmetic Act. This act was the beginning of modern food regulation. As the food supply became more highly processed, legislators, finding even the new law to be inadequate, added several amendments and modifications. The Miller Pesticide Amendment of 1954 established the procedure for determining safe levels for pesticide residues on fresh fruit, vegetables, and other agricultural commodities. Four years later, Congress passed the 1958 Food Additives Amendment. This amendment shifted the burden of proof that an additive was safe away from the government and onto the manufacturer. It requires manufacturers to test any new substance they wish to use on at least two species of animals, submit a petition to the Food and Drug Administration (FDA), and receive approval before the additives can be used. If approved, the FDA uses a measuring stick sometimes called "the philosophy of the minimum." This means that the *tolerance level*, or amount of the additive allowed, is the smallest quantity needed to produce the desired effect, even though a higher level may be safe.

The 1958 Amendment exempted two categories of additives from testing: the GRAS substances and those with prior sanction. GRAS substances are those that are *Generally Recognized As Safe* based on long-term use or widespread use without known ill effects. Prior sanctioned additives are those that had been approved by the FDA or USDA before 1958. These two categories

TABLE 9–1 Color Additives, Adulterants, and Preservatives in Use, Early 1900s

Food	Color	Adulterant	Preservative
Milk	Annatto, azo colors, caramel.	Water, skimming	Formaldehyde, boric acid, borax, sodium bicarbonate.
Condensed milk, condensed cream, cream.		Made from skimmed milk	Same as milk, also gelatin, sucrate of lime.
Cheese			Substitute for fat.
Meats		Oleomargarine or lard	Boric acid, borax, sulphurous acid, salicylic acid
Meat extracts, sausages	Red ochre, coal tar dyes, cochineal.	Cracker or bread crumbs, horse flesh	Borax, saltpeter to preserve color, borax.
Fish, oysters			Boric acid.
Baking powder	Mislabeling of, phosphate powders, alum powders, tartaric powders.	Calcium acid phosphate, an alum, tartaric acid, bitartrate of potassium, calcium sulphate.	
Noodles	Adulterant, turmeric.		Potassium fluoride.
Tea	Coal tar dyes, prussian blue, indigo, plumbago, turmeric.	Steeped leaves, foreign leaves, soapstone, gypsum, catechu, substitute of cheaper brands.	
Coffee (whole)	Scheele's green, iron oxide, yellow ochre, chrome yellow, burnt umbre, venetian red, turmeric, prussian blue, indigo.		
Coffee (ground)		Roasted peas, beans, wheat, rye, oats, chickory, brown bread, pilot bread, charcoal, red slate, bark, date stones.	
Cocoa	Iron oxide	Starch, cocoa shells, sugar when above 60 per cent, English walnut shells, Brazil nut shells, almond shells, coconut shells, date stones, spruce sawdust, oak sawdust, linseed meal, cocoa shells, red sandalwood, ground olive stones.	
Caraway seed		Exhausted seed	
Allspice		Peas, pea hulls, exhausted ginger, cayenne, olive stones, clovestems, turmeric.	
Cinnamon		Cereal starches and bark, pea hulls, nut shells, pepper, ginger, olive stones, mustard, sawdust.	
Pepper		Olive stones, turmeric, pepper, shells, buckwheat middlings, nut shells, cayenne, charcoal, rice, sand, sawdust, turmeric.	

Food	Coloring	Adulterants	Preservatives/Acids
Cayenne	Coal tar dyes	Starches, pilot bread, crackers, ginger, nutshells, rice, gypsum, buckwheat, turmeric, mustard hulls, ground redwood, red ochre.	
Ginger		Exhausted ginger, turmeric, wheat, corn, rice, sawdust.	
Mustard		Potato starch, cayenne, corn, terra alba.	
Olive oil		Cottonseed oil, peanut oil, sunflower oil, corn oil, mustard oil, poppy seed oil, rape oil, coconut oil.	
Butter	Carrot juice	Oleomargarine, renovated butter	Borax, boric acid, formaldehyde, salicylic acid, sulphurous acid.
Oleomargarine Lard		Paraffin and inferior fats. Cottonseed oil, beef stearin, peanut oil, corn oil, coconut oil, water.	
Molasses, sirups	Tin salts	Glucose which sometimes contains arsenic.	
Honey		Cane sugar and commercial glucose, gelatin.	
Candy	Coal tar dyes	Paraffin, terra alba, talc, iron oxides	
Cider	Caramel	Water, sugar, sodium carbonate	Salicylic acid, sulphurous acid, beta-napthol.
Beer		Sodium carbonate	Fluorides, salicylic acid, benzoin acid, sulphites.
Vinegar	Caramel	Water, mineral acids, artificial vinegar, accidental adulteration, copper, lead, zinc, and arsenic.	
Ketchups	Coal tar dyes	Free sulphuric acid, alum	Saccharin, borax, boric acid; salicylic acid.
Pickles	Copper salts	Turnip	Saccharin.
Horseradish (bottled) Jellies and jams	Coal tar dyes	Glucose for cane sugar, sulphuric acid, alum, citric acid, tartaric acid, starch, gelatin, agar-agar, often made from refuse pulp, artificial flavors, apple pulp	
Vanilla extract		Coumarin and vanillin substituted for vanilla, bay rum, prune juice.	
Essences	Caramel	Artificial essences of pineapple, melon, strawberry, rasberry, gooseberry, grape, apple, orange, pear, lemon, black cherry, cherry, plum, apricot, peach currant.	

Source: Congressional Record, June 21, 1906, 59th Congress, 1st Session, pp. 8891–94.

of additives were excluded from testing requirements in order for the FDA to direct its resources to the more pressing issue of new additives. The initial 1958 GRAS list contained slightly over 200 items and grew to over 600 by 1969. The safety of some substances on this list have been questioned in recent years as newer and more sensitive methods of analysis and evaluation have been developed. An example of a substance that was removed from the GRAS list after reevaluation is cyclamate.

Given the concern about the safety of the foods on this list, a review of GRAS was ordered in 1969. This intensive review is being conducted by scientists associated with the Federation of American Societies for Experimental Biology (FASEB). FASEB first reviewed 415 of the most widely used additives. The results of that review have been published, and the remainder will be reviewed over time. Of the first 415, 305 were given class I status, meaning that they are considered safe for use at current and future anticipated levels under conditions of good manufacturing practices. The 305 items will remain on the GRAS list. The review committee recommended that the other 110 items undergo further study and placed them in classes from II to IV, as shown in Table 9–2.

The most controversial section of the 1958 Food Additives Amendment was the Delaney clause, sponsored by Congressman Delaney (D-NY). The clause prohibits the use of a food additive if any quantity of it is found to induce cancer when ingested by humans or animals. In 1960 the Color Additives Amendment was passed, requiring that all color additives be shown to be safe prior to use. Color additives are prohibited where they will deceive the consumer, conceal inferiority or damage, or otherwise result in misbranding or adulteration.(2)

Who Protects the Public?

Three federal regulatory agencies are responsible for most food and nutrition policies in the United States: the Federal Trade Commission (FTC), the Food and Drug Administration (FDA), and the U.S. Department of Agriculture (USDA). Over the years a few other agencies acquired certain responsibilities; for example, the Treasury Department sets the standards for alcoholic beverages.

The FTC tries to ensure that food advertising is fair and does not deceive the public. The agency can regulate ads and promotional material but has no jurisdiction over books, pamphlets, and speeches. In these, writers can make any claims they want and are protected by the First Amendment, which guarantees freedom of speech.

Both the FDA and USDA promote food safety. The USDA monitors meat and poultry, which includes an inspection process that begins with the live animal and continues through slaughter and processing. This department also sets the standards for grading food according to quality. You may recall seeing

TABLE 9–2	Classification of GRAS Items
Class I:	Considered safe for use at current and anticipated levels under conditions of good manufacturing practices. Includes 305 ingredients such as vegetable oils, casein, tartrates, aluminum compounds, benzoates, protein hydrolyzates.
Class II:	Safe for use at current levels, but more research is needed to determine whether a significant increase in consumption would constitute a dietary hazard. Includes 68 substances such as some zinc salts, alginates, iron and some iron salts, tannic acid, sucrose, vitamins A and D.
Class III:	Additional studies recommended because of unresolved questions in research data. Includes caffeine, BHA, and BHT.
Class IV:	FDA urged to establish safer conditions or prohibit addition of the ingredient to foods. Includes 5 substances: salt and four modified starches.
Class V:	Insufficient data on which to make a recommendation. Includes 18 substances such as glycerides and certain iron salts, and carnauba wax.

Source: FDA Consumer, March 1981, p. 15.

"US Grade A" on a food product enclosed within the outline of a shield. The standards the product had to meet to receive such a grade are set by the USDA.

The FDA administers the Federal Food, Drug and Cosmetic Act of 1938 and the amendments to it, so a large proportion of the food supply falls within the domain of this agency. It makes periodic inspections of plants, investigates consumer complaints of improper labeling, and monitors food additives, colors, and pesticide residues.

Today there are few attempts at food adulteration as blatant as those in the nineteenth century. In fact, the FDA considers food-related hazards of natural origin to be a greater threat to the population than those of man-made origin. The list of dangers posed by food, as ranked by the FDA, follows in descending order of importance:(3)

1. Food-borne disease, especially botulism
2. Malnutrition
3. Environmental contaminants
4. Naturally occurring toxins
5. Pesticide residues
6. Deliberate additives

Food-borne disease refers to illness caused by microbial growth in the food. Malnutrition includes both undernutrition and overnutrition, the latter being the more pressing problem in the United States. Environmental contaminants are substances that enter food and water as a result of exposure to such factors as smoke, fumes, and dust. Naturally occurring toxins are harmful substances present as natural components of food. Scientists actually know more about the safety of substances intentionally added to food than about these naturally occurring toxins. Pesticide residues refer to substances used to control insects and other pests that destroy crops. These enter the food supply mainly when animals eat plants sprayed with pesticides and humans then eat the flesh and products of these animals. Additives are a large array of substances added to food either intentionally or accidentally. The FDA ranks these lowest in order of food hazards, yet they are of enormous concern to the public.

FOOD ADDITIVES

A food additive is a natural or synthetic substance or a mixture of substances present in a food as a result of any aspect of production, processing, storage, or packaging. This includes substances that get into food accidentally. There are some 2,800 substances intentionally added to foods to produce a desired effect. These are called intentional additives. As many as 10,000 others find their way into various foods through some aspect of processing, packaging, or storage and are called incidental additives.(4)

Manufacturers use intentional additives for specific reasons: (1) to maintain or improve nutritional quality, (2) to preserve and prevent spoilage, (3) to help in processing or preparation, and (4) to make food more appealing, often called "cosmetic purposes."

An incidental additive could be a substance such as a small piece of cellophane that enters food during packaging or processing, or it could be small amounts of insect parts in wheat flour. Indeed, a certain number of insect parts, rodent hairs, and vermin are allowed in agricultural products because it is so difficult to keep food free of them. Trace elements occur in all foods and are often a result of accidental contamination. Exposure of food to these elements occurs through dust, fumes, pesticides, feed additives, and metals used in food processing and cooking. Some historians speculate that the fall of the Roman Empire was due to the lead in the wine which, over time, resulted in a large number of cases of brain damage. There are a few recorded cases of zinc poisoning from prolonged consumption of water from galvanized pipes and vessels.(5) Several cases of severe cardiac failure in heavy beer drinkers were attributed to high levels of cobalt.(5) With increased industrialization and the release of numerous pollutants into the environment, it is difficult to determine how many of these trace minerals in modern foods originate naturally and how many from incidental contamination.

Nutritive Additives

Even among the best-fed populations in the world, nutrient deficiencies have occurred because the food supply was insufficient in the nutrients or because people made poor food choices. In order to ensure that the food supply provides all the essential nutrients, the U.S. government has designed programs whereby specific nutrients are added to popular foods. This practice is called enrichment, restoration, and fortification of foods.

Enrichment applies to the addition of four specific nutrients (thiamin, riboflavin, niacin, and iron) to bread, flour, and cereal products. The amounts are set by the government. Originally enrichment was intended to prevent iron-deficiency anemia, pellagra, and beriberi.

Restoration is quite similar to enrichment in that manufacturers restore to foods nutrients that were present originally but that have been destroyed or lost in processing. The difference between the two terms is that enrichment refers specifically to cereal products, while restoration refers to other foods.

Fortification is the addition of one or more nutrients that were not present or were present in small amounts in the natural food. Fortification not only restores nutrients lost during processing and storage, but can be used to combat deficiency diseases by providing nutrients lacking in the diet. With today's food supply, it also helps ensure that substitute foods are nutritionally balanced.(6) Actually a product such as a breakfast cereal can be said to be both enriched and fortified, because it is a cereal product with iron, niacin, thiamin, and riboflavin added, and an array of other nutrients not originally there, such as vitamins C and D, are also added.

The following are the most common practices in enriching, restoring, and fortifying foods:

- The enrichment of flour, bread, degerminated cornmeal, and white rice with thiamin, riboflavin, niacin, and iron. The restoration of thiamin, riboflavin, niacin, and iron in processed food cereals. (A comparison of whole wheat and enriched white bread is shown in Table 9–3.)

- The fortification of milk, fluid skim milk, and nonfat dry milk with vitamin D.

- The fortification of margarine, fluid skim milk, and nonfat dry milk with vitamin A.

- The fortification of table salt with iodine.

- The addition of fluoride to water in areas where the water supply has low fluoride content.

- The fortification of some fruit juices and most fruit drinks with vitamin C.

TABLE 9–3 Whole Wheat vs. Enriched White Bread

Nutrient	Whole Wheat (unenriched)	Enriched White
Thiamin (B-1)		√
Riboflavin (B-2)		√
Niacin		√
Iron	(about the same)	
Vitamin B-6	√	
Vitamin E	√	
Trace minerals	√	

√ = contains the higher percentage of the RDA per slice.

Nonnutritive additives are put into food for purposes other than the improvement of nutrient quality. Usually they preserve the food or add cosmetic appeal. Below are some of the many categories of nonnutritive additives.

Preservatives maintain appearance, palatability, and wholesomeness of food by delaying deterioration from mold, bacteria, and yeast. Sugar and salt are commonly used for these purposes. Other preservatives include sodium benzoate, sorbic acid, potassium sorbate, and nitrates.

Antioxidants prevent changes in color or flavor by binding with oxygen so it cannot react with components of the food and cause undesirable changes. Certain fruits and vegetables like apples, apricots, bananas, cherries, peaches, and potatoes have naturally occurring enzymes that cause the food to darken once exposed to air if cut or bruised. Antioxidants retard this discoloration. They also prevent fats, oils, and formulated foods containing fats from developing rancid tastes and odors.

Flavor additives make up the largest group of food additives. They include spices, both synthetic and natural; and liquid derivatives of onion, cloves, and peppermint. Since there are not enough natural flavors to satisfy demand and since those that are available are costly, manufacturers use synthetic substances to impart the flavor of such items as strawberries, grapes, and cherries. Labels must indicate whether flavors are used in products. For instance, "strawberry yogurt" means the product contains all natural strawberry flavor; "strawberry flavored yogurt" indicates that other natural flavorings have been added to the natural strawberry flavor; "artificially flavored strawberry yogurt" means the product is flavored completely by artificial flavorings or by a combination of artificial and natural flavors.(7)

Flavor enhancers such as monosodium glutamate (MSG) do not add flavor; they magnify the natural flavor of foods. Some work by deadening nerves responsible for certain unwanted flavors, allowing other flavors to be intensified.

Color additives can be synthetic or natural, but more than 90 percent now in use are synthetic because they are stronger than natural colors and can be used in smaller amounts at less cost. They are made from aniline (derived from petroleum), which in its pure or uncombined form is poisonous.(2) Dyes have complex chemical names, so the FDA has given them simplified official names consisting of primary colors, followed by *F.D. and C.* (Food, Drugs, and Cosmetics).(2) Synthetic colors are used in soft drinks, candy, frozen desserts, gelatin and puddings, maraschino cherries, meat casings, prepared mixes, and some baked goods. Natural colors include beet powder, caramel, grapeskin extract, juices of edible fruits and vegetables, paprika, saffron, cochineal extract (taken from the dried bodies of insects), and carotene.

Emulsifiers improve the uniformity, fineness of grain, smoothness, and body of such products as baked foods, ice cream, and candy. They permit the dispersion of tiny particles of globules of one liquid in another. For example, oil and vinegar used in a salad dressing will separate as soon as mixing stops. With the addition of an emulsifier, they stay combined longer, as will the components of peanut butter and mayonnaise. Many emulsifiers come from natural sources. An example is lecithin. The lecithin in milk keeps the fat and water together; egg yolks, also containing lecithin, improve the texture of ice cream and mayonnaise. Mono- and diglycerides, used to make bread soft, improve the stability of margarine, and keep the oil and peanuts from separating in peanut butter, come from vegetables or animal tallow.(7).

Stabilizers and thickeners impart smooth texture and help maintain flavor. Chocolate milk and instant breakfasts, made basically of skim milk, contain stabilizers to thicken the milk and prevent separation of the chocolate. Carageenan, a seaweed derivative, is widely used in diet milk products and infant formula. In commercial ice cream and other frozen desserts, stabilizers often are used to increase viscosity and help prevent the water in the product from freezing into crystals. Most stabilizers and thickeners are natural substances such as gelatin (from animal bones or hooves), pectin (from citrus rind), and vegetable gums (from trees, seaweed, and other plants). Common food additives and their functions are shown in Table 9–4.

Testing for Safety

In order for the FDA to approve a new additive, a manufacturer must first subject the substance to chemical tests to determine if it performs as expected. The additive is fed in large doses over an extended period of time to two species of animals, usually rodents and dogs, to see if it causes cancer, birth defects, or injury. If the additive is approved, the manufacturer can only use 1/100th of the maximum amount that was found not to produce any harmful effects in the test animals. This rule is called the *100-fold margin of safety.* So if a 100-milligram dose of an additive was the highest dose given an animal before harmful side effects occurred, the largest dose acceptable for use in foods would be 1/100th of this, or 1 milligram. If a substance causes cancer, it cannot be used at all. Once a manufacturer submits test results of the FDA, the agency decides how the additive can be used in food. GRAS and prior sanctioned substances are exempt from this procedure.

Part of the reason for greater concern over additives is that testing procedures have become so sophisticated that additives once considered safe are now being banned. Scientists must try to answer the question of whether traces of additives in infinitesimal amounts are as hazardous as when present in higher concentrations.

Risk versus Benefit

The toxicity of a substance is its ability to produce injury when tested by itself. The hazard of a substance is its ability to produce injury when used under normal circumstances. For instance, potatoes and cabbage contain toxic substances, but they are present in such small amounts that they pose little danger

TABLE 9–4 Common Food Additives

Chemical	Sources	Foods in Which Used	Function
Adipic acid	Synthetic	Gelatin desserts	Flavor
Amino acids	Natural and synthetic	Breads, cereals	Nutrition supplement
Butylated hydroxyanisole (BHA)	Synthetic	Pastries, crackers, potato chips	Antioxidant
Butylated hydroxytoluene (BHT)	Synthetic	Cereals, nuts, soup mixes	Antioxidant
Calcium propionate Sodium propionate	Synthetic	Baked goods	Mold inhibitor
Calcium silicate	Natural	Powders and crystalline substances, baking powder	Anticaking agent
Carageenan	Natural (from plants) and synthetic	Liquid diet foods, cottage cheese	Stabilizer, thickener
Citric acid	Natural (from citrus fruits) and synthetic	Candies, soft drinks, jams, gelatin desserts	Flavor
EDTA (ethylenediamine tetra acetic acid)	Synthetic	Margarine, cheeses, salad dressings	Sequestrant (prevents rancidity by combining with metallic catalysts of oxidation)
Gelatin	Natural (from bones) and synthetic	Icings, flavored milk, cheese spreads	Stabilizer, thickener
Guar gum, gum arabic	Natural and synthetic	Instant breakfast drinks, syrups, gravies	Stabilizer, thickener
Lecithin	Natural (from egg yolk and soybeans)	Salad dressings, ice cream, cakes	Emulsifier
Maltol	Synthetic	Soft drinks, jams, gelatin desserts	Flavor intensifier

Additive	Source	Found in	Function
Methyl salicylate	Synthetic	Grape, mint, and nut flavors	Flavor
Mono- and diglycerides	Synthetic	Shortenings, ice cream, baked goods	Antistaling agents, emulsifiers
Monocalcium phosphate	Natural	Baked goods	Leavening agent
Monosodium glutamate	Synthetic	Prepared meats, fish, soup mixes, canned foods, cheese spreads	Flavor intensifier
Phosphoric acid	Natural and synthetic	Candies, soft drinks, jams, gelatin desserts	Flavor
Polysorbates	Synthetic	Sherbet, soft drinks	Emulsifier
Potassium iodide	Natural	Table salt	Nutrition supplement
Propylene glycol monostearate	Synthetic	Whipped toppings, ice cream, salad dressings, candy, frostings, cakes	Emulsifier
Saccharin	Synthetic	Low-kcalorie foods	Artificial sweetener
Sodium aluminum phosphate	Natural	Baked goods	Leavening agent
Sodium sulfite	Synthetic	Sliced apples, potatoes, fruits, and vegetables	Antibrowning agent
Sorbic acid, potassium sorbate	Synthetic	Cheese, chocolate, syrups, jellies, cakes, dried fruits	Mold inhibitor
Sorbitan monostearate	Synthetic	Baked goods, salad dressings, ice cream	Emulsifier
Tocopherols	Natural (from vegetable oils)	Cereals, Butter, fats, meat products, potato chips	Antioxidant
Vitamins	Natural and synthetic	Butter, milk, breads, flours, juices, cereals, macaroni products	Nutritional supplement

under normal use. Safety requires proof of reasonable certainty that no harm will result from the proposed use of an additive; it does not require proof beyond any possible doubt that no harm will result under any circumstance. Every substance will cause harm in laboratory animals in large enough doses; there is no substance, even in small amounts, that will not cause harm to a small number of people who are sensitive to it.

At best, scientists can estimate the hazards of a substance and compare these to the benefits derived from using that substance. For example, saccharin remains on the market because diabetics and weight watchers feel their desire for a nonnutritive sweetener outweighs the potential risks of bladder cancer. Some consumers say banning potentially harmful substances is a restriction of freedom. Cigarettes and alcohol pose a greater health hazard than saccharin, but would Americans allow these products to be banned?

It can be worth taking a small degree of risk with an additive if its use increases the food supply by making the food more available or allowing it to last longer, or if it increases the nutritive value of food or drastically reduces the cost to the consumer. Improving flavor, color, or texture are much less justifiable reasons for taking risks.

Health food stores are often good sources of bulk grains and beans though many of their products, such as megadose supplements of minerals and vitamins, are of questionable value.

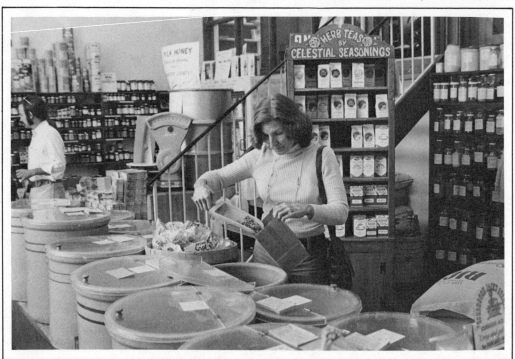

Issue

Organic, Natural, and Health Foods

How "natural" are natural foods? What allows certain foods to be called organic? And just how beneficial to health are health foods? A huge industry has developed around these special categories of food. In 1974, it was projected that organic food retail sales would reach $3 billion in 1980, a rise from $500 million in 1972.(8) Organic, natural, and health foods usually cost more than conventional foods. Such high costs can be a problem for the low-income consumer or for anyone trying to whittle down a food budget. Do organic, natural, and health foods offer enough advantages over regular foods that it is worth paying higher prices for them? Or are they no different from conventional foods?

The term *health food* is often used when referring to a food or ingredient that some people believe is beneficial in promoting physiological and psychological well-being and assuring optimal resistance to stress, infection, and disease. Rice, bran, yogurt, wheat germ oil, and royal jelly (honey) have all achieved this status at some point in time.

The term *organic* has probably been misused more than any other. The word itself technically means a substance containing carbon. All food, whether from animal or vegetable sources, is organic. In recent years the term has been loosely used to refer to "organically grown" food, meaning those foods grown without the use of any agricultural chemicals and processed without the use of food chemicals or additives. These are usually grown in soil fertilized by organic fertilizers of various types. Oregon is the only state with a legal definition of organically grown foods, and even this definition allows for a small amount of pesticide residues on foods.

Foods that are not changed in any way after agricultural production are called *natural foods*. The FTC, in a proposed Food Advertising Rule, states that for foods to be advertised as "natural," they may not contain synthetic or artificial ingredients and may not be more than "minimally processed." "Minimal processing" includes such actions as washing or peeling fruits or vegetables; homogenizing milk; canning, bottling, and freezing food; baking bread; aging and roasting meats; and grinding nuts. If the process cannot generally be done in a home kitchen or involves certain types of chemicals or sophisticated technology, then it is not a "minimal process" and if applied to a food the term "natural" cannot be used in its advertising.(8,9)

A major criticism of health, organic, or natural foods is that they are often not what they are billed to be. Health food store managers have even been found to offer the same food available in supermarkets under a different label.

- Anything added to the food supply is potentially dangerous.
- Pesticides are poisonous and Scontribute undesirable residues to food.

- Chemical fertilizers produce plants of inferior nutritional quality and in turn result in inferior nutrition for animals and humans. Conversely, organic fertilizers are superior to chemical fertilizers.

Each of these positions has an element of truth. In some, only the barest trace of validity is present; in others, a real issue exists. A closer look at the three types of foods and the movements behind them may help to clear up any confusion concerning their advantages over regular foods.

EVALUATING FOOD CLAIMS AND RISKS

Health Foods

Prior to World War II a small but stable market existed in health foods. Disease-prevention claims were passed by word of mouth or in an occasional article or book. This narrow market appealed almost exclusively to consumers who viewed the products as effective in the prevention of disease or death. This type of consumer is like the true believer of today who considers vitamins, minerals, and other supplements as natural cures for many diseases. These individuals sometimes ignore the known functions of these nutrients in the body.

Claim. Certain foods are so high in particular nutrients that they possess miracle value or have curative powers for a whole host of common and uncommon diseases and illnesses.

Response. Some nutrients have appeared to perform miracles in curing certain deficiency diseases because minute amounts do cure such illnesses as beriberi and scurvy. None of the nutrients, as far as is known, work special miracles when taken in addition to an adequate diet. Amounts in excess of physiological needs do not promote health and virility, nor do excessive amounts reverse the aging process. Promotion of foods on the basis of special curative properties is quackery. It is a dangerous practice if people substitute miracle foods for medical care or other proper attention.

Health foods are not only supposed to promote health, but are claimed to be totally safe. Many, however, contain natural toxicants. Herbal teas, for instance, contain numerous chemicals that have never been tested for safety. Traditionally, herbal teas were used in weak, diluted solutions. Now people often consume them in large amounts, unaware that many contain potentially harmful substances. Tea from the bark of the sassafras root contains safrole, known to cause liver cancer in rats. Certain herbs, like burdock and golden-seal, are toxic in high dosages. Active ingredients in herbal teas vary with the plant used, the stage of plant growth at harvest, and the growing location, so foragers should exercise caution before brewing up wild plants.

Organic Foods

The organic food movement originated during the 1940s but gained its present dimensions from the ecological and environmental movements of the 1960s. Concern over environmental pollution and the risk of toxicity from the use of chemical pesticides are two factors motivating this new consumer group.

Claim.   Pesticides (insecticides, herbicides, fungicides) and chemical fertilizers are poisonous and contribute undesirable residues to food. In addition, chemical or inorganic fertilizers produce plants of inferior nutritional quality and, in turn, inferior nutrition for animals and humans. Conversely, organic fertilizers are superior to chemical fertilizers.

Response.   Pesticides certainly have the potential to be harmful if misused, and it is important to maintain careful surveillance to keep the food supply as free of pesticide residues as possible. But the problem with organically grown foods is that there is no guarantee they are pesticide-free. Some pesticide residues remain in the soil for years after the last application on a crop. If land has been recently converted to an organic farm, chemical residues will remain in the soil and contaminate the food for a number of years. Even if a farm has been in operation for years, fresh residues from drifting sprays and dusts or from rainfall runoff from nearby farms can contaminate crops.(8) A 1972 New York state survey found pesticide residues on 30 percent of the organic foods studied and on only 20 percent of the regular supermarket foods.(10)

Do these residues make food unfit for consumption? Although no consumers have ever been harmed by pesticides used in accordance with regulations and directions,(11) accidental contamination resulting in acute toxicity has occurred on a number of occasions. The position that these substances contribute undesirable residues to food has merit; their use should be carefully evaluated and controlled. Some are poisonous and must be removed from food before it is eaten; others are nontoxic in the immediate sense, but scientists do not know about the long-term implications.

A recent report indicates that some farmers in the United States have been able to cut back substantially on use of pesticides without reducing crop yield.(12) However, eliminating the use of all pesticides would cause a drop in world food production. Insects multiply at a phenomenal rate, about 191 quadrillion offspring in a single summer. Efforts at using nonchemical means of insect control such as insect parasites, insect predators, insect disease, and sex pheromones are underway, but total biological control is years away.(3)

As plants grow, they use up nutrients in the soil that must be added back through fertilization. Farmers use fertilizers to produce high yields and to grow crops on otherwise infertile soils. Depleted soil reduces crop yield. Chemical or inorganic fertilizers are fertilizers that are synthetic and whose elements exist in simple chemical form. Organic, in the context used by advocates of such fertilizers, means that the fertilizers were not synthesized in a laboratory but were derived from a living source. Such fertilizers usually exist in a more complex chemical form, generally in association with carbon. The rationale often given for the superiority of organic fertilizers is that a substance derived from living sources can best enhance the soil's ability to support plants which yield foods of high nutritive value for humans. In fact, plants do not use organic matter but take up inorganic minerals from the soil and carbon dioxide from the air. The complex forms of nitrogen, phosphorus, and potassium from manure or other organic matter must be broken down into simple ones. This is precisely what is present in chemical fertilizers: simple, inorganic forms of the minerals required by plants. Once absorbed, plants cannot tell the difference.

Both chemical and organic fertilizers may be adequate or deficient, depending upon how well the composition of the fertilizer matches the needs of the soil. Inorganic fertilizers can be tailor-made to contain the elements in the proportions needed by a specific soil to support plant growth. Organic fertilizers such as manure or turned-under cover crops can be unbalanced and perpetuate a soil deficiency.

Organic fertilizers do add texture to the soil in a way that chemical fertilizers cannot. They build good physical soil characteristics such as tilth, aeration, and holding capacity for water and nutrients.(3) They also serve to recycle wastes. Mulches are useful in conserving moisture and controlling weeds. In addition, the energy requirements of organic farmers are less than those of conventional farmers(12) because the energy cost of producing chemical fertilizers is very great. A recent United States Department of Agriculture report on organic farming was quite favorable. It stated the following:(12)

Contrary to popular belief most organic farmers have not regressed to agriculture as it was practiced in the 1930s. While they attempt to avoid or restrict the use of chemical fertilizers and pesticides, organic farmers use modern farm machinery, recommended crop varieties, certified seed, sound methods of organic waste management, and recommended soil and water practices.

The report concluded that "the greatest opportunity for organic farming will probably be on small farms and on larger mixed crop/livestock farms with large numbers of animal units."(12)

Regardless of the type of fertilizer used, the protein, fat, carbohydrate, and vitamin composition of the plants is determined by the genetic composition of the seed and the maturity of the plant at harvest. Fertilizers affect only the mineral composition. Commercial fertilizers can be relied on to provide a specified amount of these minerals. Test trials have shown that plants grown with chemical fertilizers are equally if not more nutritious than those grown organically. For this reason, special health claims for organic foods cannot legally be put on labels, though it is legal to distribute literature and display articles next to advertisements for them.(13)

In general, organic foods look and taste like and have similar nutrient composition to regular foods. The only way to be sure a product is organic is to know the grower, distributor, and retailer and to check soil and water reports.

Natural Foods

Those desiring natural foods are motivated by three wishes. The first is a wish to return to that period of American history when daily life is believed to have been simpler and more meaningful and when the family was the central unit. These consumers have a growing interest in home activities, such as arts and crafts, as well as cooking and baking. They are willing to exchange some level of convenience in the kitchen for a sense of achievement. A second motivating factor among this group is their genuine concern over the environment and the growing importance of technology in our culture. They fear that health and the general quality of life are compromised for convenience. The third motivation is fear of food additives and a belief that food as it comes from nature is safest. Their fears increase as more and more challenges are made against substances on the GRAS list and with stronger demands that other substances be banned by enforcement of the Delaney Clause.

Claim. Foods are safer and more nutritious as they appear in nature; anything added to the food supply is potentially dangerous. There are too many chemicals in the food supply today.

Response. All additives, whether from nature or from the laboratory, are chemical. For that matter, all foods are chemical. The use of additives is not new, but the surge in their use in recent times has raised issues that place a serious responsibility on food technologists and the government.

Risks versus Benefits of Nutritive Additives

In the past, additives have been used rashly to adulterate, "upgrade," confuse the consumer, and otherwise spoil a good food. Few would argue against the elimination of additives in these cases. Few would also argue strongly against the use of additives to improve food nutritionally in cases where this serves a common good. The basic problem lies in resolving the issues between the two extremes of the obviously good and the obviously bad additives.

For example, fortification can enhance the nutritive value of foods, but critics claim that the health problems of today are linked to fats, fiber, sweets, sodium and kcalories, and will not be solved by putting vitamins and minerals in food. They feel that foods are overfortified, pointing to breakfast cereals which generally are high in sugar but so fortified with vitamins and minerals that manufacturers promote them as nutritious. They predict that manufacturers will start fortifying nutrient-poor foods like candy with vitamins and minerals in order to increase sales.

An unforeseen backlash to fortification came when consumers argued they have a right to determine whether or not their food has added nutrients. This is not a problem with products such as juices and salt which can be purchased with or without the added nutrients. In the case of fluoridated water, however, consumers have little choice unless they resort to bottled water. The case for and against water fluoridation is one of the longest-running battles between public health departments and the public.

Fluoridation of water is done as a public health measure to prevent dental caries(14). It is not a form of medication; rather, it is an adjustment of an essential nutrient to a level favorable to health. Fluoride occurs naturally in foods and water, but in some areas is present only in small amounts.

Another possible benefit of fluoridated water is that it may offer some protection against the bone loss that leads to osteoporosis, a condition common among the elderly. Fluoride in high doses, however, can cause tooth mottling or brown spots. This has occurred only in areas where fluoride is naturally present in high amounts, not from fluoridation of the water supply. In order for fluoride to be toxic, a person must consume 20 to 80 milligrams daily for years. Fluoridated water provides only about 1 milligram a day.

Benefits and Risks of Nonnutritive Additives

In 1928 the number of items offered in a typical grocery store was about 900; today that number exceeds 12,000. Some of these foods are basic items that are now available in different forms, such as canned, frozen, or dried. Others are highly processed and fabricated.

Natural food advocates fear that some additives known to cause harm in animals are allowed in the human food supply. For example, two of the most controversial antioxidants, butylated hydroxyanisole (BHA) and butylated hydroxytoluene (BHT), widely used in cereals, snack foods, and soup mixes, caused enlarged livers in laboratory rats. BHT was removed from the GRAS list in 1973 and is currently being tested for possible adverse effects on health. Ironically, these two additives are currently being investigated for their possible role in decreasing stomach cancer in the United States by their ability to inhibit certain carcinogens.

The removal of additives from the GRAS list or actual banning of those additives only recently in use creates further alarm about those remaining in use. Examples are safrole and coumarin, which were banned as flavoring agents(15) and monosodium glutamate (MSG), which was banned as a flavoring agent in infant foods. MSG, however, can still be used in other foods, although some people are sensitive to it and experience tightening of the face and neck muscles, headaches, nausea, and giddiness. This group of symptoms are together called the Chinese Restaurant Syndrome, so named because Chinese foods are typically high in MSG to bring out the flavor of the vegetables.

Color additives are the most controversial of all the additives. Opponents to their use claim they contribute nothing to nutrition, taste, safety, or ease of processing, and are used only to give products better sales appeal at the risk of increasing health hazards. In the past decade, the FDA has prohibited four colors from use in foods: a violet used to stamp meats; Red No. 2, suspected to cause cancer; Red No. 4, used in maraschino cherries and shown to cause bladder lesions in animals; and Carbon Black, used in candies such as licorice and jelly beans. Manufacturers voluntarily stopped producing Orange B, used in sausage and hotdog casings, because of possible contamination with a carcinogen. The two most widely used food colors now are Red No. 40, suspected of causing premature lymph tumors in mice, and Yellow No. 5, a substance that causes an allergic reaction in 50,000 to 90,000 Americans. Because of these adverse effects, the FDA is reviewing a petition to ban Red No. 40 and has proposed a regulation requiring manufacturers to list Yellow No. 5 on labels to warn consumers sensitive to it.(15)

Hyperactivity. A final risk that has been associated with nonnutritive additives is that they may contribute to hyperactivity in children. Hyperactivity describes a child of normal intelligence who has a short attention span and is easily distracted. The child may also have trouble with coordination and motor skills. No one knows what causes hyperactivity, but suggestions include genetics, brain damage, crowded homes, high population density, demanding parents, lead poisoning, fluorescent lights, and now diet.

Dr. Benjamin Feingold, a California pediatrician, has proposed the theory that hyperactivity in children is caused by salicylate compounds in natural foods and by artificial food flavors and colors. It is difficult to measure hyperactivity, since ratings by teachers and parents are highly subjective. Even so, seven studies involving about 190 children have been conducted to determine if food additives cause hyperactivity. The results of these studies were reviewed by a panel of medical and behavioral scientists.(16)

The panel concluded that food colors and salicylates were not the cause of hyperactivity in children, although a few children may have a rare genetic susceptibility to certain ones and show behavioral problems when they consume these additives. The panel recommended that the safety of food colors be monitored as should that of all additives, not because of the relationship to hyperactivity, but for all possible effects. They admitted that the food-additive-free diet has no harmful effects and can actually be beneficial to families because of its placebo effects. One problem with these studies is that they focused on food colors, not all food additives, so demands for more research in this area are sure to continue.

The FDA is currently involved in a cycle review program to evaluate the safety of all food and color additives, including the GRAS list, intentional additives, and incidental additives. The degree of consumer exposure to food additives based on food consumption data is also being assessed.

Issue

Junk Food/Fast Food

Americans spend $250 billion a year on food—that is about $1000 for every person in the United States.(17) Thirty percent goes to institutional and restaurant foods, with an expected increase to 50 percent by 1985.(18) To put it simply, Americans like to eat out.

With so much of the food dollar going to foods prepared outside the home, many nutrition-minded consumers wonder just what it is they are getting for their money. Parents of school-age children shudder at the thought of a school vending machine stuffed with candies, cookies, and sodas.

JUNK FOODS

Before we can debate the spread of junk foods into schools and other institutions, we have to define "junk." A few years ago, when the Federal Trade Commission tried to regulate the use of the term "nutritious" in advertising, nutritionists faced the problem of defining nutritious and, by the same token, junk. It wasn't easy.

No food by itself makes a nutritious diet. What is important is a variety of foods that combined provide all the essential nutrients and energy in amounts necessary to health but not in excess to cause fat accumulation. Whether a food is nutritious or junk varies with the context of the total diet.(19) In short, there are no junk foods, only junky diets. Is an orange nutritious if the person eating it has already met all nutrient needs except calcium? Wouldn't a calcium-rich source be more nutritious for this person? What about the athlete who has met all daily nutrient requirements but who still needs kcalories? If this person chooses to eat a pastry, is that pastry junk even though it provides the necessary kcalories? What is it that makes some foods better for you than others? Should certain items be avoided altogether because they are nutritionally worthless?

In general, the nutrient density concept (Chapter 2) is a good measure of the overall quality of foods and diets. If a diet is made up of foods with high nutrient density, it is more likely to be nutritious than one made up of low nutrient-dense foods. The Index of Nutrient Quality (INQ) equals:

$$\frac{\text{Nutrient in food} \div \text{nutrient needed daily*}}{\text{kcalories in food} \div \text{kcalories needed daily**}}$$

*(usually expressed as the U.S. RDA or RDA)
**(usually based on 2000 to 2200 kcalories)

Foods are often considered junk if they have too many kcalories with too few nutrients. These kcalories usually come from fats and sugars. If the fats or sugars add too many kcalories in proportion to other nutrients, the food will have an INQ below 1. If, despite the sugar and fat, the food still manages to keep an INQ above 1 for four or more nutrients, or above 2 for at least two nutrients, it is "holding its own" nutritionally.(19)

The idea of determining a food's value solely on its nutrient content has created some problems. Take the example of Astrofood, a cake made by ITT Continental Baking Company, which is served in school breakfast programs. This high-protein fortified food, when served with a cup of whole milk, provides one-third of the RDA for children, except for kcalories.(18) Is this food nutritious because it meets the RDA or is it junk because, by eating it, children may draw the conclusion that cake is an acceptable breakfast food?

Some nutritionists believe that when manufacturers take a basically empty kcalorie food (one containing mainly energy and few nutrients) and fortify it with four or five nutrients, they are deceiving the consumer, who believes the product is nutritious based on these added nutrients. Often fiber and trace minerals will be missing. Others hold that the worth of a food is the sum of its nutrients (whether they were present naturally or placed there by a manufacturer) as it relates to the consumer's immediate needs. Astrofood, to these nutritionists, is nutritious because it meets one-third of the RDA of children.

The philosophies behind the junk food issue are complex and confusing. In fact, there probably is no single correct position on this issue. Each food has to be evaluated in relation to the situation. But there are some practical suggestions to follow when you choose foods. Try to pick nutrient-dense foods. It is hard to keep track of your nutrient intake over the course of a day, so if you pick foods of high nutrient density you are more assured of a good diet than if you consistently choose empty kcalorie foods. Avoid large amounts of foods high in fats or sugars, or those with a high salt content. Become more aware of your overall diet. Keep a seven-day food record to assess your general pattern of eating. Table 9–5 lists some nutritious snack suggestions.

FAST FOODS

There are an estimated 140,000 fast food places in the United States.(20) A recent Gallup poll showed 33 percent of adults eating out every day, with at least 23 percent eating at fast food places.(20) Lunch is the most popular meal, but breakfasts, dinners, and snacks are also commonly eaten away from home.

The popularity of fast food restaurants stems from their ability to serve inexpensive, filling, and (to some people) tasty foods. They also offer convenience and consistency: You can't tell a Whopper in California from one in Massachusetts. The speed with which you can be served is also a big factor in a society where many people have the money to spend in restaurants and less time to prepare home-cooked meals. Critics of fast food restaurants say they are a blot on the American landscape and reduce eating to on-the-run fillups. Consumer activists condemn fast food as a threat to health. There is no accounting for taste, whether it is in designing arches or hamburgers, but there are ways to determine if fast foods are "junk" or if they have any redeeming nutritional value.

For instance, Table 9–6 compares the INQ values for specific fast food entrees. Nutrients with an INQ value greater than or equal to 1 or 2 are highlighted. The values are based on the requirements of an adult woman (men usually require more energy and nutrients except for iron). In general, these entrees provide plenty of protein, fat, and carbohydrates. The kcalories come mainly from fat, with most of the fats being unsaturated. Most of the carbohydrates are starches, not sugars, surprisingly enough. The vitamins thiamin, riboflavin, B-12, and niacin, and the minerals phosphorus and iron have high INQ values. Although they are not all shown in the table, the nutrients in short supply in fast foods are vitamins A, C, and B-6, and calcium and magnesium.(12) Sodium is high.

The major criticism of fast foods is their fat, kcalorie, and sodium content. Their nutrient pattern parallels changing American food habits: increased fat and sugars, and decreased complex carbohydrates.(20)

Eating at fast food restaurants is acceptable if you do it infrequently and as part of a well-balanced diet. One study(21) found few people relying on fast food for more than three purchases a week. Some people, however, indulged more than six

TABLE 9–5 How to Cure the Munchies

Fresh fruit

Apples	Pears
Peaches	Apricots
Plums	Cherries
Grapes	Oranges
Strawberries	Melon
Pineapple	Banana

Try apple wedges spread with soft cheese or peanut butter.

Finger foods
Nuts, sunflower seeds, pumpkin seeds
Popcorn—plain, or sprinkled with grated cheese or Brewer's yeast
Pickles or olives
Chips—corn or potato, pretzels (avoid those that are highly salted)

Beverages
Juices—any unsweetened
Milk, buttermilk
Water
Banana milk drink (beat a banana into 1 cup cold milk; add strawberries if desired)

For variety
Meat or cheese cubes on toothpicks
Eggs—hardboiled or deviled
Crackers—whole wheat; try with cheese spreads
Yogurt
Cornbread
Carrot and raisin salad
Sandwiches: peanut butter with thin apple slices; cream cheese with olives
Cheese crisp

Dips
A good cheese dip can be made by mixing 1½ cups cottage cheese and ½ cup drained crushed pineapple. Serve carrot, celery, or cucumber sticks for dipping.
Add grated or melted cheese or cottage cheese to refried beans and season to taste. Try Worcestershire sauce, catsup, chili sauce, grated onion.

Source: How to Cure the Munchies, Maricopa (Arizona) County Department of Health Services.

times a week. If you are going to eat at these restaurants, there are ways to maximize the nutrient value of your meals. To keep kcalories down, order a small cheeseburger instead of a superburger; milk instead of a thick shake; cole slaw or salad instead of French fries; and unsweetened iced tea, juice (also for the vitamin C), or water instead of soda. Limit intakes of French fries and shakes, since these greatly increase your kcalorie and sodium consumption. If you regularly eat at fast food restaurants, include in your other meals dark green leafy vegetables, yellow vegetables, fresh fruit, whole grains and cereals, and milk (low-fat or skim if you are having a hard time holding down kcalories).

TABLE 9–6 **Rating of Fast Foods by INQs**

Food	Total INQ Score	Serving Size (oz.)	Kcalories	Fat (grams)	Carbohydrates (grams)	Total Sugars (grams)	Sodium (mg)	≤⅓ daily sodium allowance	% of kcalories from fat ≤ 30
Jack-in-the-Box Jumbo Jack	★	8¼	538	28	44	7	1007		
McDonald's Big Mac	★●	7.5	591	33	46	6	963		
Wendy's Old Fashioned hamburgers	●	6.5	413	22	29	5	708		
Burger King Whopper	★	9	660	41	49	9	1083		
Roy Rogers Roast Beef Sandwich	★	5.5	356	12	34	0	610	✓	✓
Burger King chopped beef steak sandwich	★●	6¾	445	13	50	.7	966		✓
Hardee's Roast Beef sandwich	★	4.5	351	17	32	3	765		
Arby's Roast Beef sandwich	★●	5¼	370	15	36	1	869		
Long John Silver's	★	7½	483	27	27	.1	1333		
Arthur Treacher's Original	●	5¼	439	27	27	.3	421	✓	
McDonald's filet-o-fish	●	4½	383	18	38	3	613	✓	
Burger King Whaler	●	7	584	34	50	5	968		
Kentucky Fried Chicken snack box	★	6¾	405	21	16	0	728		
Arthur Treacher's Original chicken	★	5½	409	23	25	0	580	✓	
Wendy's Chili	★	10	266	9	29	9	1190		✓
Pizza Hut Pizza Supreme	★●	7¾	506	15	64	6	1281		✓
Jack-in-the-Box taco	●	5½	429	26	34	3	926		

Food	Protein	Vitamin A	Thiamin	Riboflavin	Vitamin B-6	Vitamin B-12	Niacin	Calcium	Phosphorus	Iron
Jack-in-the-Box Jumbo Jack	■		■	□		■	■		□	
McDonald's Big Mac	■					■	□			
Wendy's Old Fashioned hamburgers	■									□
Burger King Whopper	□					■	■			□
Roy Rogers Roast Beef Sandwich	■		■	□						
Burger King chopped beef steak sandwich	■		■	□	□	■	■		□	□
Hardee's Roast Beef sandwich	■		■	□		■	■		□	□
Arby's Roast Beef sandwich	■			□		■	■			□
Long John Silver's	■					■	□	□		
Arthur Treacher's Original	■					□	□			
McDonald's filet-o-fish	□		■	□		■	□			
Burger King Whaler	□					■	■			
Kentucky Fried Chicken snack box	■			□	□	■	■			
Arthur Treacher's Original chicken	■					■	■			
Wendy's Chili	■	■	□	□	□	■	□	□	□	■
Pizza Hut Pizza Supreme	■	□	■	□		□	■		□	□
Jack-in-the-Box taco	□	□								

● INQ of 1 for 4 or more nutrients   □ INQ≥1
★ INQ of 2 for 2 or more nutrients   ■ INQ≥2

Source: INQs derived from data in "Fast-Food Chains," *Consumer Reports* (September 1979), p. 509.

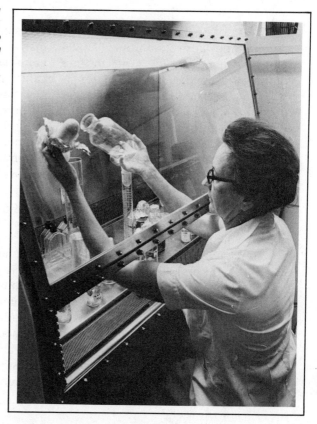

Cancer research is conducted worldwide, although much of the evidence linking diet to cancer is based on epidemiological as well as laboratory studies.

Issue

Cancer

You may think I'm nuts, but I think that a heck of a lot of the "cancer epidemic" is due to the preservatives that are put in bread...both rich and poor get cancer, and we all eat bread.

From a consumer's letter to the FDA(6)

Cancer refers to a number of diseases characterized by uncontrolled growth and spread of abnormal cells.(22) These spreading cells are called *tumors* or neoplasms. A neoplasm can be benign and simply fill a space in the body, or it can be malignant and invade the surrounding tissue by way of the blood or lymph. A carcinogen is a substance that causes malignant tumors to develop in greater incidence than would occur spontaneously.

Cancer is the second leading

cause of death, estimated to have claimed approximately 405,000 lives in 1980.(22) One in five deaths in the United States is cancer-related, and one in every four Americans will develop it.

Cancer can strike any part of the body, although at present the leading types, in decreasing order of occurrence, are cancers of the lung, large intestine, and breast (Figure 9–1). The good news is that death rates from some cancers like breast, colon, and rectum have not changed since 1930, while others, like stomach and uterine cancers, have declined. The only cancer that is on the rise is lung cancer, which is due not to food, but to cigarette smoking (Figure 9–2).

Two factors are needed for cancer to develop: a carcinogen and a susceptible host. There are as many theories on how carcinogens work as there are types of cancers.

It has been estimated that 80 to 90 percent of all human cancers are related to one or more environmental factors, making them potentially preventable.(23) These factors include drugs, alcohol, contaminants in air and water, tobacco smoke, hair dyes, radiation, and viruses. The problem with studying these factors is that it can take 20 years after a carcinogen is introduced into the environment before cancer symptoms become evident in the population.(24) After so much time has elapsed, it is difficult to separate out any other intervening variables that may have exerted an influence.

FIG. 9–1

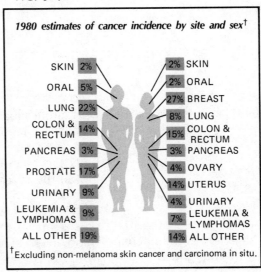

1980 estimates of cancer incidence by site and sex[†]

SKIN	2%		2%	SKIN
ORAL	5%		2%	ORAL
			27%	BREAST
LUNG	22%		8%	LUNG
COLON & RECTUM	14%		15%	COLON & RECTUM
PANCREAS	3%		3%	PANCREAS
PROSTATE	17%		4%	OVARY
			14%	UTERUS
URINARY	9%		4%	URINARY
LEUKEMIA & LYMPHOMAS	9%		7%	LEUKEMIA & LYMPHOMAS
ALL OTHER	19%		14%	ALL OTHER

[†]Excluding non-melanoma skin cancer and carcinoma in situ.

Source: Cancer Facts and Figures, 1980 (New York: American Cancer Society, 1979), p. 8.

FIG. 9-2

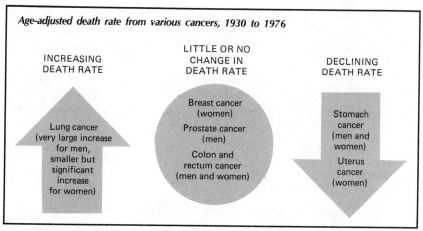

Age-adjusted death rate from various cancers, 1930 to 1976

INCREASING DEATH RATE

LITTLE OR NO CHANGE IN DEATH RATE

DECLINING DEATH RATE

Lung cancer (very large increase for men, smaller but significant increase for women)

Breast cancer (women)

Prostate cancer (men)

Colon and rectum cancer (men and women)

Stomach cancer (men and women)

Uterus cancer (women)

Source: M.W. Pariza, "Food Safety: From the Eye of a Hurricane," *Professional Nutritionist,* fall 1979, p. 14.

Evidence for a Dietary Role in Cancer

The occurrence of cancer differs among populations. Migrant studies show the cancer incidence and death rate for immigrants change from that of their native population to that of their host country even if both countries have similar rates of pollution and food contamination.(25) Japanese migrants to the United States develop less stomach and more colon cancer than native Japanese, until by the third generation their patterns become similar to those of American whites. The native Japanese diet differs from the American in having fewer kcalories and fat. Colon cancer strikes other population groups at different rates. There is a high rate among New York Jews and a low rate among Seventh-Day Adventists. Seventh-Day Adventists have much lower rates of many cancers than other Americans. Their diet contains less meat, fish, coffee, tea, and milk than the typical American diet.

The rate of cancer of the esophagus differs in various communities. The highest rates are in northern Iran, where the people eat coarse wheat, few fruits and vegetables, and drink no alcohol, and in parts of eastern and southern Africa, where consumption of home-brewed beers is high.(26)

Could these differences in the occurrence of cancer be caused by the dietary differences among the groups? Recall from Chapter 4 that these kinds of findings, called correlations, refer to two factors changing in a corresponding manner. They do not prove that one of the factors caused the other to change. Correlations, though, do point the way for research studies to determine cause and effect. Thus it is important to examine the correlations between diet and the occurrence of cancer. The occurrence of at least half of all cancers in women and one-third in men are correlated with intake of some dietary components.(25,27) The types of cancers where these correlations exist are those of the mouth, esophagus, stomach, colon, rectum, liver, bladder, and indirectly with cancers of the breast and uterus. In some cases occurrence increases with high intakes of the dietary component, while in other cases it decreases. The risk of developing a particular cancer may be increased or decreased by intake of certain substances or nutrients.

Diet is believed to influence the risk of cancer in two ways. First, food may contain a carcinogen or a co-carcinogen (a substance that enhances another substance's cancer-causing power); and second, the component of the diet may make organs more or less susceptible to carcinogens.

Dietary Carcinogens

Foods can contain carcinogens as natural ingredients, accidental additives, and rarely, as in the case of saccharin, as intentional additives. Carcinogens occurring naturally in foods include aflatoxin in corn and peanuts, solanin in potatoes, and patulin in apple juice. Natural carcinogens are banned for use as additives but allowed in their natural sources. Safrole, a natural ingredient of the sassafras root and a known carcinogen, cannot be added to root beer for flavor but occurs as a natural component of nutmeg, mace, wild ginger, laurel, and black pepper.(28)

Synthetic additives that cause cancer can enter the food supply by accident. For example, in November 1959 scientists found traces of the weed killer aminotriazole in samples of cranberries. Aminotriazole belongs to a class of substances called goitrogens which, when fed at high levels for long periods of time, can produce cancerous tumors in rats. Goitrogens also occur naturally in foods such as plants of the cabbage family.

Consumers are most skeptical of intentional food additives as potential carcinogens. Some have come to believe that everything causes cancer. There is no evidence that U.S. cancer rates have increased since 1930 because of additives and pesticides.(29) Other countries such as Poland and Czechoslovakia use different means of preserving food than those used in the United States, yet have cancer rates as high or higher than those in this country.(29) Even so, some food additives have been banned in recent years due to their ability to cause cancer in laboratory animals. These include Red Dye No. 2 and cyclamates.

Diet and Susceptibility to Carcinogens

The relationship between the nutrient composition of the diet and the occurrence of cancer is much stronger than the relationship between additives in food and occurrence of cancer.

Kcalories. Restricting kcalories in laboratory animals inhibits tumor growth and delays the time when tumors appear. Researchers first documented this effect when they observed that mice fed all day long had eight times the number of tumors as mice fed once daily. The mice were also more obese. Suggested reasons for the higher number of tumors include hormone differences; the fact that intestinal tracts of mice fed once are free of food for longer portions of the day, which may cause different types of bacteria to grow; and the fact that continuous eating schedules are unnatural to mice.

In humans, excess kcalories increase the risk of women developing cancers of the breast, ovary, gall bladder, and endometrium and of men developing colon and prostate cancers. There is a 16 percent increase in the risk of all cancers in men who are more than 20 percent overweight and a 13 percent increase in women who are this much overweight.(24)

Fat and Cholesterol. Certain cancers are associated with high-fat diets. In population studies colon cancer risk is increased with high fat consumption, especially polyunsaturated fats. Both Japan and Chile have low occurrences of colon cancer and low fat diets. In countries like Belgium, New Zealand, and the United States, where populations have high-fat diets, the occurrence of this cancer is high.(25) Epidemiological studies also show an association between fat consumption and death from breast cancer (Figure 9–3). The fat level in the diet may change the balance of hormones, so that those hormones associated with an increase incidence of cancer become more influential.(26)

Cholesterol has been linked with cancer because epidemiological studies show an association between coronary heart disease and several forms of cancer. In one study, patients given a cholesterol-lowering drug showed remission of cancer. Other studies have shown a lower cholesterol intake among colon cancer

FIG. 9–3

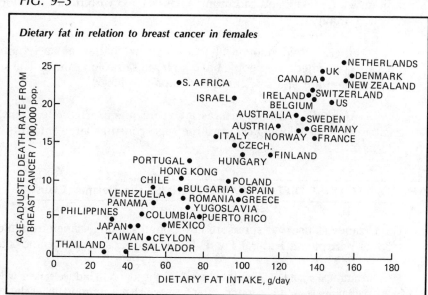

Source: E.L. Wynder, "Nutrition and Cancer," *Federation Proceedings* 35 (1976): 1309–15.

patients than among healthy persons. Such conflicting evidence needs to be studied further.

Protein.   Protein is not believed to play a direct role in tumor development, although some studies have shown fewer tumors in laboratory animals when the animals' diet contained low levels of certain amino acids.(25) In rat studies, the effect of the carcinogen aflatoxin is increased when the protein level in the diet is high. The least carcinogenic effect of aflatoxin is seen when the protein in the diet is near the RDA.(30) A number of epidemiological studies show correlations between high protein intakes and cancers of the breast, colon, prostate, and pancreas.(30)

Vitamins and Minerals.   Adequate amounts of certain vitamins and minerals can protect the body from cancer, while deficiencies or megadoses can increase the risk of the disease. For instance, vitamin C exerts a protective effect against cancer-causing nitrosamines though at megadose levels, the vitamin may be mutagenic, an indication that it may also cause cancer.(30) Recent research indicates that synthetic forms of vitamin A, called retinoids or vitamin A analogs, may be beneficial in treating cancer. This theory is still in the experimental stage.(31) Where iodine deficiency is more frequent, the incidence of thyroid cancer is high; where iron and riboflavin deficiencies are common, intestinal cancer occurs more often. The same types of relationships exist between vitamin A deficiency and the incidence of cervical cancer and between pyridoxine deficiency and liver cancer. Although vitamin deficiencies may enhance cancer risk, certain anticancer agents work by preventing tumors from getting the vitamins they need.

Excesses of certain trace minerals such as arsenic, beryllium, chromium, radium, lead, nickel, and cadmium are associated with tumor development and cancer mortality.

Fiber.   Epidemiological studies show that in areas where low-fiber diets are consumed, the people have high rates of colon cancer. The significance of these data are still unclear (see Chapter 3: Fiber).

Alcohol.   Alcohol acts as a co-carcinogen. Cigarette smokers have a greater risk of developing cancer if they also consume large amounts of alcohol.

PROTECTION AGAINST DIETARY CARCINOGENS: The Delaney Clause

The Delaney clause was sponsored by Congressman Delaney from New York in 1958 as part of the Federal Food, Drug, and Cosmetic Act and states:

That no additive shall be deemed to be safe if it is found to induce cancer when ingested by men or animals, or if it is found, after tests which are appropriate for the evaluation of the safety of food additives, to induce cancer in man or animals....

On the surface it seems simple enough (isn't everybody against cancer?), yet this short statement has caused a larger uproar in food regulation in recent years than any other issue.

The Delaney clause covers only those additives intentionally put into food, not natural ingredients or accidental additives. Its main purpose is not to ban additives already in use, but to prevent carcinogens from being added to the food supply in the first place. Opponents to the Delaney clause claim:

- It does not accept the possibility that a substance is carcinogenic at high levels but not low, or that a substance produces a tumor in one species but not another.
- Safe levels of carcinogens can be predicted from animal tests and human experience. The doses given animals are unrealistically high.
- The clause arbitrarily removes scientific judgment in deciding to ban an additive.
- The clause impedes technological progress in food production.
- Current methods of detecting traces of additives are so sensitive that foods for years considered safe are now banned. A risk-benefit analysis would be a better method of determining whether an additive should be banned.
- Even natural essential nutrients such as selenium can be carcinogenic.

Advocates counter with these arguments:

- How can you predict safe levels of carcinogens from human experience when cancers take years to develop? Even if there is a safe level of a carcinogen, humans are bombarded with a number of potential carcinogens in air, water, and food, giving a multiplying effect to their risk.
- The Delaney clause prevents a regulatory official from arbitrarily approving an additive in response to pressure from special interest groups.(32) Instead, scientific judgment is required if the tests performed on the substance were appropriate, including factors such as experimental design, route of administration, and number of animals tested.
- Few of the chemicals affected by the Delaney clause could be considered essential to the diet. Why take the risk of developing cancer?
- Naturally occurring substances that are essential for health but that may be carcinogens must be accepted in exchange for their biological functions. Even though carcinogens exist within the body, it is still important to eliminate the risk from carcinogens purposely added to the food supply.

In 1979 Congress began a major review of the food laws, giving particular attention to the Delaney clause. The ban on saccharin, proposed in 1978, was still under a moratorium because of consumer and industry efforts to retain the sweetener. The FDA was studying the possibility of banning nitrite and certain animal drugs, and pressures against the clause mounted. Industry and farmers said it was too rigid and ignored economic constraints. Without nitrite, they warned, meat prices would rise; and without saccharin, soft drink costs would soar. Consumer advocates said the clause had too many loopholes. They argued that it does not state when a ban must go into effect if the carcinogen also protects against another serious health risk. The classic case of this situation is *nitrite*.

Nitrites are present naturally in carrots, lettuce, and celery leaves, and other vegetables, and in drinking water. Manufacturers added nitrites to processed meats, poultry, fish, and certain imported cheeses to impart a distinctive flavor, color, and texture. Later they found that nitrites prevented the growth of botulism spores that survive heat processing.(33) Nitrites come not only from these processed sources but are present in human saliva, formed in the body by bacteria during digestion, and from natural food sources.

When nitrites combine with amines, one of the breakdown products of protein, they form *nitrosamines;* some nitrosamines cause cancer in test animals. The nitrite issue is complicated because nitrosamines are not the substances added to foods. Nitrites are not only naturally present in saliva, but have not been shown to cause cancer. Also, if the FDA bans nitrites, what will prevent consumers from getting botulism, the most serious form of food poisoning? Nitrite opponents argue that manufacturers use nitrites primarily for the color and flavor they impart to meats, not for preserving food, and that other methods of preservation are available. At present the FDA and USDA have submitted a plan to Congress that would gradually phase out the use of nitrite, allowing manufacturers time to switch to other means of preserving these products.

The controversies over nitrites and saccharin have led to considerable pressure to replace the Delaney clause with a risk-benefit analysis of an additive. It will be some time before the issue of the Delaney clause is finally decided. If the risk-benefit advocates win, it will be an equally long time before scientists and legislators decide how to judge the benefits of a substance against its ability to cause cancer.

Dietary Recommendations

No, everything does not cause cancer.

Yes, certain imbalances in the diet have been implicated with an increased risk of certain cancers.

What can you do to reduce your risk? There are no diets guaranteed to protect you from cancer. There are, however, several guidelines to follow to avoid increasing your chances of contracting cancer:

- Maintain ideal body weight by balancing kcalorie intake and proper exercise.
- Avoid a high intake of fat, both saturated and polyunsaturated, and cholesterol.
- Include a generous, but not excessive, intake of fiber.
- Maintain a nutritionally balanced and varied diet, with plenty of fruits and vegetables to ensure an adequate intake of vitamins and minerals.
- Consume alcoholic beverages only in moderation.

These guidelines can be met by increasing consumption of whole grain cereals and breads, vegetables, and fruits, and decreasing intake of fatty foods. Such a diet is also in keeping with the prudent diet recommended for lowering risk of heart disease.

REFERENCES

1. V.S. Packard, Jr. "Natural? Organic? What Do They Really Mean?" *Professional Nutritionist,* 10 (Summer 1978), pp. 1–3.

2. H. Hopkins, "The Color Additive Scoreboard," *FDA Consumer,* March 1980, pp. 24–27.

3. IFT Expert Panel and CPI, "Organic Foods: A Scientific Summary," *Food Technology,* January 1974, pp. 71–74.

4. P. Lehmann, "More Than You Ever Thought You Would Know about Food Additives—Part I," *FDA Consumer,* April 1979, pp. 10–16.

5. E.J. Underwood, "Trace Elements." In Food and Nutrition Board, Committee on Food Protection, National Academy of Sciences, *Toxicants Naturally Occurring in Foods,* 2nd ed. (Washington, D.C.: National Academy of Sciences, 1973), pp. 43–87.

6. P. Lehmann, "More Than You Ever Thought You Would Know About Food Additives— Part II," *FDA Consumer,* May 1979, pp. 18–23.

7. T.H. Jukes, "The Predicament of Food and Nutrition," *Food Technology,* October 1979, pp. 42–51.

8. "FTC Defines 'Natural'," *FDA Consumer,* January 1981, p. 2.

9. J. Mayer, "How Natural Should You Get?" *Family Health,* April 1979, pp. 20–23.

10. T.H. Jukes, "Pesticides Reported Used in Growing 'Health Foods,'" *AIN Nutrition Notes,* June 1979, p. 6.

11. T.H. Jukes, "The 'Organic Food' Fad," *Nutrition and the M.D.,* May 1976, p. 1.

12. L.J. Carter, "Organic Farming Becomes 'Legitimate'," *Science* 209(1980):254–56.

13. T.H. Jukes, "The Organic Food Myth," *Journal of the American Medical Association* 230 (1974):276–77.

14. E.R. Schlesinger, D.E. Overton, H.C. Chase, and K.T. Cantwell, "Newburgh-Kingston Caries-Fluorine Study; 12: Pediatric Findings after Ten Years," *Journal of the American Dental Association* 52 (1956):296–306.

15. P. Lehmann. "More Than You Ever Thought You Would Know About Food Additives—Part III," *FDA Consumer,* June 1979.

16. The National Advisory Committee on Hyperkinesis and Food Additives, *Final Report to the Nutrition Foundation* (Washington, D.C.: The Nutrition Foundation, October 1980), pp. 12–19.

17. M. Moskowitz, M. Katz, and R. Levering, eds., *Everybody's Business: An Almanac* (New York: Harper & Row, 1980).

18. C.K. Sherck, "Changes in Food Consumption Patterns," *Food Technology* 25 (September 1971):914–16.

19. H.A. Guthrie, "Junk Food: A Scientific Evaluation," *Professional Nutritionist* (Winter 1980), 12–14.

20. "Fast-Food Chains," *Consumer Reports* (September 1979), 508–13.

21. C. Greecher and B. Shannon, "Impact of Fast Food Meals on Nutrient Intake of Two Groups," *Journal of the American Dietetic Association* 70(1977):368–72.

22. American Cancer Society, *Cancer Facts and Figures,* 1980.

23. National Dairy Council, "Nutrition, Diet, and Cancer," *Dairy Council Digest* 46 (1975):25–30.

24. F.J. Roe, "Food and Cancer," *Journal of Human Nutrition* 33 (1979):405–15.

25. G.B. Gori, "Diet and Cancer," *Journal of the American Dietetic Association* 71 (1977):375–92.

26. "Food and Cancer," *Nutrition Reviews* 36 (1978):313–14.

27. E.L. Wynder, "Nutrition and Cancer," *Federation Proceedings* 35(1976):1309–15.

28. R.L. Hall, "Toxicants Occurring Naturally in Spices and Flavors." In Food and Nutrition Board, Committee on Food Protection, National Academy of Sciences, *Toxicants Naturally Occurring in Foods,* 2nd ed. (Washington, D.C.: National Academy of Sciences, 1973), pp. 448–63.

29. American Council on Science and Health, *Cancer in the United States: Is There an Epidemic?* December 1978.

30. T. Colin Campbell, "More Is Not Necessarily Better," *Natural History,* May 1981, pp. 12–16.

31. "Vitamin A, Tumor Initiation and Tumor Promotion," *Nutrition Reviews* 37 (1979):153–56.

32. S.S. Epstein, "The Delaney Amendment," *Preventive Medicine* 2(1973):140–49.

33. N. Glick, "Bringing Home the (Nitrite-Less) Bacon," *FDA Consumer,* May 1979, pp. 25–26.

Glossary

A

A

acid A chemical substance that contains hydrogen atoms and is capable of releasing these as hydrogen ions in solution. Acids usually taste sour, turn blue litmus paper red, and unite with bases (alkalis) to form salts.

adenosine triphosphate (ATP) A high energy compound containing three phosphate groups. When the third phosphate group is split from the compound, energy is released for fueling.

aerobic Living, functioning, or occurring in the presence of oxygen. An aerobic reaction is one that can occur only in the presence of oxygen.

aerobic exercise Exercise fueled by energy utilized in the presence of inspired oxygen. Such exercise can be maintained for sustained periods and increases endurance and heart, lung, and circulatory capacity.

alkali (base) A substance capable of accepting hydrogen ions; turns red litmus paper blue. Strong alkalis feel slippery and are corrosive to human tissue.

amino acids The small units that compose proteins; each includes an acid group and a nitrogen containing amino group.

amniotic fluid The liquid contained in the sac that envelops the developing fetus. It protects the fetus from injury, helps maintain an even temperature, and prevents formation of adhesions of the sac to the skin of the fetus.

amphetamine A synthetic drug that stimulates the central nervous system, increases blood pressure, represses appetite, and reduces nasal congestion.

anerobic Living, functioning, or occurring in the absence of oxygen; the opposite of aerobic.

anemia A condition in which there is a deficiency of hemoglobin in red blood cells (and sometimes a deficiency in the number of red blood cells), or the red blood cells are not of normal size, or both.

angina pectoris Severe pain radiating from the heart to the left shoulder and down the left arm; caused by an insufficient supply of blood to the heart.

anorexia Lack or loss of appetite for food.

anorexia nervosa A state characterized by extreme emaciation resulting from self-starvation, usually occurring in young women.

antacid A substance that will neutralize acidity, especially in the digestive tract. Common antacids include calcium carbonate, aluminum hydroxide, aluminum carbonate, magnesium carbonate, magnesium oxide, and sodium bicarbonate.

antibiotic Any of a group of substances that inhibit the growth of or destroy microorganisms; used widely to treat infectious diseases in humans, animals, and plants.

antibody   One of many specific substances produced in the body in response to a foreign or antagonistic substance known as an antigen.

anticoagulant   A substance that slows down or prevents blood clotting by interfering with the processes that bring about clotting.

anticonvulsant   An agent that prevents or relieves a convulsion or involuntary muscle contractions and relaxations.

antioxidant   A substance that can protect other substances from uniting with oxygen and losing their chemical and physical properties. The antioxidant itself combines with oxygen, thus protecting other substances.

appetite   A learned response that causes one to seek food for the purpose of tasting and enjoying it.

aqueous   Watery in nature.

arrhythmia   Irregularity in rhythm; irregular heart beat when used in relation to the heart.

arteriosclerosis   A number of pathological conditions in which there is a thickening, hardening, and loss of elasticity of the arteries.

asthma   Sudden, periodic attacks of labored or difficult breathing accompanied by sounds caused by spasm of the bronchial tubes or by swelling of their mucous membranes.

atherosclerosis   A type of arteriosclerosis that most often produces serious consequences and may involve the arteries of the heart, legs, or brain; it results when the inner lining of the arteries becomes thickened by deposits of fat, protein, cholesterol, and cell debris.

B

barbiturates   Substances derived from barbituric acid that depress the central nervous system and are thus sedatives.

basal metabolic rate   The energy required for basal metabolism; expressed per unit of time and usually per square meter of body surface area or per unit of body weight.

basal metabolism   Energy used for internal or cellular work while the body is at physical, emotional, and digestive rest.

beikost   Semisolid foods other than milk or formula that are given to infants, preferably after the infant is 4 to 6 months old; also referred to as ''baby food.''

bile   A fluid secreted by the liver into the intestine which mixes with intestinal and pancreatic secretions and helps digest fats.

bile salts   Substances made in the liver and stored in the gall bladder that are necessary to break up fat into tiny particles so it can be more easily digested; the salts of bile acids.

bifidus factor   A substance in breast milk that enhances the growth of the microorganism *Lactobaccilus bifidus*, increases breast-feeding infants' resistance to intestinal pathogens.

bioavailability   The rate and extent of absorption of a nutrient from the gastrointestinal tract.

blanching   Exposing food to boiling or steaming water to inactivate enzymes that cause unwanted changes in color, flavor, and nutritive value during storage.

buffer   A substance that helps preserve the original acidity or alkalinity of a solution when acid or alkali is added.

C

calorie   See *kilocalorie*.

carcinogen   A cancer-causing agent or substance.

cardiovascular disease (CVD)   The combination of heart and blood vessel problems that include heart attacks, stroke, and gangrene from blocked arteries.

caries   A condition in which a hole or cavity is produced in the surface of a tooth; decay of the teeth.

carotene   The precursor of vitamin A; present in foods of plant origin.

chylomicron   A special kind of lipoprotein composed of tiny droplets of lipids coated with a thin layer of protein. The initial transport form of much fat immediately after its digestion and absorption.

chyme   The mixture of partly digested food and stomach secretions that occur in the stomach and small intestine during digestion of food.

ciliated   Possessing cilia, which are hairlike projections on the cells that line body cavities.

cirrhosis   A chronic disease of the liver in which liver cells degenerate and are replaced by fibrous connective tissue and fatty deposits.

collagen   Protein that forms the main component of connective tissue and the organic substance of teeth and bones.

colostrum Yellowish fluid secreted from the breasts of lactating mammals in the first few days after giving birth before the mature milk comes in.

coma An abnormal state of deep unconsciousness occurring in illness or as a result of it or injury.

conception The union of the male sperm and the female ovum (egg).

congenital malformation Abnormally formed features or organ systems present at birth.

cornea The exposed and transparent portion of the eyeball.

cretinism A condition occurring in fetal life and early infancy caused by lack of thyroid hormones during the fetal period and afterward. Results in arrested physical and mental development, dry skin, chubby hands, large protruding tongue and abdomen, and low basal metabolism.

crude fiber The residue from foods of plant origin left after a food is treated with hot acid and hot alkali. This procedure destroys much dietary fiber.

D

Daily Food Guide Also called the *Five Food Groups*. This guide is the Basic Four Food Groups with the addition of a fifth group that includes foods such as fats, sweets, and alcohol with kcalories and few nutrients.

deficiency diseases Diseases caused by inadequacy of one or more nutrients in the diet.

degenerative diseases Diseases associated with the deterioration or impairment of an organ or tissues. The degenerative diseases most commonly related to nutrition are cardiovascular disease, diabetes, and cancer.

dentition The type, number, and arrangement of teeth in the mouth; also refers to eruption of teeth.

diabetes (Diabetes mellitus) A disorder in which the body's ability to utilize carbohydrates is impaired because of inadequate production or poor utilization of the hormone insulin. When the condition occurs suddenly in childhood (Type I diabetes), there is usually an insufficiency of insulin and the condition is unstable and difficult to regulate. When the

condition occurs in middle age (Type II diabetes), the problem is often due more to poor utilization of insulin than an insufficiency, and symptoms may be alleviated with dietary modification.

diabetic An individual afflicted with diabetes mellitus.

diastolic pressure The blood pressure that occurs when the ventricles of the heart are not forcing blood out into blood vessels, the pressure during the resting phase.

dietary fiber Also called *roughage*. The component in foods of plant origin that is resistant to human digestive enzymes. It is important for regulating the passage of food through the gastrointestinal tract.

digestion The process (mechanical and chemical) of breaking down food and releasing nutrients in a form suitable for absorption.

disaccharide A type of simple carbohydrate containing 2 sugar units, which can be broken down to form two "simple sugars."

diuretic A substance that increases the secretion of urine.

diverticular disease A disease of the lower intestine, especially the colon, characterized by outpouchings of the mucous membrane through gaps or weak spots in the circular muscles of the colon. These outpouchings are called diverticula. If they are not inflamed the condition is called diverticulosis; if they are inflamed it is called diverticulitis.

E

edema The accumulation of abnormally large amounts of body fluid in a part of or in the entire body, causing swelling of the part or the body in general.

electrolyte An element (or molecule) that becomes ionized (takes on a positive or negative charge) when dissolved.

emaciation Abnormal leanness due to wasting of the body.

endemic A disease always present in a community but occurring in small numbers.

enrichment The addition of thiamin, riboflavin, niacin, and iron to bread, flour, and cereal products.

enzyme A protein produced by living tissues that catalyzes the chemical reactions in living organisms.

epidemiological Having to do with the relationships of factors that determine the frequency and distribution of a disease in a human community.

esophagus　The hollow muscular tube extending from the pharynx (throat area) to the stomach; serves as a passageway for food.

essential fatty acid　A fatty acid that cannot be made by the body and must be obtained through food.

essential (indispensable) amino acids　Amino acids that the body cannot synthesize at the rate required for health and growth; must be obtained through the diet.

Essentials of an Adequate Diet　Also called the *Basic Four Food Groups*. This guide places food with similar nutrient composition into four food groups: meat and meat substitutes, milk and milk products, fruits and vegetables, and breads and cereals.

Exchange System　Originally designed for diabetics who had to control their carbohydrate intake, this guide groups foods in lists according to carbohydrate, protein, fat, and energy content.

extracellular fluid　The fluid outside of cells.

F

fatty acid　A molecule consisting of a chain of carbons, with attached hydrogens, and an acid group at one end.

feces　The material excreted from the intestines, which consists of food residue, bacteria, mucus, cells sloughed off the intestinal wall, and intestinal secretions.

fermentation　The enzyme-catalyzed breakdown of carbohydrates in the absence or near absence of oxygen.

fetus　The developing offspring in the uterus, after it passes the embryonic stages, about the second to the ninth months in humans.

flatulence　Distention of the stomach ·or intestine by air or gas.

fortification　The addition to a food of one or more nutrients that were not present or present in only small amounts in the natural food.

fuel nutrient　Any of the three nutrients—carbohydrates, fats, proteins—that can be broken down to provide energy to the body.

G

gallstones　Stonelike structures in the gall bladder or duct leading from the gall bladder into the small intestine.

gastrointestinal tract　The digestive tract, including the stomach and intestines.

genitals　Reproductive organs.

gestation　The period from conception to birth when the offspring develops within the mother's uterus.

goiter　An enlargement of the thyroid gland; one type is caused by a dietary deficiency of iodine.

goitrogen　A substance that produces goiter (enlargement of the thyroid gland); occurs in certain foods, including turnips, rutabaga, and cabbage.

gout　A disease in which uric acid levels in the blood become excessive. Uric acid deposits form in the joints, causing them to be swollen and inflamed; usually begins in the knee or foot.

H

hemoglobin　The oxygen-carrying pigment of red blood cells. Its main function is to carry oxygen from the lungs to the tissues and transport carbon dioxide back to the lungs.

hemorrhage　Internal or external bleeding from blood vessels or capillaries.

hemorrhoids　Enlarged, twisted veins (varicose veins) in the lower part of the colon and surrounding the region of the anus.

hepatitis　Inflammation of the liver; usually causes jaundice (yellow coloration of the skin), fever, and sometimes enlargement of the liver.

hiatus hernia　A protrusion of the stomach up through the passageway where the esophagus passes through the diaphragm.

hormone　A chemical substance produced by groups of cells or an organ called an endocrine gland that is released directly into the blood or body fluids and transported to another organ or tissues, where it performs specific regulatory actions.

humus　Organic material in soils produced by decomposition of plant or animal matter; essential for fertility and for holding moisture.

hunger　The sensation that occurs when

there is a physiological need for food.

hydrogenation   The process by which hydrogens are added to unsaturated oils so they become more saturated and are solidified.

hydrolysis   A chemical reaction in which a molecule is split to form two new ones; involves the adding in of water.

hypertension   High blood pressure, which is the persistent elevation of blood pressure above normal.

hyperthyroidism   An oversecretion of the thyroid hormones which results in an elevated basal metabolic rate and weight loss.

hypoglycemia   A condition in which the pancreas consistently releases too much insulin resulting in low blood sugar levels and feelings of faintness, hunger, and anxiety.

hypothalamus   The area of the brain that lies below the thalamus. It regulates many functions basic to life, such as body temperature, body fluid levels, and appetite.

hypothyroidism   An undersecretion of the thyroid gland hormones which results in a lowered basal metabolic rate and tendency toward weight gain.

ischemia   An insufficiency of blood in a part of the body due to a constriction or obstruction of a blood vessel.

K

ketones   The collective term given to several intermediate products formed during the breakdown of fatty acids.

ketosis   A condition in which ketones accumulate in the body generally due to carbohydrate deficiency or inadequate utilization of carbohydrate(s).

kilocalorie   A measurement of heat. In nutrition *calorie* is commonly used although the correct term is **kilocalorie.** A **kilocalorie** is the amount of heat required to raise the temperature of one kilogram of water one degree centigrade.

Kwashiorkor   A condition of undernutrition resulting primarily from a diet that is deficient in protein but provides energy; most common among small children.

I

immunization   Becoming immune (resistant to disease), or the process of making a person immune.

index of nutrient quality (INQ)   A mathematical expression of a food's nutrient density. The INQ of a nutrient is calculated by dividing the percent of the requirement for the nutrient that a food supplies by the percent of the energy requirement supplied by that same food.

insulin   The hormone secreted by certain cells of the pancreas that is essential for proper metabolism of blood sugar.

intracellular fluid   The fluid in cells.

intrinsic factor   A substance normally present in the juices secreted by the stomachs of humans that is required for adequate absorption of vitamin B-12.

ions   An atom or group of atoms carrying an electric charge.

inorganic   Substances such as minerals that occur in nature independent of living things. In nutrition, inorganic usually refers to substances that do not contain carbon.

L

lactation   The secretion of milk or the period when milk is formed and secreted by all mammals.

Laetrile (amygdalin, vitamin B-17)   A substance present in the seeds of such fruits as peaches, plums, and apricots which can release cyanide in the presence of certain enzymes; promoted as a cancer cure.

leach   To remove a constituent of a substance or mixture by washing or soaking with a liquid that dissolves the constituent.

legumes   The fruit or seed of a pod-bearing plant—peas, beans, lentils, peanuts.

lesion   An injury, wound, or any loss of biochemical or physical function in the body.

linoleic acid   An essential fatty acid.

lipids   Fats and fatlike substances that are insoluble in water but soluble in fat-solvents like ether, acetone, and chloroform.

lipoprotein   A combination of protein and lipids (fatty acids, cholesterol, or triglycerides); the form in which fat is carried through the bloodstream.

M

macronutrient The nutrients carbohydrates, fats, protein, and water which are required in relatively large amounts (grams) by the body.

malignant Harmful, resisting treatment; used to describe cancerous growths such as malignant tumors.

malnutrition A condition in which the body receives too much or too little of a nutrient or energy for health.

marasmus A severe condition of undernutrition resulting primarily from an inadequacy of both protein and energy; causes extreme wasting of body tissue.

megadose Quantities of a substance, such as a vitamin, that are massive compared to the amount required for physiological function.

megaloblastic anemia A condition of the blood in which the red blood cells do not mature normally; are larger than normal, mature red blood cells; and retain the nucleus.

menarche Onset of menstruation, usually between ages 10 and 17.

menopause The period in the life cycle of women when menstruation ceases permanently; occurs between 35 and 58 years of age.

menstruation The monthly flow of blood from the uterus of women during their reproductive years—that is, from puberty to menopause.

metabolism The sum of the chemical changes that occur in the body from the time nutrients are absorbed and utilized (for building body substances or for energy) or excreted as wastes.

micronutrient The nutrients, vitamins and minerals which are required in relatively small amounts (milligrams and micrograms) by the body.

molecule A chemical combination of two or more atoms that form a specific chemical substance with properties different from those of the component atoms.

monosaccharide A type of simple carbohydrate containing only a single sugar unit, a "simple sugar."

monounsaturated fatty acid A fatty acid with one double bond.

mucus A viscous fluid secreted by mucous membranes and glands.

mulch Material such as straw, leaves, or loose earth that is spread on the ground to conserve moisture and protect the roots of newly planted plants.

mutation A change or transformation in genetic material capable of being transmitted to offspring.

N

neoplasm A new and abnormal formation of tissue that serves no useful function, but grows at the expense of the healthy organism.

neurotransmitter A substance that serves as a chemical link for communication between nerve cells.

nonessential (dispensable) amino acids Amino acids that the body cannot synthesize at the rate required for health and growth; must be obtained through the diet.

nucleic acids An important group of complex molecular substances found in cells. The two general types are deoxyribonucleic acid (DNA), which carries the hereditary information of the organism, and ribonucleic acid (RNA), which is responsible for the synthesis of proteins.

nucleus The vital structure within a living cell that contains the cell's heredity material and controls its metabolism, growth, and reproduction.

nutrient density The relationship of the nutrient a food provides to the energy it provides. Foods that meet a high percentage of the requirement for several nutrients but a low percentage of the kcalories needed is considered nutrient dense.

O

obesity Excessive body fat. An individual is considered obese when body weight is 20 percent or more above the desirable level. Overweight, which can be due to an unusually large amount of muscle mass, is not necessarily the same as obesity.

organic Any substance that contains carbon in its chemical structure such as carbohydrates, proteins, and fats. The term is sometimes used to describe foods grown without pesticides or chemical fertilizers.

osteomalacia (adult rickets) A condition in which there is a reduction in the mineral content of bones, causing them to be flexible and brittle and leading to deformities; generally caused by lack of exposure to sunlight, coupled with diet deficient in vitamin D.

osteoporosis   A condition in which there is a loss of bone. The remaining bone is of normal composition but it is weaker and fractures easily. Occurs most frequently in elderly, white women.

overweight   Weight in excess of some arbitrary standard; does not necessarily indicate excessive body fatness.

oxidize   To combine chemically with oxygen; to increase the positive charges of an atom or molecule through loss of electrons.

P

palpitations   Rapid, violent, or throbbing pulsations, such as an abnormally rapid throbbing or fluttering heart.

paralysis   Temporary or permanent loss of function, especially loss of sensation or the ability to move.

pasteurizing   Heating a substance to a moderate temperature which kills some of the microorganisms that cause food spoilage and illness.

pathogenic   Capable of causing disease.

peptic ulcer   An ulcer of the lining of the stomach or duodenum (upper segment of the small intestine); usually causes a "gnawing" pain in the region over the pit of the stomach about one to three hours after a meal.

peristalsis   Part of the mechanical action of digestion in which the muscles of the stomach wall contract, kneading and churning food, mixing it with stomach secretions to form chyme.

pesticide   A substance used to destroy pests of any sort; includes fungicides, insecticides, and rodenticides.

pheromone   A substance that provides for chemical communication between animals and some insects, usually of the same species. It is probably detected by smell and may influence development, reproduction, or behavior.

photosynthesis   The process by which green plants trap the sun's energy and use it to convert carbon dioxide from the air and water from the air and soil into carbohydrate.

pica   The practice of eating nonfood items such as laundry starch and clay.

placebo   An inactive substance that has no effect but cannot be differentiated in appearance and taste from a substance being tested.

placebo effect   An effect having nothing to do with the substance being given to a patient or individual in a study; a psychological effect that occurs because it is expected.

placenta   The structure that develops on the wall of the uterus during pregnancy and to which the developing fetus is attached by means of the umbilical cord. Nourishment is transferred from maternal blood to fetal blood, and wastes in the reverse direction, through the placenta, but the material and fetal blood are separated by thin membranes across which nutrients and wastes must pass.

plasma   The liquid part of blood and lymph; the portion that remains when cells have been removed.

polysaccharide   Also called complex carbohydrates or starches; these carbohydrates contain many molecules of glucose.

polyunsaturated fatty acid (PUFA)   A fatty acid with more than one double bond.

postpartum   Occurring after childbirth.

preservatives   Additives that maintain the appearance, palatability, and wholesomeness of food by delaying deterioration due to oxidation or microorganisms.

progestin   A term used to cover a large group of synthetic drugs that have properties similar to the natural hormone, progesterone, which prepares the uterus for the fertilized egg.

protein-energy malnutrition (PEM)   An insufficiency of both protein and energy; causes retarded growth, weight loss, listlessness; the primary form of undernutrition in developing countries.

prothrombin   A protein in the blood required for normal blood clotting.

provitamins (vitamin precursors)   Substances, chemically related to certain vitamins, which can be converted by the body to the active form of the vitamins.

P/S ratio   The ratio of polyunsaturated fats to saturated fats in a given food or diet.

R

rancid   Having an offensive taste and/or smell due to partial decomposition, as happens with decomposition of fat.

reduce   To decrease the positive charge of

an atom or molecule through the gain of electrons.

restoration The addition of nutrients to food that were generally present in the food but destroyed or lost in processing.

risk factors Factors such as personal habits and inherited or acquired traits that describe an individual's potential for developing a disease; indicative of a relationship only and not cause and effect.

S

satiety Feeling of fullness or of being satisfied.

saturated fat Fat composed of a high proportion of saturated fatty acids, which are molecules having all the carbons in the chain linked to hydrogen so that only single bonds exist. Fats from animal sources are usually saturated.

saturated fatty acid A fatty acid in which the carbons within the chain have all available bonds filled (saturated) with hydrogens.

scrotum The external pouch of the male that encloses the testes; found in most mammals.

serum The watery, clear portion of blood that separates from the blood cells after clotting.

sterols One of a group of complex molecular substances related to fat and found in animals and plants. Cholesterol is the most familiar sterol found only in animals.

stroke The common term used for sudden brain injury generally caused by rupture of a blood vessel in the brain.

subclinical Period before the appearance of typical symptoms of a disease.

subcutaneous fat Fat located just beneath the skin.

substrate A substance on which an enzyme acts.

symbiosis (symbiotic relationship) The living together, in close association, of two organisms.

systolic pressure The blood pressure that occurs during contraction of the ventricles, which are the muscular portions of the heart that force blood out into the blood vessels.

T

thoracic duct The main lymph-conducting vessel of the body. It receives lymph from all parts of the body except the right side of the head, neck, and thorax and right shoulder and arm; it empties into the blood on the left side of the neck.

thyroid gland An endocrine gland in the neck that secretes the iodine-containing hormones.

tilth The physical condition of soil as it relates to plant growth.

toxemia of pregnancy A broad term referring to a continuum of symptoms called pre-eclampsia and eclampsia which can occur during pregnancy. In pre-eclampsia the woman experiences high blood pressure, protein losses in her urine, and edema. In later stages, eclampsia, she goes into convulsions and/or coma.

triglycerides Compounds composed of one glycerol molecule combined with three fatty acids; the most common form of fat in the diet.

U

underweight Weight less than 90 percent of that which is ideal for height, age, and body build.

unsaturated fatty acid A fatty acid in which the carbon chain contains one or more double bonds; that is, some carbons are not saturated with hydrogens.

urea The major nitrogen-containing end product of protein breakdown in the body.

uric acid The end product formed when substances called purines are broken down in the human body. The purines may come from food or from the breakdown of body tissues.

U.S. Recommended Daily Allowances (USRDA) A nutrient standard developed for labeling purposes representing the highest RDA (from the 1969 RDA table) for the various age-sex groups excluding pregnant and lactating women. The USRDA for calcium and phosphorus are exceptions in that they represent the RDA for adult men rather than the much higher value for adolescent boys.

uterus The hollow, muscular, pear-shaped structure of the female in which the fertilized egg is implanted and the developing offspring nourished until birth.

V

varicose veins Enlarged, twisted veins that may occur almost anywhere in the body but are most common in the lower legs.
villi Small, finger-like projections found on some membraneous surfaces, such as the surface of the small intestine.
vitamin precursor (provitamin) The forerunner of a vitamin; a substance very similar to a vitamin that can be converted to the actual vitamin by the body.

W

whey The liquid left after milk has coagulated.

X

xerophthalmia A condition of the eyeball in which it becomes dry and lusterless, followed by inflammation and infection leading to ulceration, softening, and blindness. May be caused by severe vitamin A deficiency.

Professional Nutrition Organizations

B

American College of Nutrition (ACN)

100 Manhattan Ave. #1606
Union City, NJ 07087
(201) 866–3518

Publication: Annual meeting proceedings

The more than 230 members of the ACN, a nonprofit education society, are dedicated to the dissemination of nutrition knowledge, including continuing education of the health care team and interchange of nutrition research information between academic and clinical nutritionists. Annual meetings are held to facilitate this interchange. ACN activity is supported by membership dues and grants from industry.

The American Dietetics Association (ADA)

430 North Michigan Ave.
Chicago, IL 60611
(312) 280–5000

Publications: *Journal of the American Dietetics Association* (monthly), *Courier* (bimonthly for members only)

The ADA is the professional organization of registered dietitians. Its 39,000 members work as nutritional health care professionals in medicine, public health, education, food ser-

vice and industry. The association establishes educational standards for the profession of dietetics and maintains continuing education programs for practitioners, as well as nutrition education programs and materials for the public, including annual sponsorship of National Nutrition Week.

The American Heart Association (AHA)

7320 Greenville Ave.
Dallas, TX 75231
(214) 750–5300

Publications: *Circulation* (monthly), *Circulation Research* (monthly), *Stroke—Journal of Cerebral Circulation* (bimonthly), *Hypertension* (bimonthly), Other educational materials, published continuously

The goal of the AHA is to reduce premature death and disability from heart disease, and it supports research and education toward this end. Thousands of medical and nonmedical volunteers work in the AHA chapters nationwide. The National Center in Dallas provides guidelines and supports community programs implemented locally. Contributions and fundraising activities are the AHA's major sources of revenue.

Source: Updated from Professional Nutritionist 12, *spring 1980.*

The American Home Economics Association (AHEA)

2010 Massachusetts Ave., NW
Washington, DC 20036
(202) 862–8300

Publications: *Journal of Home Economics* (five times a year), *AHEA Action* (newsletter), *Home Economics Research Journal* (quarterly), *AHEA Publications List* (two times a year), *Washington Dateline* (monthly newsletter)

The AHEA represents 50,000 home economists who work in education and business, with more than 10,000 members in its Food and Nutrition Section. It promotes professional standards and conduct, and works to strengthen the environment in which families function. The association is funded by member dues and program-related sources.

American Institute of Nutrition (AIN)

9650 Rockville Pike
Bethesda, MD 20014
(301) 530–7050

Publications: *Journal of Nutrition* (monthly), *AIN Notes* (quarterly newsletter)

Most of the 1,900 members of the AIN conduct nutrition research and teach in departments of nutrition or other related sciences. They work primarily in universities, industrial research laboratories, colleges, and medical schools. Membership is limited to persons who have, in the opinion of their scientific peers, demonstrated expertise in well-designed and executed research.

American Public Health Association (APHA)

1015 Fifteenth St., NW
Washington, DC 20005
(202) 789–5600

Publications: *American Journal of Public Health* (monthly), *The Nation's Health* (monthly newspaper)

The APHA represents the interests of its 50,000 members at federal, state, and local levels of government, as well as to industry and the general public. It provides summaries of health-related legislative activities and policy issues to its members and publishes numerous materials reflecting the latest findings in public health. It is funded primarily through membership dues.

The American Society for Clinical Nutrition, Inc. (ASCN)

9650 Rockville Pike
Bethesda, MD 20014
(301) 530–7110

Publication: *The American Journal of Clinical Nutrition* (monthly)

ASCN, the clinical branch of the AIN, is composed of 400 nutritionists, most of whom are physicians. They are active in research and graduate and undergraduate education in biological sciences. ASCN holds an annual meeting in conjunction with other professional societies. Funding is provided principally by membership dues.

The American Society for Parenteral and Enteral Nutrition (ASPEN)

6110 Executive Blvd., Suite 810
Rockville, MD 20852
(301) 881–4626

Publications: *Journal of Parenteral and Enteral Nutrition* (bimonthly), *ASPEN Update* (monthly newsletter)

ASPEN's 3,000 members are health care professionals dedicated to the fostering of good nutritional support of patients during hospitalization and rehabilitation by promoting the team approach and by helping educate professionals at all levels. ASPEN holds an annual clinical congress, sponsors numerous regional meetings, and conducts continuing education courses in all nutrition-related disciplines.

Center for Science in the Public Interest (CSPI)

1755 S Street, NW
Washington, DC 20009
(202) 332–9110

Publications: *Nutrition Action* (monthly), *CSPI Newsletter*, also many books and posters

Although concerned with the effect of technology on society in general, the CSPI focuses primarily on technology's effect on food and nutrition. Its major activities include public education through its various publications and monitoring federal agencies involved in food safety, trade, and nutrition. The CSPI has 15,000 members, both professionals and consumers, and is funded through publication sales, donations, and grants.

The Children's Foundation (CF)

1420 New York Avenue, NW
Suite 800
Washington, DC 20005
(202) 347–3300

Publications: Fact sheets, bulletins and newsletters

CF is an antihunger advocacy organization which works to: (1) inform eligible Americans of their rights to food assistance, (2) monitor federal, state and local administration of federal food programs, and (3) correct abuses of the system that prevent aid to the poor. Toward this end, the foundation pushes for improved food aid legislation and works with poor communities to oversee wise appropriation of funds. CF is supported by contributions.

Community Nutrition Institute (CNI)

1146 19th St., NW
Washington, DC 20036
(202) 833–1730

Publications: *CNI Weekly Report, CFNP Report* (Community Food & Nutrition Program) (bimonthly), assorted papers, brochures, and manuals

CNI is a nonmembership advocacy organization which seeks to ensure a safe, affordable food supply for all consumers. The Hunger and Action Division trains community organizations in nutrition; The Consumer Division is active in government testimony and training consumers in public participation; and The Training Center works with senior citizens to improve nutrition. The institute is funded primarily by foundation grants, government contracts, and publication sales.

Food and Nutrition Board (FNB)

2101 Constitution Ave, NW
Washington, DC 20418
(202) 389–6366

Publications: Various committee reports published as completed

The FNB serves under the terms of the charter of the National Academy of Sciences as an advisory body to federal agencies and, on its own initiative, to the general public on science as related to nutrition. It is the advisory board that established the Recommended Dietary Allowances (RDA). It evaluates the safety of additives for the FDA's GRAS list. The purity specifications for certain chemicals are found in the Board's *Food Chemical Codex*. The FNB is composed of approximately 16 members, with rotating appointments.

Food Protein Council (FPC)

1800 M St., NW
Washington, DC 20036
(202) 467–6610

Publications: Brochures including "Vegetable Protein: Products and the Future," and "Soy Protein: Improving Our Food Systems"

Fourteen companies that deal in vegetable protein products have joined together to form the FPC. It works to build public awareness of the nutritional properties of vegetable protein. The FPC participates in the formulation of U.S. nutrition policies and promotes greater reliance on vegetable protein in the world's food supply.

Food Research and Action Center (FRAC)

2011 I St., NW
Washington, DC 20006
(202) 452–8250

Publications: Periodic mailings explaining food programs and welfare reform

FRAC is a public interest law firm organized to help end hunger and malnutrition among the poor in the U.S. It monitors national programs and policies so that it can influence legislation, and assists the poor to benefit from federal food programs through various communications programs. Funding comes primarily through the Community Services Administration.

The Institute of Food Technologists (IFT)

221 N. La Salle St.
Chicago, IL 60601
(312) 782–8424

Publications: *Food Technology* (monthly), *The Journal of Food Science* (bimonthly)

The IFT is a professional scientific society with 18,000 members, 60 percent of whom work for food or food ingredient processing companies. To implement its interest in the development of improved food sources, products, and processing and their proper use by industry, the institute has a program of publications, scientific meetings, and educational activities for members and the public. Costs of these activities are supported by dues, convention revenue, and publication sales.

La Leche League International, Inc. (LLLI)

9616 Minneapolis Ave.
Franklin Park, IL 60131
(312) 455–7730

Publications: *LLL News* (bimonthly journal for members), *Leaven* (bimonthly for league leaders), many small pamphlets and brochures

LLLI was founded to give help, encouragement, and personal instruction to mothers who wish to breastfeed their babies. LLLI also has family nutrition education programs. The League reaches a million women annually in 43 countries. It has group meetings, information centers, and many publications available to the public. It is often referred to mothers by pediatricians and obstetricians. LLLI is funded by dues, contributions, and sales of publications.

The March of Dimes Birth Defects Foundation (MOD)

1275 Mamaroneck Ave.
White Plains, NY 10605
(914) 428–7100

Publications: Education materials on birth defects and prenatal care

Some 900 chapters nationwide make up the March of Dimes network. Staffed by professionals and volunteers, MOD's main concern is the prevention of birth defects. It recognizes the role nutrition plays in the outcome of pregnancy, and seeks to educate the public accordingly. MOD conducts various educational nutrition programs, and provides a grant to the Food and Nutrition Board for developing guidelines for nutrition services for normal and high-risk mothers and babies.

Meals for Millions/Freedom From Hunger Foundation (MFM)

1800 Olympic Blvd.
P.O. Drawer 680
Santa Monica, CA 90406
(213) 829–5337

Publication: Annual report, newsletter (3–4 times/year)

MFM is a worldwide self-help organization dedicated to strengthening the capabilities of developing communities to solve their own food and nutrition problems. To achieve this goal, MFM has two primary programs: (1) Food and Nutrition Institute, a training center for community level workers, food technologists, and nutritionists from the less developed nations; and (2) Applied Nutrition Programs, nutrition-oriented rural education development programs. MFM also offers seminars for field-focused professionals. The foundation is funded through donations, grants, and government aid.

National Dairy Council (NDC)

6300 N. River Road
Rosemont, IL 60018
(312) 696–1020

Publications: *Focus* (monthly), full catalog listing of educational materials

The NDC is the nutrition research and education arm of the United Dairy Industry. Its comprehensive nutrition education program covers the four food groups and is directed to all ages. In addition, the NDC produces syndicated radio and newspaper reports on nutrition. Research focuses on the role of dairy products in diet and health. NDC materials are available by contacting the council or any of its 34 regional affiliates.

National Nutrition Consortium, Inc. (NNC)
24 Third St. NE, Suite 200
Washington, DC 20002
(202) 547–4819

Publications: *Public Affair Alerts* (15–20 issues/year), *Report from the Consortium* (printed in member organization journals 4 times/year)
Sponsor Societies
American Dietetic Association
American Institute of Nutrition
American Society for Clinical Nutrition
American Society for Parenteral and Enteral Nutrition
Institute of Food Technologists
Society for Nutrition Education
Liaison Organizations
American Association of Cereal Chemists
American College of Nutrition
The NNC is a nonprofit organization comprising major professional societies in food, nutrition, and dietetics. It serves as a clearinghouse for information on nutrition and aims to offer the public and policy makers access to a spectrum of opinions. In addition, it sponsors a fellowship for graduate students. It is supported by dues and contributions.

The Nutrition Foundation
888 17th Street, NW
Washington, DC 20006
(202) 872–0778

Publications: *Nutrition Reviews* (monthly), other books and pamphlets for professionals, teachers, and the public
The foundation is a group of more than 50 companies in food and related industries. Its goal is to advance the science and knowledge of food and nutrition to promote good health. It sponsors nutrition research, and educational and career development programs. The foundation also provides support to several nutrition-related organizations and advises government agencies and Congress on nutrition and food safety.

Nutrition Today Society
703 Giddings Ave.
Annapolis, MD 21401
(301) 267–8616

Publication: *Nutrition Today* (bimonthly)
The Nutrition Today Society's goal is to increase and disseminate nutrition knowledge through its magazine, teaching aids, and other nutrition material. It also organizes "nutrition tours," allowing members to fly to nutrition conferences at reduced cost. Its members are professionals in health fields, home economics, and the food industry. The society is funded through membership dues and contributions.

The Society for Nutrition Education (SNE)
1736 Franklin St.
Oakland, CA 94612
(415) 444–7133

Publications: *Journal of Nutrition Education* (quarterly), *Communicator* (quarterly)
The SNE's overall goal is nutritional well-being for all people through education, communication, and education-related research. The SNE actively promotes policies to ensure optimum nutritional health for the public. It develops policy statements relative to legislation, regulations for TV ads, food labeling, and nutrition education programs. SNE's 5,500 members are professional nutritionists, educators, and students. Funding is provided primarily through membership dues.

Nutrition Periodicals

C

ACSH News and Views

A bimonthly newsletter for professionals. Presents current issues in health and safety, book reviews, interviews, and guest editorials by well-known food and nutrition scientists.

From: American Council on Science and Health, 1995 Broadway, New York, NY 10023

$35/yr for individuals; $175/yr for institutions

Agenda

A magazine published 10 times/year for the general public and professionals. Presents information about U.S. policy and programs regarding economic and social development in the third world.

From: Agency for International Development, Office of Public Affairs, Washington, DC 20523

Free; subscriptions limited to the U.S.

American Journal of Clinical Nutrition

A monthly journal for professionals and college-level students.

Regularly features nutrition surveys, original communications, comments in nutrition, perspectives in nutrition, methods in nutrition, nutrition education, diet therapy.

From: AJCN, 9650 Rockville Pike, Bethesda, MD 20014

$40/yr for individuals; $55/yr for institutions; $17.50/yr for students

American Journal of Public Health

A monthly journal for professionals and college-level students.

Features reports of original research and other papers covering the broad aspects of public health, including nutrition, epidemiology, maternal/child health, environmental health.

From: APHA, 1015 15 St. NW, Washington, DC 20005

$40/yr regular membership; $60/yr contributing membership; $20/yr student membership

Apple Press

A newsletter published 8 times a year for teachers, children, and the general public.

Features recipes, ideas, and information to provide nutrition education, support, and alternatives to parents, schools, and the community.

From: Apple Press, 1404 Sunnymeade, South Bend, IN 46615

$3/yr; bulk rates available on request

Cajanus

A quarterly journal for professionals.

Contains articles dealing with nutrition issues of the Caribbean.

From: Caribbean Food and Nutrition Institute, P.O. Box 140, Kingston 7, Jamaica

Free to subscribers in developing countries; $12/yr in U.S. and other countries

California Council against Health Fraud Newsletter

A monthly newsletter for professionals, college-level students, and the general public.

Contains information concerning nutrition misinformation, food faddism, and health fraud. Reports of the CCAHF activities.

From: CCAHF, Box 1276, Loma Linda, CA 92354

$10/yr regular membership; $25/yr supporting membership; $2/yr student membership; $50/yr institutional membership

CNI Weekly Report

A weekly newsletter for the general public, professional, and college-level students.

Monitors food program and policy developments from a consumer viewpoint.

From: Community Nutrition Institute, 1146 19th St. NW, Washington, DC 20036

$35/yr; $25/yr for multiple and introductory subscriptions

Consumers Union News Digest

A bimonthly newsletter for the general public, professionals, and college-level students.

Contains information on subjects ranging from health to ecology, money, nutrition, advertising. Prepared by the library staff of Consumer Reports magazine.

Consumers Union of United States, Inc., Mount Vernon, NY 10550

$36/yr

Consumer Reports

A monthly magazine for the general public, professionals, and college-level students.

Gives product ratings, information, and counsel on consumer goods and services.

From: Consumers Union, Orangeburg, NY 10962

$14/yr, $24/2 yrs, $34/3 yrs, $54/4 yrs, Canada, add $1/yr, other countries, add $2/yr.

Currents in Food, Nutrition and Health

A quarterly newsletter for the general public and professionals.

Contains concise information from leading food, nutrition, and health experts on relationships between what we eat and good health.

From: Cereal Institute, 1111 Plaza Dr., Schaumburg, IL 60195

Free

Dairy Council Digest

A bimonthly newsletter for professionals, and college-level students.

Contains information on current nutrition research

From: National Dairy Council, 6300 N. River Rd., Rosemont, IL 60018

$2.50/yr.

Diabetes—The Journal of the American Diabetes Association

A monthly journal for professionals.

Publishes major scientific papers and review articles dealing with diabetes and related endocrine disorders.

From: ADA, 2 Park Ave., New York, NY 10016

$50/yr for individual; $37.50/yr for institution

Diabetes Care

A bimonthly journal for professionals.

Aimed at improving the care of diabetic patients by professionals.

From: ADA, 2 Park Ave., New York, NY 10016

$25/yr for individual; $35/yr for institution

Ecology of Food and Nutrition: An International Journal

A journal, 8 issues per year, for college-level students and professionals.

An international journal of the nutritional sciences with a particular emphasis on foods and their utilization in the nutritional needs of people, but extending also to nonfood contributions to obesity and leanness malnutrition, vitamin requirements, and mineral needs.

From: Gordon and Breach Science Publishers, 42 William IV St., London WC2, England

$398/yr

Environmental Nutrition

A newsletter published 10 times a year for the general public, professionals, and college-level students.

Contains reviews of current issues in nutrition, books, and a readers forum.

From: Environmental Nutrition, Inc., 52 Riverside Dr., Suite 15–A, New York, NY 10024

$18/yr

Family Economics Review

A quarterly periodical for professionals.

Reports on the research relating to economic aspects of family living.

From: Family Economics Research Group, SEA, Rm. 338, Federal Bldg., Hyattsville, MD 20782

Single copies free, mailing list limited to professional workers in home economics and related fields

FDA Consumer

A monthly magazine for the general public, professionals, and college-level students.

Contains articles on the latest actions and concerns of the Food and Drug Administration.

From: Superintendent of Documents, U.S. Government Printing Office, Washington, DC 20402

$12/yr domestic; $15/yr Foreign

Free Kids—It's the Law!

A monthly newsletter for professionals.

Contains general food program news, overview of current regulatory and legislative action,

stories from communities around the country concerning the Child Nutrition Programs.

From: The Children's Foundation, 1420 New York Ave., NW, Suite 800, Washington, DC 20005

$4/yr community groups and individuals; $8/yr agencies

Food and Nutrition

A bimonthly periodical for the general public, professionals, and college-level students. Prepared by the USDA/FNS.

From: Superintendent of Documents, Government Printing Office, Washington, DC 20402

$4/yr domestic; $5/yr foreign

Food and Nutrition News

A newsletter for professionals and college-level students; published 5 times/academic year.

Features articles on nutrition and related topics; also book reviews, scientific abstracts, items on food, nutrition, and health.

From: National Live Stock and Meat Board, 444 N. Michigan Ave., Chicago, IL 60611

In U.S. and its territories: free to nutrition, health, and home economics professionals; foreign subscriptions: $2/yr

Food Facts and Findings

An annual newsletter for professionals.

Newsletter of the International Committee for the Anthropology of Food and Food Habits.

From: Wilson Museum, Catine, ME 04421

Send request with return postage.

Food for Thought

A quarterly newsletter for the general public and professionals.

Contains nutrition information on a variety of topics in a nontechnical style.

From: Food for Thought, 2400 Reading Rd., Cincinnati, OH 45202

$2/yr

Food Technology

A monthly journal for professionals

Official journal of the Institute of Food Technologists; presents original papers and articles concerned with food science.

From: Institute of Food Technologists, 221 North LaSalle St., Chicago, IL 60601

$40/yr domestic, Canada, Mexico; $45/yr foreign

The Harvard Medical School Health Letter

A monthly newsletter for the general public, professionals, and college-level students.

Medical news and information on preventive health care; monthly column entitled "Medical Forum" by Harvard medical doctors.

From HMSHL, 79 Garden St., Cambridge, MA 02138

$12/yr

Health Education

A bimonthly journal for professionals.

Presents recent advances in the area of health education; journal of the Association for the Advancement of Health Education.

From: Health Education, 1201 16th St., NW, Washington, DC 20036

$35/yr

Health Fact Tips

A quarterly fact sheet (usually 20 pages) for the general public and professionals.

Fact sheet on current issues in health.

From: Health Education Foundation, 600 New Hampshire Ave., NW, Washington, DC 20037

$2/issue

HEF News

A quarterly newsletter for the general public and professionals.

Records current and updated information on trends and knowledge as it relates to health and life style.

From: Health Education Foundation, 600 New Hampshire Ave., NW, Washington, DC 20037

$10/yr

Home Economics Research Journal

A quarterly journal for college-level students and professionals that records and reports scientific methods and applications of home economics research; facilitates scholarly interchange between home economists and other professionals concerned with the well-being of families.

From: American Home Economics Association, 2010 Massachusetts Ave., NW, Washington, DC 20036

$35/yr

Hunger Notes

A monthly newsletter for the general public and professionals concerned with issues in world hunger and domestic food programs.

From: World Hunger Education Service, 2000 P St., NW, Washington, DC 20036

$7.50/yr individual; $12/yr libraries; bulk rates available

Illinois Teacher of Home Economics

A bimonthly journal for teachers and professionals. Contains a variety of articles for home economics teachers, dealing with teaching techniques, societal problems, nutrition, women's rights.

From: Illinois Teacher of Home Economics, 351 College of Education, University of Illinois, Urbana, IL 61801

$7.50/yr

Journal of Food Science

A bimonthly journal for professionals and college-level students. Contains research articles on recent advances in food science.

From: Institute of Food Technologists, 221 North LaSalle St., Chicago, IL 60601

$45/yr in U.S., Canada, and Mexico; $50/yr all other countries

Journal of Home Economics

A quarterly journal for professionals and college-level students. Contains articles concerning nutrition, families, environment, home economics, consumerism.

From: American Home Economics Association, 2101 Massachusetts Ave., NW, Washington, DC 20036

$16/yr

Journal of Nutrition for the Elderly

A quarterly journal for professionals and college-level students. Focus is on recommendations and their implementation to provide better nutrition for older persons.

$19/yr individuals; $38/yr institutions; $48/yr library/subscription agencies

Journal of Nutrition

A monthly journal for professionals and college-level students. Reports of original research bearing on the nature of food nutrients and their function in a variety of organisms, and articles that report on developments in nutritional concepts.

From: American Institute of Nutrition, 9650 Rockville Pike, Bethesda, MD 20014

$30/yr for members of AIN, $55/yr for nonmembers; $65/yr institutions; $18/yr students

Journal of Nutrition Education

A quarterly journal for professionals. Contains original articles, educational materials, reviews, editorials, and other information to assist nutrition educators to be up-to-date and effective in teaching, counseling, and communicating.

From: Subscription Dept., Society for Nutrition Education, 1736 Franklin St., Oakland, CA 94612

$25/yr individuals, U.S.; $27/yr all other countries; $30/yr institutions U.S.; $32/yr all other countries

LaLeche League News

A newsletter for the general public. Contains articles and stories submitted by parents sharing their experiences on breastfeeding.

From: LaLeche League, 9616 Minneapolis Ave., Franklin Park, IL 60131

$3/yr

National Food Review

A quarterly magazine for professionals. Reviews the latest developments in food programs, consumption, prices, government action, and legislation.

From: Superintendent of Documents, U.S. Government Printing Office, Washington, DC 20402

$5.50/yr U.S.; $6.90/ foreign

Newsletter—Office of Health, Nutrition, and Physical Education, Archdiocese of Chicago

A quarterly newsletter for professionals and the general public. Contains the latest information and research in health, nutrition, and physical education.

From: Office of Health, Nutrition and Physical Education, 730 North LaSalle St., Chicago, IL 60610

$5/yr

Nutrition and Cancer: An International Journal

A quarterly journal for professionals. Contains reviews, reports, and original papers containing the results of experimental, clinical, or statistical studies relating nutrition with the etiology, therapy, and prevention of cancer.

From: The Franklin Institute Press, Box 2266, Philadelphia, PA 19103

$60/yr U.S., Canada, and Mexico; $70/yr foreign

Nutrition and Food Science

A bimonthly magazine for professionals and the general public. Contains authoritative articles on all aspects of nutrition and food science, with special application to nutrition education in schools and colleges.

From: Forbes Publications, Ltd., Hartree House, Queensway, London W2, 4SH England

$30/yr in U.S. and Mexico

Nutrition and the M.D.

A monthly newsletter for professionals and college-level students. Contains brief articles on topics of interest to nutrition professionals and medical doctors. Also contains reviews on the latest books and materials.

From: Nutrition and the M.D., P.O. Box 2160, Van Nuys, CA 91405

$30/yr; $20/yr for students

Nutrition News

A quarterly newsletter for professionals. Contains articles on nutrition-related research and development; and tools and techniques in teaching nutrition.

From: National Dairy Council, 6300 N. River Rd., Rosemont, IL 60018

$2/yr

Nutrition Notes

A quarterly newsletter for professionals. Contains nutrition information, written in non-technical terms, taken from standard medical and scientific publications.

From: United Fresh Fruit and Vegetable Association, North Washington at Madison, Alexandria, VA 22314

$5/yr

Nutrition and Health

A bimonthly newsletter for professionals and the general public. Presents the most important medical facts as well as the dietary considerations covering a variety of health topics.

From: Nutrition and Health, Columbia University, 701 West 168th St., New York, NY 10032

$10/yr

Nutrition Intelligence

A monthly newsletter for professionals. Contains information on nutrition policy and public safety.

From: Nutrition Intelligence, Suite 303, 1750 Pennsylvania Ave., NW, Washington, DC 20006

$165/yr

Nutrition Planning

A quarterly abstract journal for professionals and college-level students. Contains abstracts of studies designed to combat malnutrition, especially in developing countries. Includes documents, proceedings, journal articles, books.

From: Nutrition Planning, P.O. Box 8080, Ann Arbor, MI 48107

$45/yr for surface postage; $55/yr for air postage

Nutrition Reviews

A monthly journal for professionals and college-level students. Features articles by international scientists and interpretive summaries of important clinical and experimental research in biochemistry, food science, public health, toxicology, dentistry, and nutrition.

From: The Nutrition Foundation, 888 17th St., NW, Suite 300, Washington, DC 20006

$15/yr; $7.50/yr, students

Nutrition Today

A bimonthly magazine for professionals and college-level students. Contains articles on current issues in nutrition.

From: Nutrition Today, 703 Giddings Ave., Annapolis, MD 21404

$14.75/yr

Pediatrics

A monthly journal for professionals and college-level students. Contains research articles on recent advances in pediatric medicine. Topics include nutrition.

From: American Academy of Pediatrics, 1300 N. 17th St., Suite 350, Arlington, VA 22209

$24/yr in U.S., Canada, Central and South America; $30/yr all other countries; $16/yr student rate

Pan American Health

A quarterly magazine for professionals and college-level students. Contains articles on public health.

From: Pan American Health Organization, 525 23rd St. NW, Washington, DC 20037

$4/yr

Penny Power

A monthly magazine for children, grades 4 to 6. Contains consumer information on nutrition, products, and services used by children.

From: Penny Power, Consumers Union, 256 Washington St., Mt. Vernon, NY 10550

$7.50/yr individual subscription; bulk rates available

Public Affairs Alerts

A fact sheet prepared by the National Nutrition Consortium staff as nutrition issues arise or documents become available.

From: National Nutrition Consortium, 24 Third St. NE, Suite 200, Washington, DC 20002

$20/yr for members in NNC organizations; $30/yr for others

Of Consuming Interest

A biweekly newsletter for professionals and college-level students. Reports and analyzes federal and state legislation and regulation concerning consumer issues—energy, food and drug, finance

From: Federal-State Reports, Inc. 5203 Leesburg Pike, Suite 1201, Falls Church, VA 22041

$85/yr

Rise and Shine

A bimonthly newsletter for professionals and college-level students. Offers school breakfast success stories, local problems and solutions, plus the latest on regulations.

From: The Children's Foundation, 1420 New York Ave., NW, Suite 800, Washington, DC 20005

$6/yr for agencies; $4/yr for community groups and individuals

Summer Food Bulletin

A quarterly newsletter for professionals. Contains the latest information on the Summer Food Service Program for children. Gives national overview of the program, analysis of issues, and legislative updates.

From: The Children's Foundation, 1420 New York Ave., NW, Suite 800, Washington, DC 20005

$6/yr for agencies; $4/yr for community groups and individuals

School Food Service Research Review

A semi-annual journal for professionals. Contains articles on research findings in nutrition applicable to school food service.

From: American School Food Service Association, 4101 E. Iliff Ave., Denver, CO 80222

$8/yr

Weight Watchers Magazine

A monthly magazine for the general public. Contains recipes, nutrition information, physical fitness advice for those interested in weight control.

From: Weight Watcher's Magazine, P.O. Box 2555, Boulder, CO 80322

$9/yr U.S.; add $3/yr for Canada and Mexico; add $4/yr foreign

Food
Exchange
Lists
D

MILK EXCHANGE

Each contains 12 g carbohydrates, 8 g protein, 80 kcalories.

Nonfat fortified milk	*1 Exchange*
Skim or nonfat milk	1 cup
Powdered (nonfat dry, before adding liquid)	⅓ cup
Canned, evaporated—skim milk	½ cup
Buttermilk made from skim milk	1 cup
Yogurt made from skim milk (plain, unflavored)	1 cup

Low-Fat fortified milk	
1% fat fortified milk (uses ½ fat exchange)	1 cup
2% fat fortified milk (uses 1 fat exchange)	1 cup
Yogurt (plain, unflavored) made from 2% fortified milk (uses 1 fat exchange)	1 cup
Fruit-flavored yogurt (uses 1½ bread exchanges and 1 fat exchange)	1 cup

Whole milk (each uses 2 fat exchanges)	
Whole milk	1 cup
Canned, evaporated whole milk	½ cup
Buttermilk made from whole milk	1 cup
Yogurt made from whole milk (plain, unflavored)	1 cup
Fruit-flavored yogurt made from whole milk (uses 1½ bread exchanges)	1 cup

The exchange lists are based on material in the *Exchange Lists for Meal Planning* prepared by Committees of the American Diabetes Association, Inc. and the American Dietetic Association in cooperation with the National Institute of Arthritis, Metabolism and Digestive Diseases and the National Heart and Lung Institute, National Institutes of Health, Public Health Service, U.S. Department of Health, Education and Welfare.

MEAT EXCHANGE

Each exchange contains 7 g protein, 3 g fat, plus added fat; 55 kcalories plus kcalories for added fat. There are 3 meat exchange lists: low-fat, medium-fat (each exchange uses ½ fat exchange), and high-fat (each exchange uses 1 fat exchange).

Low-fat meat and other protein-rich foods

Beef
Baby beef (very lean), chipped beef, chuck, flank steak, tenderloin, plate ribs, plate skirt steak, round (bottom, top), all cuts rump, spare ribs, tripe .... 1 ounce

Lamb
Leg, rib sirloin, loin (roast and chops), shank, shoulder .... 1 ounce

Pork
Leg (whole rump, center shank), ham, smoked (center slices) ... 1 ounce

Veal
Leg, loin, rib, shank, shoulder, cutlets .... 1 ounce

Poultry .... 1 ounce
Meat without skin of chicken, turkey, cornish hen, guinea hen, pheasant

Fish
Any fresh or frozen .... 1 ounce
Canned lobster, salmon, tuna, mackerel, or crab .... ¼ cup
Clams, oysters, scallops, shrimp .... 5 or 1 ounce
Sardines, drained .... 3 ounces

Cheeses
Cottage, dry and 2% butterfat .... ¼ cup
Cottage, low-fat .... ¼ cup
Soft-spread cheese food .... 1 ounce
Whipped cheese food .... 1 ounce
Sliced cheese food .... 1 ounce
Farmer's cheese or pot cheese, low-fat .... 1 ounce
Dried beans and peas, cooked (uses 1 bread exchange) .... ½ cup

Medium-fat meat and other protein-rich foods. Each meat exchange in this list uses ½ fat exchange

Beef
Ground (diet lean 15% fat), corned beef (canned), rib eye, round (ground commercial) .... 1 ounce

Fish
Breaded and deep-fat fried (uses ½ bread exchange and ½ additional fat exchange) .... 1 ounce

Pork
Loin (all cuts tenderloin), shoulder arm, shoulder blade, Boston butt, Canadian bacon, boiled ham .... 1 ounce

Organ meats
Liver, heart, kidneys, and sweetbreads (these are high in cholesterol) .... 1 ounce

Cheeses
Cottage, creamed .... ¼ cup
Mozzarella (made with skim milk), ricotta, farmer's, neufchatel .... 1 ounce

Parmesan	3 tablespoons
Egg (high in cholesterol)	1
Peanut butter (uses 2 additional fat exchanges)	2 tablespoons

High-fat meat and other protein-rich foods. Each meat exchange in this list uses 1 fat exchange.

Beef	1 ounce
Brisket, corned beef, ground beef, hamburger, chuck, roasts, steaks, soy bean extended ground beef	
Lamb	
Breast	1 ounce
Pork	
Spare ribs, loin, pork (ground), country-style ham, deviled ham	1 ounce
Veal	
Breast	1 ounce
Poultry	
Capon, duck, goose	1 ounce
Breaded and deep-fat fried (uses ½ bread exchange and 1 additional fat exchange)	1 ounce
Cheeses	
American, blue, brick, camembert, cheddar, gouda, limburger, muenster, swiss (all types), all processed cheeses	1 ounce
Cold cuts	4½″ × ⅛″ slice
Frankfurter	1 small
Sausage	
Braunschweiger (uses 1 additional fat exhange)	1 ounce
Salami, dry type (uses 1 and ½ additional fat exchanges)	1 ounce

VEGETABLE EXCHANGE

Each exchange contains 5 g carbohydrate, 2 g protein, 25 kcalories; (Each exchange = ½ cup)

Asparagus	Kale
Bean sprouts	Mustard
Beets	Spinach
*Broccoli	Turnip
*Brussels sprouts	Mushrooms
Cabbage	Okra
*Carrots	Onions
Cauliflower	Rhubarb
Celery	Rutabaga
Cucumber	Sauerkraut
Eggplant	Squash, summer
*Green pepper	String beans: green or yellow
*Greens:	*Tomatoes
Beet	Tomato juice
Chard	Turnips
Collards	Vegetable juice cocktail
Dandelion	Zucchini

The following raw vegetables may be eaten as desired:

Chicory
Chinese cabbage
Endive
*Escarole

Lettuce
*Parsley
Radishes
*Watercress

*These vegetables are high in vitamin A; include at least 1 serving of one of these each day.

FRUIT EXCHANGE

Each exchange contains 10 g carbohydrate, 40 kcalories.

Apple (2″ diameter)	1 small
Apple juice	⅓ cup
Applesauce (unsweetened)	½ cup
Apricots, fresh	2 medium
Apricots, dried	4 halves
Banana	½ small
Berries	
Blackberries	½ cup
Blueberries	½ cup
Raspberries	½ cup
Strawberries	¾ cup
*Cantaloupe (6″ diameter)	¼ cup
Cherries	10 large
Cider	⅓ cup
Dates	2
Figs, fresh	1
Figs, dried	1
*Grapefruit	½
*Grapefruit juice	½ cup
Grapes	12
Grape juice	¼ cup
*Honeydew melon (7″ diameter)	⅛
Mango	½ small
Nectarine	1 small
*Orange	1 small
*Orange juice	½ cup
Papaya	¾ cup
Peach	1 medium
Pear	1 small
Persimmon (native)	1 medium
Pineapple	½ cup
Pineapple juice	⅓ cup
Plums	2 medium
Prunes, dried	2
Prune juice	¼ cup
Raisins	2 tablespoons
*Tangerine	1 medium
Watermelon	1 cup

*These fruits are rich sources of vitamin C; include at least 1 serving of one of these each day.

BREAD EXCHANGE

Includes bread, cereal, and starchy vegetables. Each contains 15 g carbohydrate, 2 g protein, and 70 kcalories.

Bread
White (including French and Italian) — 1 slice
Whole wheat — 1 slice
Rye or pumpernickel — 1 slice
Raisin — 1 slice
Bagel, small — ½
English muffin, small — ½
Plain roll, bread — 1
Frankfurter roll — ½
Hamburger bun — ½
Dried bread crumbs — 3 tablespoons
Tortilla, 6″ — 1

Cereal
Bran flakes — ½ cup
Other ready-to-eat unsweetened cereal — ¾ cup
Puffed cereal (unfrosted) — 1 cup
Cereal (cooked) — ½ cup
Grits (cooked) — ½ cup
Rice or barley (cooked) — ½ cup
Pasta (cooked), spaghetti, noodles, macaroni — ½ cup
Popcorn (popped, no fat added, large kernel) — 3 cups
Cornmeal (dry) — 2 tablespoons
Flour — 2½ tablespoons
Wheat germ — ¼ cup

Crackers
Arrowroot — 3
Graham, 2½″ square — 2
Matzoth, 4″ × 6″ — ½
Oyster — 20
Pretzels, 3 ⅛″ long × ⅛″ diameter — 25
Rye wafers, 2″ × 3½″ — 3
Saltines — 6
Soda, 2½″ square — 4

Dried Beans, Peas, Lentils
Beans, peas, lentils (dried and cooked) — ½ cup
Baked beans, no pork (canned) — ¼ cup

Starchy Vegetables
Corn — ⅓ cup
Corn on cob — 1 small
Lima beans — ½ cup
Parsnips — ⅔ cup
Peas, green (canned or frozen) — ½ cup
Potato, white — 1 small
Potato (mashed) — ½ cup
Winter squash, acorn or butternut — ½ cup
Yam or sweet potato — ¼ cup

Prepared Foods
Biscuit, 2″ diameter (uses 1 fat exchange) — 1
Corn bread, 2″ × 2″ × 1″ (uses 1 fat exchange) — 1
Corn muffin, 2″ diameter (uses 1 fat exchange) — 1
Crackers, round butter type (uses 1 fat exchange) — 5
Muffin, plain small (uses 1 fat exchange) — 1
Potatoes, french fried, length 2″ to 3½″ (uses 1 fat exchange) — 8
Potato or corn chips (uses 2 fat exchanges) — 15
Pancake, 5″ × ½″ (uses 1 fat exchange) — 1
Waffle, 5″ × ½″ (uses 1 fat exchange) — 1

FAT EXCHANGES

This list shows the kinds and amounts of fat-containing foods to use for one fat exchange. Each exchange contains 5 g fat and 45 kcalories.

*Margarine, soft, tub or stick	1 teaspoon
**Avocado (4" in diameter)	⅛
Oil, corn, cottonseed, safflower, soy, sunflower	1 teaspoon
**Oil, olive	1 teaspoon
**Oil, peanut	1 teaspoon
**Olives	5 small
**Almonds	10 whole
**Pecans	2 large whole
**Peanuts	
Spanish	20 whole
Virginia	10 whole
Walnuts	6 small
**Nuts, other	6 small
Margarine, regular stick	1 teaspoon
Butter	1 teaspoon
Bacon fat	1 teaspoon
Bacon, crisp	1 strip
Cream, light	2 tablespoons
Cream, sour	2 tablespoons
Cream, heavy	1 tablespoon
Cream cheese	1 tablespoon
***French dressing	1 tablespoon
***Italian dressing	1 tablespoon
Lard	1 teaspoon
***Mayonnaise	1 teaspoon
***Salad dressing, mayonnaise type	2 teaspoons
Salt pork	¾" cube

*Made with corn, cottonseed, safflower, soy or sunflower oil only.
**Fat content is primarily monounsaturated.
***If made with corn, cottonseed, safflower, soy, or sunflower oil, can be used on fat-modified diet.

BEVERAGE, SEASONING AND CONDIMENT EXCHANGES

These foods may be used as desired unless the physician finds a special reason to limit them. They contain no appreciable carbohydrate, fat, or protein if used in ordinary amounts.

Coffee	Lemon
Tea	Mustard
Clear broth	Nutmeg
Bouillon, without fat	Onion seasoning
Gelatin, unsweetened	Parsley seasoning
Rennet tablets	Pepper
Celery seasoning	Saccharin, sucaryl, and other noncaloric sweetners
Cinnamon	Vinegar
Garlic	Pickles (sour or unsweetened dill)

Energy Expenditure in Household, Recreational, and Sports Activities (in kcal/min)

E

HOW TO USE THIS TABLE

Refer to the column that comes closest to your present body weight. Multiply the number in this column by the number of minutes you spend in an activity. For example, suppose an individual weighs 157 pounds and spends 30 minutes playing a casual game of table tennis. To determine the kcal cost of participation, multiply the caloric value of 4.8 kcal obtained in the table by 30 to obtain a total energy expenditure of 144 kcal. If the same individual drives a tractor for 45 minutes the energy expended would be calculated as 2.6 kcal × 45 min or 117 kcal.

Activity	Kcal/min·kg	kg lb	50 110	53 117	56 123	59 130	62 137	65 143	68 150
Archery	0.065		3.3	3.4	3.6	3.8	4.0	4.2	4.4
Badminton	0.097		4.9	5.1	5.4	5.7	6.0	6.3	6.6
Bakery, general (F)	0.035		1.8	1.9	2.0	2.1	2.2	2.3	2.4
Basketball	0.138		6.9	7.3	7.7	8.1	8.6	9.0	9.4
Billiards	0.042		2.1	2.2	2.4	2.5	2.6	2.7	2.9
Bookbinding	0.038		1.9	2.0	2.1	2.2	2.4	2.5	2.6
Boxing									
in ring	0.222		6.9	7.3	7.7	8.1	8.6	9.0	9.4
sparring	0.138		11.1	11.8	12.4	13.1	13.8	14.4	15.1
Canoeing									
leisure	0.044		2.2	2.3	2.5	2.6	2.7	2.9	3.0
racing	0.103		5.2	5.5	5.8	6.1	6.4	6.7	7.0
Card playing	0.025		1.3	1.3	1.4	1.5	1.6	1.6	1.7
Carpentry, general	0.052		2.6	2.8	2.9	3.1	3.2	3.4	3.5
Carpet sweeping (F)	0.045		2.3	2.4	2.5	2.7	2.8	2.9	3.1
Carpet sweeping (M)	0.048		2.4	2.5	2.7	2.8	3.0	3.1	3.3
Circuit-training	0.185		9.3	9.8	10.4	10.9	11.5	12.0	12.6
Cleaning (F)	0.062		3.1	3.3	3.5	3.7	3.8	4.0	4.2
Cleaning (M)	0.058		2.9	3.1	3.2	3.4	3.6	3.8	3.9
Climbing hills									
with no load	0.121		6.1	6.4	6.8	7.1	7.5	7.9	8.2
with 5-kg load	0.129		6.5	6.8	7.2	7.6	8.0	8.4	8.8
with 10-kg load	0.140		7.0	7.4	7.8	8.3	8.7	9.1	9.5
with 20-kg load	0.147		7.4	7.8	8.2	8.7	9.1	9.6	10.0
Coal mining									
drilling coal, rock	0.094		4.7	5.0	5.3	5.5	5.8	6.1	6.4
erecting supports	0.088		4.4	4.7	4.9	5.2	5.5	5.7	6.0
shoveling coal	0.108		5.4	5.7	6.0	6.4	6.7	7.0	7.3
Cooking (F)	0.045		2.3	2.4	2.5	2.7	2.8	2.9	3.1
Cooking (M)	0.048		2.4	2.5	2.7	2.8	3.0	3.1	3.3

Activity	71 157	74 163	77 170	80 176	83 183	86 190	89 196	92 203	95 209	98 216
Archery	4.6	4.8	5.0	5.2	5.4	5.6	5.8	6.0	6.2	6.4
Badminton	6.9	7.2	7.5	7.8	8.1	8.3	8.6	8.9	9.2	9.5
Bakery, general (F)	2.5	2.6	2.7	2.8	2.9	3.0	3.1	3.2	3.3	3.4
Basketball	9.8	10.2	10.6	11.0	11.5	11.9	12.3	12.7	13.1	13.5
Billiards	3.0	3.1	3.2	3.4	3.5	3.6	3.7	3.9	4.0	4.1
Bookbinding	2.7	2.8	2.9	3.0	3.2	3.3	3.4	3.5	3.6	3.7
Boxing										
in ring	9.8	10.2	10.6	11.0	11.5	11.9	12.3	12.7	13.1	13.5
sparring	15.8	16.4	17.1	17.8	18.4	19.1	19.8	20.4	21.1	21.8
Canoeing										
leisure	3.1	3.3	3.4	3.5	3.7	3.8	3.9	4.0	4.2	4.3
racing	7.3	7.6	7.9	8.2	8.5	8.9	9.2	9.5	9.8	10.1
Card playing	1.8	1.9	1.9	2.0	2.1	2.2	2.2	2.3	2.4	2.5
Carpentry, general	3.7	3.8	4.0	4.2	4.3	4.5	4.6	4.8	4.9	5.1
Carpet sweeping (F)	3.2	3.3	3.5	3.6	3.7	3.9	4.0	4.1	4.3	4.4
Carpet sweeping (M)	3.4	3.6	3.7	3.8	4.0	4.1	4.3	4.4	4.6	4.7
Circuit-training	13.1	13.7	14.2	14.8	15.4	15.9	16.5	17.0	17.6	18.1
Cleaning (F)	4.4	4.6	4.8	5.0	5.1	5.3	5.5	5.7	5.9	6.1
Cleaning (M)	4.1	4.3	4.5	4.6	4.8	5.0	5.2	5.3	5.5	5.7
Climbing hills										
with no load	8.6	9.0	9.3	9.7	10.0	10.4	10.8	11.1	11.5	11.9
with 5-kg load	9.2	9.5	9.9	10.3	10.7	11.1	11.5	11.9	12.3	12.6
with 10-kg load	9.9	10.4	10.8	11.2	11.6	12.0	12.5	12.9	13.3	13.7
with 20-kg load	10.4	10.9	11.3	11.8	12.2	12.6	13.1	13.5	14.0	14.4
Coal mining										
drilling coal, rock	6.7	7.0	7.2	7.5	7.8	8.1	8.4	8.6	8.9	9.2
erecting supports	6.2	6.5	6.8	7.0	7.3	7.6	7.8	8.1	8.4	8.6
shoveling coal	7.7	8.0	8.3	8.6	9.0	9.3	9.6	9.9	10.3	10.6
Cooking (F)	3.2	3.3	3.5	3.6	3.7	3.9	4.0	4.1	4.3	4.4
Cooking (M)	3.4	3.6	3.7	3.8	4.0	4.1	4.3	4.4	4.6	4.7

Note: Symbols (M) and (F) denote experiments for males and females, respectively.

Source: Frank I. Katch and William D. McArdle, *Nutrition, Weight Control, and Exercise* (Boston: Houghton Mifflin, 1977), Appendix B, p. 348.

Recommended Daily Dietary Allowances

F

Recommended Daily Dietary Allowances, (Revised 1980)[a]

| | | Weight | | Height | | | Fat-Soluble Vitamins | | |
| | | | | | | | Vita-min A | Vita-min D | Vita-min E |
	Age (years)	(kg)	(lb)	(cm)	(in)	Protein (g)	(μg RE)[b]	(μg)[c]	(mg α-TE)[d]
Infants	0.0−0.5	6	13	60	24	kg × 2.2	420	10	3
	0.5−1.0	9	20	71	28	kg × 2.0	400	10	4
Children	1−3	13	29	90	35	23	400	10	5
	4−6	20	44	112	44	30	500	10	6
	7−10	28	62	132	52	34	700	10	7
Males	11−14	45	99	157	62	45	1000	10	8
	15−18	66	145	176	69	56	1000	10	10
	19−22	70	154	177	70	56	1000	7.5	10
	23−50	70	154	178	70	56	1000	5	10
	51+	70	154	178	70	56	1000	5	10
Females	11−14	46	101	157	62	46	800	10	8
	15−18	55	120	163	64	46	800	10	8
	19−22	55	120	163	64	44	800	7.5	8
	23−50	55	120	163	64	44	800	5	8
	51+	55	120	163	64	44	800	5	8
Pregnant						+30	+200	+5	+2
Lactating						+20	+400	+5	+3

[a] The allowances are intended to provide for individual variations among most normal persons as they live in the United States under usual environmental stresses. Diets should be based on a variety of common foods in order to provide other nutrients for which human requirements have been less well defined.

[b] Retinol equivalents, 1 retinol equivalent = 1 μg retinol or 6 μg β carotene.

[c] As cholecalciferol. 10 μg cholecalciferol = 400 IU of vitamin D.

[d] α-tocopherol equivalents. 1 mg d-α tocopherol = 1 α-TE. See text for variation in allowances and calculation of vitamin E activity of the diet as α-tocopherol equivalents.

Water-Soluble Vitamins

	Vitamin C (mg)	Thiamin (mg)	Riboflavin (mg)	Niacin (mg NE)[e]	Vitamin B-6 (mg)	Folacin (µg)	Vitamin B-12 (µg)
Infants	35	0.3	0.4	6	0.3	30	0.5[g]
	35	0.5	0.6	8	0.6	45	1.5
Children	45	0.7	0.8	9	0.9	100	2.0
	45	0.9	1.0	11	1.3	200	2.5
	45	1.2	1.4	16	1.6	300	3.0
Males	50	1.4	1.6	18	1.8	400	3.0
	60	1.4	1.7	18	2.0	400	3.0
	60	1.5	1.7	19	2.2	400	3.0
	60	1.4	1.6	18	2.2	400	3.0
	60	1.2	1.4	16	2.2	400	3.0
Females	50	1.1	1.3	15	1.8	400	3.0
	60	1.1	1.3	14	2.0	400	3.0
	60	1.1	1.3	14	2.0	400	3.0
	60	1.0	1.2	13	2.0	400	3.0
	60	1.0	1.2	13	2.0	400	3.0
Pregnant	+20	+0.4	+0.3	+2	+0.6	+400	+1.0
Lactating	+40	+0.5	+0.5	+5	+0.5	+100	+1.0

[e] 1 NE (niacin equivalent) is equal to 1 mg of niacin or 60 mg of dietary tryptophan.

[f] The folacin allowances refer to dietary sources as determined by *Lactobacillus casei* assay after treatment with enzymes (conjugases) to make polyglutamyl forms of the vitamin available to the test organism.

[g] The recommended dietary allowance for vitamin B-12 in infants is based on average concentration of the vitamin in human milk. The allowances after weaning are based on energy intake (as recommended by the American Academy of Pediatrics) and consideration of other factors, such as intestinal absorption.

Minerals

	Calcium (mg)	Phosphorus (mg)	Magnesium (mg)	Iron (mg)	Zinc (mg)	Iodine (µg)
Infants	360	240	50	10	3	40
	540	360	70	15	5	50
Children	800	800	150	15	10	70
	800	800	200	10	10	90
	800	800	250	10	10	120
Males	1200	1200	350	18	15	150
	1200	1200	400	18	15	150
	800	800	350	10	15	150
	800	800	350	10	15	150
	800	800	350	10	15	150
Females	800	800	300	18	15	150
	1200	1200	300	18	15	150
	1200	1200	300	18	15	150
	800	800	300	18	15	150
	800	800	300	10	15	150
Pregnant	+400	+400	+150	[h]	+5	+25
Lactating	+400	+400	+150	[h]	+10	+50

[h] The increased requirement during pregnancy cannot be met by the iron content of habitual American diets nor by the existing iron stores of many women; therefore the use of 30–60 mg of supplemental iron is recommended. Iron needs during lactation are not substantially different from those of nonpregnant women, but continued supplementation of the mother for 2–3 months after parturition is advisable in order to replenish stores depleted by pregnancy.

Source: Committee on Dietary Allowances, Food and Nutrition Board, National Research Council, *Recommended Dietary Allowances*, 9th rev. ed., 1980 (Washington, D.C.: National Academy of Sciences, 1980).

Estimated Daily Dietary Intakes: Selected Vitamins and Minerals

G

Estimated Safe and Adequate Daily Dietary Intakes of Selected Vitamins and Minerals[a]				
		Vitamins		
	Age (years)	*Vitamin K (μg)*	*Biotin (μg)*	*Panto-thenic Acid (mg)*
Infants	0–0.5	12	35	2
	0.5–1	10–20	50	3
Children	1–3	15–30	65	3
and	4–6	20–40	85	3–4
adolescents	7–10	30–60	120	4–5
	11+	50–100	100–200	4–7
Adults		70–140	100–200	4–7

				Trace Elements[b]			
	Age (years)	*Copper (mg)*	*Man-ganese (mg)*	*Fluoride (mg)*	*Chromium (mg)*	*Selenium (mg)*	*Molyb-denum (mg)*
Infants	0–0.5	0.5–0.7	0.5–0.7	0.1–0.5	0.01–0.04	0.01–0.04	0.03–0.06
	0.5–1	0.7–1.0	0.7–1.0	0.2–1.0	0.02–0.06	0.02–0.06	0.04–0.08
Children	1–3	1.0–1.5	1.0–1.5	0.5–1.5	0.02–0.08	0.02–0.08	0.05–0.1
and	4–6	1.5–2.0	1.5–2.0	1.0–2.5	0.03–0.12	0.03–0.12	0.06–0.15
adolescents	7–10	2.0–2.5	2.0–3.0	1.5–2.5	0.05–0.2	0.05–0.2	0.10–0.3
	11+	2.0–3.0	2.5–5.0	1.5–2.5	0.05–0.2	0.05–0.2	0.15–0.5
Adults		2.0–3.0	2.5–5.0	1.5–4.0	0.05–0.2	0.05–0.2	0.15–0.5

	Age (years)	Electrolytes		
		Sodium (mg)	Potassium (mg)	Chloride (mg)
Infants	0–0.5	115–350	350–925	275–700
	0.5–1	250–750	425–1275	400–1200
Children	1–3	325–975	550–1650	500–1500
and	4–6	450–1350	775–2325	700–2100
adolescents	7–10	600–1800	1000–3000	925–2775
	11 +	900–2700	1525–4575	1400–4200
Adults		1100–3300	1875–5625	1700–5100

[a] Because there is less information on which to base allowances, these figures are not given in the main table of RDA and are provided here in the form of ranges of recommended intakes.

[b] Since the toxic levels for many trace elements may be only several times usual intakes, the upper levels for the trace elements given in this table should not be habitually exceeded.

Source: Committee on Dietary Allowances, Food and Nutrition Board, National Research Council, *Recommended Dietary Allowances,* 9th rev. ed., 1980 (Washington, D.C.: National Academy of Sciences, 1980).

United States Recommended Daily Allowances (U.S. RDA)*

H

	Adults and children 4 or more years of age (For use in labeling conventional foods and also for "special dietary foods")	Infants	Children under 4 years of age (For use only with "special dietary foods")	Pregnant or lactating women
*Nutrients which **must** be declared on the label (in the order below)*				
Protein[†]	45 g "high quality protein" 65 g "proteins in general"	—	—	
Vitamin A	5000 IU	1500 IU	2500 IU	8000 IU
Vitamin C (or ascorbic acid)	60 mg	35 mg	40 mg	60 mg
Thiamin (or vitamin B-1)	1.5 mg	0.5 mg	0.7 mg	1.7 mg
Riboflavin (or vitamin B-2)	1.7 mg	0.6 mg	0.8 mg	2.0 mg
Niacin	20 mg	8 mg	9 mg	20 mg
Calcium	1.0 g	0.6 g	0.8 g	1.3 g
Iron	18 mg	15 mg	10 mg	18 mg
*Nutrients which **may** be declared on the label (in the order below)*				
Vitamin D	400 IU	400 IU	400 IU	400 IU
Vitamin E	30 IU	5 IU	10 IU	30 IU
Vitamin B-6	2.0 mg	0.4 mg	0.7 mg	2.5 mg
Folic acid (or folacin)	0.4 mg	0.1 mg	0.2 mg	0.8 mg

* Note: The U.S. RDA are the amounts of proteins, vitamins, and minerals established by the Food and Drug Administration as standards for nutrition labeling. These allowances were derived from the RDA set by the Food and Nutrition Board. The U.S. RDA for most nutrients approximates the highest RDA of the sex-age categories in this table, excluding the allowances for pregnant and lactating females. Therefore, a diet that furnishes the U.S. RDA for a nutrient will furnish the RDA for most people and more than the RDA for many. U.S. RDA are protein, 45 grams (eggs, fish, meat, milk, poultry), 65 grams (other foods); vitamin A, 5,000 International Units; thiamin, 1.5 milligrams; riboflavin, 1.7 milligrams; niacin, 20 milligrams; ascorbic acid, 60 milligrams; calcium, 1 gram; phosphorus, 1 gram; iron, 18 milligrams. For additional information on U.S. RDA, see the *Federal Register*, 38 (March 14, 1973): 6959–60, and Agriculture Information Bulletin 382, *Nutritional Labeling–Tools for Its Use.*

	Adults and children 4 or more years of age (For use in labeling conventional foods and also for "special dietary foods")	Infants	Children under 4 years of age	Pregnant or lactating women
			(For use only with "special dietary foods")	
Vitamin B-12	6 μg	2 μg	3 μg	8 μg
Phosphorus	1.0 g	0.5 g	0.8 g	1.3 g
Iodine	150 μg	45 μg	70 μg	150 μg
Magnesium	400 mg	70 mg	200 mg	450 mg
Zinc	15 mg	5 mg	8 mg	15 mg
Copper[‡]	2 mg	0.5 mg	1 mg	2 mg
Biotin[‡]	0.3 mg	0.15 mg	0.15 mg	0.3 mg
Pantothenic acid[‡]	10 mg	3 mg	5 mg	10 mg

[†] "High-quality protein" is defined as having a protein efficiency ratio (PER) equal to or greater than that of casein; "proteins in general" are those with a PER less than that of casein. Total protein with a PER less than 20% that of casein are considered "not a significant source of protein" and would not be expressed on the label in terms of the U.S. RDA but only as amount per serving.

[‡] There are no NAS-NRC RDA for biotin, pantothenic acid, and copper.

Nutritive Value of Foods

I

A table of nutritive values for household measures of commonly used foods makes up the greater part of this bulletin. First published in 1960, the bulletin was revised in 1964, 1970, 1971, 1977, and 1978. In this revision, values for breakfast cereals have been updated. Recent information is provided on the dairy products group; on the enrichment levels of white bread and rolls, white flour, self-rising flour, and products prepared with these enriched flours; and on the fatty acid content of the foods.

EXPLANATION OF THE TABLES

Some helpful volume and weight equivalents are shown in Table 1.

Table 2 shows the food values in 730 foods commonly used.

Foods Listed.   Foods are grouped under the following main headings:

- Dairy products
- Eggs
- Fats and oils
- Fish, shellfish, meat, and poultry
- Fruits and fruit products

By Catherine F. Adams and Martha Richardson, Consumer Nutrition Center, United States Department of Agriculture, Science and Education Administration. Home and Garden Bulletin 72.

- Grain products
- Legumes (dry), nuts, and seeds
- Sugars and sweets
- Vegetables and vegetable products
- Miscellaneous items

Most of the foods listed are in ready-to-eat form. Some are basic products widely used in food preparation, such as flour, fat, and cornmeal.

The weight in grams for an approximate measure of each food is shown. A footnote indicates if inedible parts are included in the description and the weight. For example, item 246 is half a grapefruit with peel having a weight of 241 grams. A footnote to this item explains that the 241 grams include the weight of the peel.

The approximate measure shown for each food is in cups, ounces, pounds, some other well-known unit, or a piece of certain size. The cup measure refers to the standard measuring cup of 8 fluid ounces or one-half liquid pint. The ounce refers to one-sixteenth of a pound avoirdupois, unless fluid ounce is indicated. The weight of a fluid ounce varies according to the food measured.

TABLE 1 Equivalents by Volume and Weight

Volume	
Level measure	*Equivalent*
1 gallon (3.786 liters; 3,786 milliliters)	4 quarts
1 quart (0.946 liter; 946 milliliters)	4 cups
1 cup (237 milliliters)	8 fluid ounces 1/2 pint 16 tablespoons
2 tablespoons (30 milliliters)	1 fluid ounce
1 tablespoon (15 milliliters)	3 teaspoons
1 pound regular butter or margarine	4 sticks 2 cups
1 pound whipped butter or margarine	6 sticks Two 8-ounce containers 3 cups

Weight	
Avoirdupois weight	*Equivalent*
1 pound (16 ounces)	453.6 grams
1 ounce	28.35 grams
3 1/2 ounces	100 grams

Food Values.   Table 2 also shows values for protein, fat, total saturated fatty acids, two unsaturated fatty acids (oleic acid and linoleic acid), total carbohydrates, four minerals (calcium, iron, phosphorus, and potassium), and five vitamins (vitamin A, thiamin, riboflavin, niacin, and ascorbic acid or vitamin C). Food energy is in kcalories. The kcalorie is the unit of measurement for the energy furnished the body by protein, fat, and carbohydrate.

Those values can be used to compare kinds and amounts of nutrients in different foods. They sometimes can be used to compare different forms of the same food.

Water content is included because the percentage of moisture present is needed for identification and comparison of many food items.

The values for food energy (kcalories) and nutrients shown in Table 2 are the amounts present in the edible part of the item, that is, in only that portion customarily eaten—corn without cob, meat without bone, potatoes without skin, European-type grapes without seeds. If additional parts are eaten—the potato skin, for example—amounts of some nutrients obtained will be somewhat greater than those shown.

Values for thiamin, riboflavin, and niacin in white flours and white bread and rolls are based on the increased enrichment levels put into effect for those products by the Food and Drug Administration in 1974. Iron values for those products and the values for enriched cornmeals, pastas, farina, and rice (except riboflavin) represent the minimum levels of enrichment promulgated under the Federal Food, Drug, and Cosmetic Act of 1955. Riboflavin values of rice are for unenriched rice, as the levels for added riboflavin have not been approved. Thiamin, riboflavin, and niacin values for products prepared with white flours represent the use of flours enriched at the 1974 levels and iron at the 1955 levels. Enriched flour is predominately used in home-prepared and commercially prepared baked goods.

Fatty acid values are given for dairy products, eggs, meats, some grain products, nuts, and soups. The values are based on comprehensive research by USDA to update and extend tables for fatty acid content for foods.

Niacin values are for preformed niacin occurring naturally in foods. The values do not include additional niacin that the body may form from tryptophan, an essential amino acid in the protein of most foods. Among the better sources of tryptophan are milk, meats, eggs, legumes, and nuts.

Values have been calculated from the ingredients in typical recipes for many of the prepared items such as biscuits, corn muffins, macaroni and cheese, custard, and many dessert-type items.

Values for toast and cooked vegetables are without fat added, either during preparation or at the table. Some destruction of vitamins, especially ascorbic acid, may occur when vegetables are cut or shredded. Since such losses are variable, no deduction has been made.

For meat, values are for meat cooked and drained of the drippings. For many cuts, two sets of values are shown: meat including fat and meat from which the fat has been removed either in the kitchen or on the plate.

A variety of manufactured items—some of the milk products, ready-to-eat breakfast cereals, imitation cream products, fruit drinks, and various mixes—are included in Table 2. Frequently those foods are fortified with one or more nutrients. If nutrients are added, this information is on the label. Values shown here for those foods are usually based on products from several manufacturers and may differ somewhat from the values provided by any one source.

FURTHER INFORMATION

A number of other publications of the Science and Education Administration, U.S. Department of Agriculture, give helpful information about nutrients and foods in which they are found.

Agriculture Handbook No. 8, *Composition of Foods...Raw, Processed, Prepared,* is a more technical publication with data for a much more extensive list of foods. In it data are presented for the nutrients in 100 grams of edible portion and 1 pound of food as purchased. Nutrients in household measures and market units for many foods are in Agriculture Handbook No. 456, *Nutritive Value of American Foods in Common Units.*

Information about nutrition labeling and the percent of the U.S. RDA of eight nutrients furnished by several household measures of foods may be found in Agriculture Information Bulletin No. 382 *Nutrition Labeling—Tools for Its Use.*

These publications may be purchased from the Superintendent of Documents, U.S. Government Printing Office, Washington, D.C. 20402, or any U.S. Government Printing Office bookstore.

TABLE 2 Nutritive Values of the Edible Part of Foods

Item No. (A)	Foods, approximate measures, units, and weight (edible part unless footnotes indicate otherwise) (B)		Water (C)	Food energy (D)	Protein (E)	Fat (F)	Fatty Acids Saturated (total) (G)	Unsaturated Oleic (H)	Unsaturated Linoleic (I)	Carbohydrate (I)	Calcium (K)	Phosphorus (L)	Iron (M)	Potassium (N)	Vitamin A value (O)	Thiamin (P)	Riboflavin (Q)	Niacin (R)	Ascorbic acid (S)
		Grams	Per cent	Kcalories	Grams	Grams	Grams	Grams	Grams	Grams	Milligrams	Milligrams	Milligrams	Milligrams	International units	Milligrams	Milligrams	Milligrams	Milligrams

DAIRY PRODUCTS (CHEESE, CREAM, IMITATION CREAM, MILK; RELATED PRODUCTS)

Butter. See Fats, oils; related products, items 103–108.

Cheese:
Natural:

Item No. (A)	Foods (B)	Grams	Water % (C)	Food energy (D)	Protein (E)	Fat (F)	Saturated (G)	Oleic (H)	Linoleic (I)	Carbo-hydrate (I)	Calcium (K)	Phosphorus (L)	Iron (M)	Potassium (N)	Vitamin A (O)	Thiamin (P)	Riboflavin (Q)	Niacin (R)	Ascorbic acid (S)
1	Blue	1 oz	28	42	100	6	8	5.3	1.9	0.2	1	150	110	0.1	73	200	.01	.11	0.3	0
2	Camembert (3 wedges per 4-oz container).	1 wedge	38	52	115	8	9	5.8	2.2	.2	Trace	147	132	.1	71	350	.01	.19	.2	0
	Cheddar:																			
3	Cut pieces	1 oz	28	37	115	7	9	6.1	2.1	.2	Trace	204	145	.2	28	300	.01	.11	Trace	0
4		1 cu in	17.2	37	70	4	6	3.7	1.3	.1	Trace	124	88	.1	17	180	Trace	.06	Trace	0
5	Shredded	1 cup	113	37	455	28	37	24.2	8.5	.7	1	815	579	.8	111	1,200	.03	.42	.1	0
	Cottage (curd not pressed down):																			
	Creamed (cottage cheese, 4% fat):																			
6	Large curd	1 cup	225	79	235	28	10	6.4	2.4	.2	6	135	297	.3	190	370	.05	.37	.3	Trace
7	Small curd	1 cup	210	79	220	26	9	6.0	2.2	.2	6	126	277	.3	177	340	.04	.34	.3	Trace
8	Low fat (2%)	1 cup	226	79	205	31	4	2.8	1.0	.1	8	155	340	.4	217	160	.05	.42	.3	Trace
9	Low fat (1%)	1 cup	226	82	165	28	2	1.5	.5	.1	6	138	302	.3	193	80	.05	.37	.3	Trace
10	Uncreamed (cottage cheese dry curd, less than 1/2% fat).	1 cup	145	80	125	25	1	.4	.1	Trace	3	46	151	.3	47	40	.04	.21	.2	0
11	Cream	1 oz	28	54	100	2	10	6.2	2.4	.2	1	23	30	.3	34	400	Trace	.06	Trace	0
	Mozzarella, made with—																			
12	Whole milk	1 oz	28	48	90	6	7	4.4	1.7	.2	1	163	117	.1	21	260	Trace	.08	Trace	0
13	Part skim milk	1 oz	28	49	80	8	5	3.1	1.2	.1	1	207	149	.1	27	180	.01	.10	Trace	0
	Parmesan, grated:																			
14	Cup, not pressed down	1 cup	100	18	455	42	30	19.1	7.7	.3	4	1,376	807	1.0	107	700	.05	.39	.3	0
15	Tablespoon	1 tbsp	5	18	25	2	2	1.0	.4	Trace	Trace	69	40	Trace	5	40	Trace	.02	Trace	0
16	Ounce	1 oz	28	18	130	12	9	5.4	2.2	.1	1	390	229	.3	30	200	.01	.11	.1	0
17	Provolone	1 oz	28	41	100	7	8	4.8	1.7	.1	1	214	141	.1	39	230	.01	.09	Trace	0
	Ricotta, made with—																			
18	Whole milk	1 cup	246	72	430	28	32	20.4	7.1	.7	7	509	389	.9	257	1,210	.03	.48	.3	0
19	Part skim milk	1 cup	246	74	340	28	19	12.1	4.7	.5	13	669	449	1.1	308	1,060	.05	.46	.2	0
20	Romano	1 oz	28	31	110	9	8	–	–	–	1	302	215	–	–	160	–	.11	Trace	0

Dashes (–) denote lack of reliable data for a constituent believed to be present in measurable amount.

NUTRIENTS IN INDICATED QUANTITY

Item No. (A)	Foods, approximate measures, units, and weight (edible part unless footnotes indicate otherwise) (B)	Measure	Grams	Water Per-cent (C)	Food energy Calories (D)	Protein Grams (E)	Fat Grams (F)	Saturated (total) Grams (G)	Unsaturated Oleic Grams (H)	Linoleic Grams (I)	Carbohydrate Grams (I)	Calcium Milligrams (K)	Phosphorus Milligrams (L)	Iron Milligrams (M)	Potassium Milligrams (N)	Vitamin A value International units (O)	Thiamin Milligrams (P)	Riboflavin Milligrams (Q)	Niacin Milligrams (R)	Ascorbic acid Milligrams (S)
21	Swiss	1 oz	28	37	105	8	8	5.0	1.7	.2	1	272	171	Trace	31	240	.01	.10	Trace	0
	Pasteurized process cheese:																			
22	American	1 oz	28	39	105	6	9	5.6	2.1	.2	Trace	174	211	.1	46	340	.01	.10	Trace	0
23	Swiss	1 oz	28	42	95	7	7	4.5	1.7	.1	1	219	216	.2	61	230	Trace	.08	Trace	0
24	Pasteurized process cheese food, American	1 oz	28	43	95	6	7	4.4	1.7	.1	2	163	130	.2	79	260	.01	.13	Trace	0
25	Pasteurized process cheese spread, American	1 oz	28	48	80	5	6	3.8	1.5	.1	2	159	202	.1	69	220	.01	.12	Trace	0
	Cream, sweet:																			
26	Half-and-half (cream and milk)	1 cup	242	81	315	7	28	17.3	7.0	.6	10	254	230	.2	314	260	.08	.36	.2	2
27		1 tbsp	15	81	20	Trace	2	1.1	.4	Trace	1	16	14	Trace	19	20	.01	.02	Trace	Trace
28	Light, coffee, or table	1 cup	240	74	470	6	46	28.8	11.7	1.0	9	231	192	.1	292	1,730	.08	.36	.1	2
29		1 tbsp	15	74	30	Trace	3	1.8	.7	.1	1	14	12	Trace	18	110	Trace	.02	Trace	Trace
	Whipping, unwhipped (volume about double when whipped):																			
30	Light	1 cup	239	64	700	5	74	46.2	18.3	1.5	7	166	146	0.1	231	2,690	0.06	0.30	0.1	1
31		1 tbsp	15	64	45	Trace	5	2.9	1.1	.1	Trace	10	9	Trace	15	170	Trace	.02	Trace	Trace
32	Heavy	1 cup	238	58	820	5	88	54.8	22.2	2.0	7	154	149	.1	179	3,500	.05	.26	.1	1
33		1 tbsp	15	58	80	Trace	6	3.5	1.4	.1	Trace	10	9	Trace	11	220	Trace	.02	Trace	Trace
34	Whipped topping, (pressurized)	1 cup	60	61	155	2	13	8.3	3.4	.3	7	61	54	Trace	88	550	.02	.04	Trace	0
35		1 tbsp	3	61	10	Trace	1	.4	.2	Trace	Trace	3	3	Trace	4	30	Trace	Trace	Trace	0
36	Cream, sour	1 cup	230	71	495	7	48	30.0	12.1	1.1	10	268	195	.1	331	1,820	.08	.34	.2	2
37		1 tbsp	12	71	25	Trace	3	1.6	.6	.1	1	14	10	Trace	17	90	Trace	.02	Trace	Trace
	Cream products, imitation (made with vegetable fat):																			
	Sweet:																			
	Creamers:																			
38	Liquid (frozen)	1 cup	245	77	335	2	24	22.8	.3	Trace	28	23	157	.1	467	[1]220	0	0	0	0
39		1 tbsp	15	77	20	Trace	2	1.4	Trace	0	2	1	10	Trace	29	[1]10	0	0	0	0
40	Powdered	1 cup	94	2	515	5	33	30.6	.9	Trace	52	21	397	Trace	763	[1]190	0	[1].16	0	0
41		1 tsp	2	2	10	Trace	1	.7	Trace	0	1	Trace	8	Trace	16	[1]Trace	0	[1]Trace	0	0
	Whipped topping:																			
42	Frozen	1 cup	75	50	240	1	19	16.3	1.0	.2	17	5	6	.1	14	[1]650	0	0	0	0
43		1 tbsp	4	50	15	Trace	1	.9	.1	Trace	1	Trace	Trace	Trace	1	[1]30	0	0	0	0
44	Powdered, made with whole milk	1 cup	80	67	150	3	10	8.5	.6	.1	13	72	69	Trace	121	[1]290	.02	.09	Trace	1
45		1 tbsp	4	67	10	Trace	Trace	.4	Trace	Trace	1	4	3	Trace	6	[1]10	Trace	Trace	Trace	Trace
46	Pressurized	1 cup	70	60	185	1	16	13.2	1.4	.2	1	4	13	Trace	13	[1]330	Trace	Trace	Trace	Trace
47		1 tbsp	4	60	10	Trace	1	.8	.1	Trace	Trace	Trace	1	Trace	1	[1]20	0	0	0	0
48	Sour dressing (imitation sour cream) made with nonfat dry milk	1 cup	235	75	415	8	39	31.2	4.4	1.1	11	266	205	.1	380	[1]20	.09	.38	.2	2
49		1 tbsp	12	75	20	Trace	2	1.6	.2	.1	1	14	10	Trace	19	[1]Trace	.01	.02	Trace	Trace

[1] Vitamin A value is largely from beta-carotene used for coloring. Riboflavin value for items 40–41 apply to products with added riboflavin.

NUTRIENTS IN INDICATED QUANTITY

Item No. (A)	Foods, approximate measures, units, and weight (edible part unless footnotes indicate otherwise) (B)		Water Per cent (C)	Food energy Kcal-ories (D)	Protein Grams (E)	Fat Grams (F)	Fatty Acids Saturated (total) Grams (G)	Unsaturated Oleic Grams (H)	Unsaturated Linoleic Grams (I)	Carbohydrate Grams (I)	Calcium Milligrams (K)	Phosphorus Milligrams (L)	Iron Milligrams (M)	Potassium Milligrams (N)	Vitamin A value International units (O)	Thiamin Milligrams (P)	Riboflavin Milligrams (Q)	Niacin Milligrams (R)	Ascorbic acid Milligrams (S)
	Ice cream. See Milk desserts, frozen (items 75–80).																		
	Ice milk. See Milk desserts, frozen (items 81–83).																		
	Milk:																		
	Fluid:																		
50	Whole (3.3% fat)	1 cup	244	88	150	8	5.1	2.1	.2	11	291	228	.1	370	[2]310	.09	.40	.2	2
	Lowfat (2%):																		
51	No milk solids added	1 cup	244	89	120	8	5	2.9	1.2	.1	12	297	232	.1	377	500	.10	.40	.2	2
	Milk solids added:																		
52	Label claim less than 10 g of protein per cup.	1 cup	245	89	125	9	5	2.9	1.2	.1	12	313	245	.1	397	500	.10	.42	.2	2
53	Label claim 10 or more grams of protein per cup (protein fortified).	1 cup	246	88	135	10	5	3.0	1.2	.1	14	352	276	.1	447	500	.11	.48	.2	3
	Lowfat (1%):																		
54	No milk solids added	1 cup	244	90	100	8	3	1.6	.7	.1	12	300	235	.1	381	500	.10	.41	.2	2
	Milk solids added:																		
55	Label claim less than 10 g of protein per cup.	1 cup	245	90	105	9	2	1.5	.6	.1	12	313	245	.1	397	500	.10	.42	.2	2
56	Label claim 10 or more grams of protein per cup (protein fortified).	1 cup	246	89	120	10	3	1.8	.7	.1	14	349	273	.1	444	500	.11	.47	.2	3
	Nonfat (skim):																		
57	No milk solids added	1 cup	245	91	85	8	Trace	.3	.1	Trace	12	302	247	.1	406	500	.09	.34	.2	2
	Milk solids added:																		
58	Label claim less than 10 g of protein per cup.	1 cup	245	90	90	9	1	0.4	0.1	Trace	12	316	255	0.1	418	500	0.10	0.43	0.2	2
59	Label claim 10 or more grams of protein per cup (protein fortified).	1 cup	246	89	100	10	1	.4	.1	Trace	14	352	275	.1	446	500	.11	.48	.2	3
60	Buttermilk	1 cup	245	90	100	8	2	1.3	.5	Trace	12	285	219	.1	371	[3]80	.08	.38	.1	2
	Canned:																		
	Evaporated, unsweetened:																		
61	Whole milk	1 cup	252	74	340	17	19	11.6	5.3	0.4	25	657	510	.5	764	[3]610	.12	.80	.5	5
62	Skim milk	1 cup	255	79	200	19	1	.3	.1	Trace	29	738	497	.7	845	[4]1,000	.11	.79	.4	3

[2] Applies to product without added vitamin A. With added vitamin A, value is 500 International Units (I.U.).
[3] Applies to product without added vitamin A.
[4] Applies to product with added vitamin A. Without added vitamin A, value is 20 International Units (I.U.).

Item No. (A)	Foods, approximate measures, units, and weight (edible part unless footnotes indicate otherwise) (B)		Water Per cent (C)	Food energy Kcalories (D)	Protein Grams (E)	Fat Grams (F)	Fatty Acids			Carbohydrate Grams (I)	Calcium Milligrams (K)	Phosphorus Milligrams (L)	Iron Milligrams (M)	Potassium Milligrams (N)	Vitamin A value International units (O)	Thiamin Milligrams (P)	Riboflavin Milligrams (Q)	Niacin Milligrams (R)	Ascorbic acid Milligrams (S)
							Saturated (total) Grams (G)	Unsaturated Oleic Grams (H)	Linoleic Grams (I)										
63	Sweetened, condensed	1 cup	306	27	980	24	27	16.8	6.7	.7	166	868	775	.6	1,136	[3]1,000	.28	1.27	.6	8
	Dried:																			
64	Buttermilk	1 cup	120	3	465	41	7	4.3	1.7	.2	59	1,421	1,119	.4	1,910	[3]260	.47	1.90	1.1	7
	Nonfat instant:																			
65	Envelope, net wt., 3.2 oz[5]	1 envelope	91	4	325	32	1	.4	.1	Trace	47	1,120	896	.3	1,552	[6]2,160	.38	1.59	.8	5
66	Cup[7]	1 cup	68	4	245	24	Trace	.3	.1	Trace	35	837	670	.2	1,160	[6]1,610	.28	1.19	.6	4
	Milk beverages:																			
	Chocolate milk (commercial):																			
67	Regular	1 cup	250	82	210	8	8	5.3	2.2	.2	26	280	251	.6	417	[3]300	.09	.41	.3	2
68	Lowfat (2%)	1 cup	250	84	180	8	5	3.1	1.3	.1	26	284	254	.6	422	500	.10	.42	.3	2
69	Lowfat (1%)	1 cup	250	85	160	8	3	1.5	.7	.1	26	287	257	.6	426	500	.10	.40	.2	2
70	Eggnog (commercial)	1 cup	254	74	340	10	19	11.3	5.0	.6	34	330	278	.5	420	890	.09	.48	.3	4
	Malted milk, home-prepared with 1 cup of whole milk and 2 to 3 heaping tsp of malted milk powder (about 3/4 oz):																			
71	Chocolate	1 cup of milk plus 3/4 oz of powder.	265	81	235	9	9	5.5	—	—	29	304	265	.5	500	330	.14	.43	.7	2
72	Natural	1 cup of milk plus 3/4 oz of powder.	265	81	235	11	10	6.0	—	—	27	347	307	.3	529	380	.20	.54	1.3	2
	Shakes, thick:[8]																			
73	Chocolate, container, net wt., 10.6 oz.	1 container	300	72	355	9	8	5.0	2.0	.2	63	396	378	.9	672	260	.14	.67	.4	0
74	Vanilla, container, net wt., 11 oz.	1 container	313	74	350	12	9	5.9	2.4	.2	56	457	361	.3	572	360	.09	.61	.5	0
	Milk desserts, frozen:																			
	Ice cream:																			
	Regular (about 11% fat):																			
75	Hardened	1/2 gal	1,064	61	2,155	38	115	71.3	28.8	2.6	254	1,406	1,075	1.0	2,052	4,340	.42	2.63	1.1	6
76		1 cup	133	61	270	5	14	8.9	3.6	.3	32	176	134	.1	257	540	.05	.33	.1	1
77		3-fl oz container	50	61	100	2	5	3.4	1.4	.1	12	66	51	Trace	96	200	.02	.12	.1	Trace
78	Soft serve (frozen custard)	1 cup	173	60	375	7	23	13.5	5.9	.6	38	236	199	.4	338	790	.08	.45	.2	1
79	Rich (about 16% fat), hardened	1/2 gal	1,188	59	2,805	33	190	118.3	47.8	4.3	256	1,213	927	.8	1,771	7,200	.36	2.27	.9	5
80		1 cup	148	59	350	4	24	14.7	6.0	.5	32	151	115	.1	221	900	.04	.28	.1	1

[5]Yields 1 qt of fluid milk when reconstituted according to package directions.
[6]Applies to product with added vitamin A.
[7]Weight applies to product with label claim of 1 1/3 cups equal 3.2 oz.
[8]Applies to products made from thick shake mixes and that do not contain added ice cream. Products made from thick shake mixes are higher in fat and usually contain added ice cream.

NUTRIENTS IN INDICATED QUANTITY

Item No. (A)	Foods, approximate measures, units, and weight (edible part unless footnotes indicate otherwise) (B)		Water (C) Per cent	Food energy (D) Kcal-ories	Protein (E) Grams	Fat (F) Grams	Fatty Acids Saturated (total) (G) Grams	Unsaturated Oleic (H) Grams	Unsaturated Linoleic (I) Grams	Carbo-hydrate (J) Grams	Calcium (K) Milli-grams	Phos-phorus (L) Milli-grams	Iron (M) Milli-grams	Potas-sium (N) Milli-grams	Vita-min A value (O) International units	Thia-min (P) Milli-grams	Ribo-flavin (Q) Milli-grams	Nia-cin (R) Milli-grams	Ascor-bic acid (S) Milli-grams
	Ice milk:		Grams																
81	Hardened (about 4.3% fat)	1/2 gal	1,048 / 69	1,470	41	45	28.1	11.3	1.0	232	1,409	1,035	1.5	2,117	1,710	.61	2.78	.9	6
82		1 cup	131 / 69	185	5	6	3.5	1.4	.1	29	176	129	.1	265	210	.08	.35	.1	1
83	Soft serve (about 2.6% fat)	1 cup	175 / 70	225	8	5	2.9	1.2	.1	38	274	202	.3	412	180	.12	.54	.2	1
84	Sherbet (about 2% fat)	1/2 gal	1,542 / 66	2,160	17	31	19.0	7.7	.7	469	827	594	2.5	1,585	1,480	.26	.71	1.0	31
85		1 cup	193 / 66	270	2	4	2.4	1.0	.1	59	103	74	.3	198	190	.03	.09	.1	4
	Milk desserts, other: From home recipe:																		
86	Custard, baked	1 cup	265 / 77	305	14	15	6.8	5.4	.7	29	297	310	1.1	387	930	.11	.50	.3	1
	Puddings: Starch base:																		
87	Chocolate	1 cup	260 / 66	385	8	12	7.6	3.3	.3	67	250	255	1.3	445	390	.05	.36	.3	1
88	Vanilla (blancmange)	1 cup	255 / 76	285	9	10	6.2	2.5	.2	41	298	232	Trace	352	410	.08	.41	.3	2
89	Tapioca cream	1 cup	165 / 72	220	8	8	4.1	2.5	.5	28	173	180	.7	223	480	.07	.30	.2	2
	From mix (chocolate) and milk:																		
90	Regular (cooked)	1 cup	260 / 70	320	9	8	4.3	2.6	.2	59	265	247	.8	354	340	.05	.39	.3	2
91	Instant	1 cup	260 / 69	325	8	7	3.6	2.2	.3	63	374	237	1.3	335	340	.08	.39	.3	2
	Yogurt: With added milk solids: Made with lowfat milk:																		
92	Fruit-flavored[9]	1 container, net wt., 8 oz	227 / 75	230	10	3	1.8	.6	.1	42	343	269	.2	439	[10]120	.08	.40	.2	1
93	Plain	1 container, net wt., 8 oz	227 / 85	145	12	4	2.3	.8	.1	16	415	326	.2	531	[10]150	.10	.49	.3	2
94	Made with nonfat milk	1 container, net wt., 8 oz	227 / 85	125	13	Trace	.3	.1	Trace	17	452	355	.2	579	[10]20	.11	.53	.3	2
	Without added milk solids:																		
95	Made with whole milk	1 container, net wt., 8 oz	227 / 88	140	8	7	4.8	1.7	.1	11	274	215	.1	351	280	.07	.32	.2	1
	EGGS																		
	Eggs, large (24 oz per dozen): Raw:																		
96	Whole, without shell	1 egg	50 / 75	80	6	6	1.7	2.0	.6	1	28	90	1.0	65	260	.04	.15	Trace	0
97	White	1 white	33 / 88	15	3	Trace	0	0	0	Trace	4	4	Trace	45	0	Trace	.09	Trace	0
98	Yolk	1 yolk	17 / 49	65	3	6	1.7	2.1	.6	Trace	26	86	.9	15	310	.04	.07	Trace	0
	Cooked:																		
99	Fried in butter	1 egg	46 / 72	85	5	6	2.4	2.2	.6	1	26	80	.9	58	290	.03	.13	Trace	0
100	Hard-cooked, shell removed	1 egg	50 / 75	80	6	6	1.7	2.0	.6	1	28	90	1.0	65	260	.04	.14	Trace	0
101	Poached	1 egg	50 / 74	80	6	6	1.7	2.0	.6	1	28	90	1.0	65	260	.04	.13	Trace	0
102	Scrambled (milk added) in butter. Also omelet.	1 egg	64 / 76	95	6	7	2.8	2.3	.6	1	47	97	.9	85	310	.04	.16	Trace	0

[9] Content of fat, vitamin A, and carbohydrate varies. Consult the label when precise values are needed for special diets.
[10] Applies to product made with milk containing no added vitamin A.

FATS, OILS; RELATED PRODUCTS

Item No. (A)	Foods, approximate measures, units, and weight (edible part unless footnotes indicate otherwise) (B)		Weight Grams	Water Per cent (C)	Food energy Kcalories (D)	Protein Grams (E)	Fat Grams (F)	Fatty Acids Saturated (total) Grams (G)	Unsaturated Oleic Grams (H)	Unsaturated Linoleic Grams (I)	Carbohydrate Grams (I)	Calcium Milligrams (K)	Phosphorus Milligrams (L)	Iron Milligrams (M)	Potassium Milligrams (N)	Vitamin A value International units (O)	Thiamin Milligrams (P)	Riboflavin Milligrams (Q)	Niacin Milligrams (R)	Ascorbic acid Milligrams (S)
	Butter:																			
	Regular (1 brick or 4 sticks per lb):																			
103	Stick (1/2 cup)	1 stick	113	16	815	1	92	57.3	23.1	2.1	Trace	27	26	.2	29	[11]3,470	.01	.04	Trace	0
104	Tablespoon (about 1/8 stick).	1 tbsp	14	16	100	Trace	12	7.2	2.9	.3	Trace	3	3	Trace	4	[11]430	Trace	Trace	Trace	0
105	Pat (1 in square, 1/3 in high; 90 per lb).	1 pat	5	16	35	Trace	4	2.5	1.0	.1	Trace	1	1	Trace	1	[11]150	Trace	Trace	Trace	0
	Whipped (6 sticks or two 8-oz containers per lb).																			
106	Stick (1/2 cup)	1 stick	76	16	540	1	61	38.2	15.4	1.4	Trace	18	17	.1	20	[11]2,310	Trace	.03	Trace	0
107	Tablespoon (about 1/8 stick).	1 tbsp	9	16	65	Trace	8	4.7	1.9	.2	Trace	2	2	Trace	2	[11]290	Trace	Trace	Trace	0
108	Pat (1 1/4 in square, 1/3 in high; 120 per lb).	1 pat	4	16	25	Trace	3	1.9	.8	.1	Trace	1	1	Trace	1	[11]120	0	Trace	Trace	0
109	Fats, cooking (vegetable shortenings).	1 cup	200	0	1,770	0	200	48.8	88.2	48.4	0	0	0	0	0	—	0	0	0	0
110	Lard	1 tbsp	13	0	110	0	13	3.2	5.7	3.1	0	0	0	0	0	—	0	0	0	0
111		1 cup	205	0	1,850	0	205	81.0	83.8	20.5	0	0	0	0	0	0	0	0	0	0
112		1 tbsp	13	0	115	0	13	5.1	5.3	1.3	0	0	0	0	0	0	0	0	0	0
	Margarine:																			
	Regular (1 brick or 4 sticks per lb):																			
113	Stick (1/2 cup)	1 stick	113	16	815	1	92	16.7	42.9	24.9	Trace	27	26	.2	29	[12]3,750	.01	.04	Trace	0
114	Tablespoon (about 1/8 stick)-	1 tbsp	14	16	100	Trace	12	2.1	5.3	3.1	Trace	3	3	Trace	4	[12]470	Trace	Trace	Trace	0
115	Pat (1 in square, 1/3 in high; 90 per lb).	1 pat	5	16	35	Trace	4	.7	1.9	1.1	Trace	1	1	Trace	1	[12]170	Trace	Trace	Trace	0
116	Soft, two 8-oz containers per lb.	1 container	227	16	1,635	1	184	32.5	71.5	65.4	Trace	53	52	.4	59	[12]7,500	.01	.08	.1	0
117	Whipped (6 sticks per lb):	1 tbsp	14	16	100	Trace	12	2.0	4.5	4.1	Trace	3	3	Trace	4	[12]470	Trace	Trace	Trace	0
118	Stick (1/2 cup)	1 stick	76	16	545	Trace	61	11.2	28.7	16.7	Trace	18	17	.1	20	[12]2,500	Trace	.03	Trace	0
119	Tablespoon (about 1/8 stick).	1 tbsp	9	16	70	Trace	8	1.4	3.6	2.1	Trace	2	2	Trace	2	[12]310	Trace	Trace	Trace	0

[11] Based on year-round average.
[12] Based on average vitamin A content of fortified margarine. Federal specifications for fortified margarine require a minimum of 15,000 International Units (I.U.) of vitamin A per pound.

NUTRIENTS IN INDICATED QUANTITY

Item No. (A)	Foods, approximate measures, units, and weight (edible part unless footnotes indicate otherwise) (B)	Grams	Water Per-cent (C)	Food energy Kcal-ories (D)	Pro-tein Grams (E)	Fat Grams (F)	Fatty Acids Satu-rated (total) Grams (G)	Unsaturated Oleic Grams (H)	Lino-leic Grams (I)	Carbo-hy-drate Grams (J)	Cal-cium Milli-grams (K)	Phos-pho-rus Milli-grams (L)	Iron Milli-grams (M)	Potas-sium Milli-grams (N)	Vita-min A value Inter-national units (O)	Thia-min Milli-grams (P)	Ribo-flavin Milli-grams (Q)	Nia-cin Milli-grams (R)	Ascor-bic acid Milli-grams (S)
	Oils, salad or cooking:																		
120	Corn 1 cup	218	0	1,925	0	218	27.7	53.6	125.1	0	0	0	0	—	—	0	0	0	0
121	1 tbsp	14	0	120	0	14	1.7	3.3	7.8	0	0	0	0	—	—	0	0	0	0
122	Olive 1 cup	216	0	1,910	0	216	30.7	154.4	17.7	0	0	0	0	—	—	0	0	0	0
123	1 tbsp	14	0	120	0	14	1.9	9.7	1.1	0	0	0	0	—	—	0	0	0	0
124	Peanut 1 cup	216	0	1,910	0	216	37.4	98.5	67.0	0	0	0	0	—	—	0	0	0	0
125	1 tbsp	14	0	120	0	14	2.3	6.2	4.2	0	0	0	0	—	—	0	0	0	0
126	Safflower 1 cup	218	0	1,925	0	218	20.5	25.9	159.8	0	0	0	0	—	—	0	0	0	0
127	1 tbsp	14	0	120	0	14	1.3	1.6	10.0	0	0	0	0	—	—	0	0	0	0
128	Soybean oil, hydro-genated (partially hardened). 1 cup	218	0	1,925	0	218	31.8	93.1	75.6	0	0	0	0	—	—	0	0	0	0
129	1 tbsp	14	0	120	0	14	2.0	5.8	4.7	0	0	0	0	—	—	0	0	0	0
130	Soybean-cottonseed oil blend, hydrogenated. 1 cup	218	0	1,925	0	218	38.2	63.0	99.6	0	0	0	0	—	—	0	0	0	0
131	1 tbsp	14	0	120	0	14	2.4	3.9	6.2	0	0	0	0	—	—	0	0	0	0
	Salad dressings: **Commercial:**																		
	Blue cheese:																		
132	Regular 1 tbsp	15	32	75	1	8	1.6	1.7	3.8	1	12	11	Trace	6	30	Trace	.02	Trace	Trace
133	Low calorie (5 Cal per tsp) 1 tbsp	16	84	10	Trace	1	.5	.3	Trace	1	10	8	Trace	5	30	Trace	.01	Trace	Trace
	French:																		
134	Regular 1 tbsp	16	39	65	Trace	6	1.1	1.3	3.2	3	2	2	.1	13	—	—	—	—	—
135	Low calorie (5 Cal per tsp) 1 tbsp	16	77	15	Trace	1	.1	.1	.4	2	2	2	.1	13	—	—	—	—	—
	Italian:																		
136	Regular 1 tbsp	15	28	85	Trace	9	1.6	1.9	4.7	1	2	1	Trace	2	Trace	Trace	Trace	Trace	—
137	Low calorie (2 Cal per tsp) 1 tbsp	15	90	10	Trace	1	.1	.1	.4	Trace	Trace	1	Trace	2	Trace	Trace	Trace	Trace	—
138	Mayonnaise 1 tbsp	14	15	100	Trace	11	2.0	2.4	5.6	Trace	3	4	.1	5	40	Trace	.01	Trace	—
	Mayonnaise type:																		
139	Regular 1 tbsp	15	41	65	Trace	6	1.1	1.4	3.2	2	2	4	Trace	1	30	Trace	Trace	Trace	—
140	Low calorie (8 Cal per tsp) 1 tbsp	16	81	20	Trace	2	.4	.4	1.0	2	3	4	Trace	1	40	Trace	Trace	Trace	—
141	Tartar sauce, regular 1 tbsp	14	34	75	Trace	8	1.5	1.8	4.1	1	3	4	.1	11	30	Trace	Trace	Trace	Trace
	Thousand Island:																		
142	Regular 1 tbsp	16	32	80	Trace	8	1.4	1.7	4.0	2	2	3	.1	18	50	Trace	Trace	Trace	Trace
143	Low calorie (10 Cal per tsp) 1 tbsp	15	68	25	Trace	2	.4	.4	1.0	2	2	3	.1	17	50	Trace	Trace	Trace	Trace
	From home recipe:																		
144	Cooked type[13] 1 tbsp	16	68	25	1	2	.5	.6	.3	2	14	15	.1	19	80	.01	.03	Trace	Trace

[13]Fatty acid values apply to product made with regular-type margarine.

Item No. (A)	Foods, approximate measures, units, and weight (edible part unless footnotes indicate otherwise) (B)		Water Per-cent (C)	Food energy Kcal-ories (D)	Pro-tein Grams (E)	Fat Grams (F)	Fatty Acids Saturated (total) Grams (G)	Unsaturated Oleic Grams (H)	Unsaturated Linoleic Grams (I)	Carbo-hy-drate Grams (J)	Cal-cium Milli-grams (K)	Phos-pho-rus Milli-grams (L)	Iron Milli-grams (M)	Potas-sium Milli-grams (N)	Vita-min A value Inter-national units (O)	Thia-min Milli-grams (P)	Ribo-flavin Milli-grams (Q)	Nia-cin Milli-grams (R)	Ascor-bic acid Milli-grams (S)
	FISH, SHELLFISH, MEAT, POULTRY; RELATED PRODUCTS																		
	Fish and shellfish:																		
145	Bluefish, baked with butter or margarine.	3 oz	68	135	22	4	—	—	—	0	25	244	0.6	—	40	.09	.08	1.6	—
	Clams:																		
146	Raw, meat only	3 oz	82	65	11	1	—	—	—	2	59	138	5.2	154	90	.08	.15	1.1	8
147	Canned, solids and liquid	3 oz	86	45	7	1	0.2	Trace	Trace	2	47	116	3.5	119	—	.01	.09	.9	
148	Crabmeat (white or king), canned, not pressed down.	1 cup	77	135	24	3	.6	0.4	0.1	1	61	246	1.1	149	—	.11	.11	2.6	—
149	Fish sticks, breaded, cooked, frozen (stick, 4 by 1 by 1/2 in).	1 fish stick or 1 oz	66	50	5	3	—	—	—	2	3	47	.1	—	0	.01	.02	.5	—
150	Haddock, breaded, fried[14]	3 oz	66	140	17	5	1.4	2.2	1.2	5	34	210	1.0	296	—	.03	.06	2.7	2
151	Ocean perch, breaded, fried[14]	1 fillet	59	195	16	11	2.7	4.4	2.3	6	28	192	1.1	242	—	.10	.10	1.6	—
152	Oysters, raw, meat only (13–19 medium Selects).	1 cup	85	160	20	4	1.3	.2	.1	8	226	343	13.2	290	740	.34	.43	6.0	—
153	Salmon, pink, canned, solids and liquid.	3 oz	71	120	17	5	.9	.8	.1	0	[15]167	243	.7	307	60	.03	.16	6.8	—
154	Sardines, Atlantic, canned in oil, drained solids.	3 oz	62	175	20	9	3.0	2.5	.5	0	372	424	2.5	502	190	.02	.17	4.6	—
155	Scallops, frozen, breaded, fried, reheated.	6 scallops	60	175	16	8	—	—	—	9	—	—	—	—	—	—	—	—	—
156	Shad, baked with butter or margarine, bacon.	3 oz	64	170	20	10	—	—	—	0	20	266	.5	320	30	.11	.22	7.3	—
	Shrimp:																		
157	Canned meat	3 oz	70	100	21	1	.1	.1	Trace	1	98	224	2.6	104	50	.01	.03	1.5	—
158	French fried[16]	3 oz	57	190	17	9	2.3	3.7	2.0	9	61	162	1.7	195	—	.03	.07	2.3	—
159	Tuna, canned in oil, drained solids.	3 oz	61	170	24	7	1.7	1.7	.7	0	7	199	1.6	—	70	.04	.10	10.1	—
160	Tuna salad[17]	1 cup	70	350	30	22	4.3	6.3	6.7	7	41	291	2.7	—	590	.08	.23	10.3	2
	Meat and meat products:																		
161	Bacon, (20 slices per lb, raw), broiled or fried, crisp.	2 slices	8	85	4	8	2.5	3.7	.7	Trace	2	34	.5	35	0	.08	.05	.8	

[14] Dipped in egg, milk or water, and breadcrumbs; fried in vegetable shortening.
[15] If bones are discarded, value for calcium will be greatly reduced.
[16] Dipped in egg, breadcrumbs, and flour or batter.
[17] Prepared with tuna, celery, salad dressing (mayonnaise type), pickle, onion, and egg.

NUTRIENTS IN INDICATED QUANTITY

Item No. (A)	Foods, approximate measures, units, and weight (edible part unless footnotes indicate otherwise) (B)		Water (C)	Food energy (D)	Protein (E)	Fat (F)	Fatty Acids			Carbohydrate (I)	Calcium (K)	Phosphorus (L)	Iron (M)	Potassium (N)	Vitamin A value (O)	Thiamin (P)	Riboflavin (Q)	Niacin (R)	Ascorbic acid (S)
							Saturated (total) (G)	Unsaturated											
								Oleic (H)	Linoleic (I)										
			Per cent	Kcalories	Grams	Grams	Grams	Grams	Grams	Grams	Milligrams	Milligrams	Milligrams	Milligrams	International units	Milligrams	Milligrams	Milligrams	Milligrams
	Beef,18 cooked:																		
	Cuts braised, simmered or pot roasted:																		
162	Lean and fat (piece, 2 1/2 by 2 1/2 by 3/4 in).	3 oz	53	245	23	16	6.8	6.5	.4	0	10	114	2.9	184	30	.04	.18	3.6	—
163	Lean only from item 162	2.5 oz	62	140	22	5	2.1	1.8	.2	0	10	108	2.7	176	10	.04	.17	3.3	—
	Ground beef, broiled:																		
164	Lean with 10% fat	3 oz or patty 3 by 5/8 in	60	185	23	10	4.0	3.9	.3	0	10	196	3.0	261	20	.08	.20	5.1	—
165	Lean with 21% fat	2.9 oz or patty 3 by 5/8 in	54	235	20	17	7.0	6.7	.4	0	9	159	2.6	221	30	.07	.17	4.4	—
	Roast, oven cooked, no liquid added:																		
	Relatively fat, such as rib:																		
166	Lean and fat (2 pieces, 4 1/8 by 2 1/4 by 1/4 in).	3 oz	40	375	17	33	14.0	13.6	.8	0	8	158	2.2	189	70	.05	.13	3.1	—
167	Lean only from item 166	1.8 oz	57	125	14	7	3.0	2.5	.3	0	6	131	1.8	161	10	.04	.11	2.6	—
	Relatively lean, such as heel of round:																		
168	Lean and fat (2 pieces, 4 1/8 by 2 1/4 by 1/4 in).	3 oz	62	165	25	7	2.8	2.7	.2	0	11	208	3.2	279	10	.06	.19	4.5	—
169	Lean only from item 168	2.8 oz	65	125	24	3	1.2	1.0	0.1	0	10	199	3.0	268	Trace	.06	.18	4.3	—
	Steak:																		
	Relatively fat-sirloin, broiled:																		
170	Lean and fat (piece, 2 1/2 by 2 1/2 by 3/4 in).	3 oz	44	330	20	27	11.3	11.1	.6	0	9	162	2.5	220	50	.05	.15	4.0	—
171	Lean only from item 170	2.0 oz	59	115	18	4	1.8	1.6	.2	0	7	146	2.2	202	10	.05	.14	3.6	—
	Relatively lean-round, braised:																		
172	Lean and fat (piece, 4 1/8 by 2 1/4 by 1/2 in).	3 oz	55	220	24	13	5.5	5.2	.4	0	10	213	3.0	272	20	.07	.19	4.8	—
173	Lean only from item 172	2.4 oz	61	130	21	4	1.7	1.5	.2	0	9	182	2.5	238	10	.05	.16	4.1	—
	Beef, canned:																		
174	Corned beef	3 oz	59	185	22	10	4.9	4.5	.2	0	17	90	3.7	—	—	.01	.20	2.9	—

18 Outer layer of fat on the cut was removed to within approximately 1/2 in. of the lean. Deposits of fat within the cut were not removed.

NUTRIENTS IN INDICATED QUANTITY

Item No. (A)	Foods, approximate measures, units, and weight (edible part unless footnotes indicate otherwise) (B)	Measure	Grams	Water Per-cent (C)	Food energy Kcal-ories (D)	Protein Grams (E)	Fat Grams (F)	Saturated (total) Grams (G)	Oleic Grams (H)	Linoleic Grams (I)	Carbo-hydrate Grams (I)	Calcium Milli-grams (K)	Phos-phorus Milli-grams (L)	Iron Milli-grams (M)	Potas-sium Milli-grams (N)	Vitamin A value Inter-national units (O)	Thia-min Milli-grams (P)	Ribo-flavin Milli-grams (Q)	Nia-cin Milli-grams (R)	Ascor-bic acid Milli-grams (S)
175	Corned beef hash	1 cup	220	67	400	19	25	11.9	10.9	.5	24	29	147	4.4	440	—	.02	.20	4.6	0
176	Beef, dried, chipped	2 1/2-oz jar	71	48	145	24	4	2.1	2.0	.1	0	14	287	3.6	142	—	.05	.23	2.7	—
177	Beef and vegetable stew	1 cup	245	82	220	16	11	4.9	4.5	.2	15	29	184	2.9	613	2,400	.15	.17	4.7	17
178	Beef potpie (home recipe), baked[19] (piece, 1/3 of 9-in diam. pie).	1 piece	210	55	515	21	30	7.9	12.8	6.7	39	29	149	3.8	334	1,720	.30	.30	5.5	6
179	Chili con carne with beans, canned.	1 cup	255	72	340	19	16	7.5	6.8	.3	31	82	321	4.3	594	150	.08	.18	3.3	—
180	Chop suey with beef and pork (home recipe).	1 cup	250	75	300	26	17	8.5	6.2	.7	13	60	248	4.8	425	600	.28	.38	5.0	33
181	Heart, beef, lean, braised	3 oz	85	61	160	27	5	1.5	1.1	.6	1	5	154	5.0	197	20	.21	1.04	6.5	1
	Lamb, cooked: Chop, rib (cut 3 per lb with bone), broiled:																			
182	Lean and fat	3.1 oz	89	43	360	18	32	14.8	12.1	1.2	0	8	139	1.0	200	—	.11	.19	4.1	—
183	Lean only from item 182	2 oz	57	60	120	16	6	2.5	2.1	.2	0	6	121	1.1	174	—	.09	.15	3.4	—
	Leg, roasted:																			
184	Lean and fat (2 pieces, 4 1/8 by 2 1/4 by 1/4 in).	3 oz	85	54	235	22	16	7.3	6.0	.6	0	9	177	1.4	241	—	.13	.23	4.7	—
185	Lean only from item 184	2.5 oz	71	62	130	20	5	2.1	1.8	.2	0	9	169	1.4	227	—	.12	.21	4.4	—
	Shoulder, roasted:																			
186	Lean and fat (3 pieces, 2 1/2 by 2 1/2 by 1/4 in).	3 oz	85	50	285	18	23	10.8	8.8	.9	0	9	146	1.0	206	—	.11	.20	4.0	—
187	Lean only from item 186	2.3 oz	64	61	130	17	6	3.6	2.3	.2	0	8	140	1.0	193	—	.10	.18	3.7	—
188	Liver, beef, fried[20] (slice, 6 1/2 by 2 3/8 by 3/8 in).	3 oz	85	56	195	22	9	2.5	3.5	.9	5	9	405	7.5	323	[21]45,390	.22	3.56	14.0	23
	Pork, cured, cooked:																			
189	Ham, light cure, lean and fat, roasted (2 pieces, 4 1/8 by 2 1/4 by 1/4 in).[22]	3 oz	85	54	245	18	19	6.8	7.9	1.7	0	8	146	2.2	199	0	.40	.15	3.1	—
	Luncheon meat:																			
190	Boiled ham, slice (8 per 8-oz pkg.).	1 oz	28	59	65	5	5	1.7	2.0	.4	0	3	47	.8	—	0	.12	.04	.7	—

[19] Crust made with vegetable shortening and enriched flour.
[20] Regular-type margarine used.
[21] Value varies widely.
[22] About one-fourth of the outer layer of fat on the cut was removed. Deposits of fat within the cut were not removed.

NUTRIENTS IN INDICATED QUANTITY

Item No. (A)	Foods, approximate measures, units, and weight (edible part unless footnotes indicate otherwise) (B)		Water (C) Per-cent	Food energy (D) Kcalories	Protein (E) Grams	Fat (F) Grams	Saturated (total) (G) Grams	Oleic (H) Grams	Linoleic (I) Grams	Carbo-hydrate (J) Grams	Calcium (K) Milligrams	Phos-phorus (L) Milligrams	Iron (M) Milligrams	Potassium (N) Milligrams	Vita-min A value (O) International units	Thiamin (P) Milligrams	Ribo-flavin (Q) Milligrams	Niacin (R) Milligrams	Ascorbic acid (S) Milligrams
	Canned, spiced or unspiced:																		
191	Slice, approx. 3 by 2 by 1/2 in.	1 slice	60	175	9	15	5.4	6.7	1.0	1	5	65	1.3	133	0	.19	.13	1.8	—
	Pork, fresh,18 cooked:																		
	Chop, loin (cut 3 per lb with bone), broiled:																		
192	Lean and fat	2.7 oz	42	305	19	25	8.9	10.4	2.2	0	9	209	2.7	216	0	.75	.22	4.5	—
193	Lean only from item 192	2 oz	53	150	17	9	3.1	3.6	.8	0	7	181	2.2	192	0	.63	.18	3.8	—
	Roast, oven cooked, no liquid added:																		
194	Lean and fat (piece, 2 1/2 by 2 1/2 by 3/4 in).	3 oz	46	310	21	24	8.7	10.2	2.2	0	9	218	2.7	233	0	.78	.22	4.8	—
195	Lean only from item 194	2.4 oz	55	175	20	10	3.5	4.1	.8	0	9	211	2.6	224	0	.73	.21	4.4	—
	Shoulder cut, simmered:																		
196	Lean and fat (3 pieces, 2 1/2 by 2 1/2 by 1/4 in).	3 oz	46	320	20	26	9.3	10.9	2.3	0	9	118	2.6	158	0	.46	.21	4.1	—
197	Lean only from item 196	2.2 oz	60	135	18	6	2.2	2.6	.6	0	8	111	2.3	146	0	.42	.19	3.7	—
	Sausages (see also Luncheon meat (items 190-191)):																		
198	Bologna, slice (8 per 8-oz pkg.).	1 slice	56	85	3	8	3.0	3.4	.5	Trace	2	36	.5	65	—	.05	.06	.7	—
199	Braunschweiger, slice (6 per 6-oz pkg.).	1 slice	53	90	4	8	2.6	3.4	.8	1	3	69	1.7	—	1,850	.05	.41	2.3	—
200	Brown and serve (10-11 per 8-oz pkg.), browned.	1 link	40	70	3	6	2.3	2.8	.7	Trace	—	—	—	—	—	—	—	—	—
201	Deviled ham, canned	1 tbsp	51	45	2	4	1.5	1.8	.4	0	1	12	.3	—	0	.02	.01	.2	—
202	Frankfurter (8 per 1-lb pkg.), cooked (reheated).	1 frankfurter	57	170	7	15	5.6	6.5	1.2	1	3	57	.8	—	—	.08	.11	1.4	—
203	Meat, potted (beef, chicken, turkey), canned.	1 tbsp	61	30	2	2	—	—	—	0	—	—	—	—	—	Trace	.03	.2	—
204	Pork link (16 per 1-lb pkg.), cooked.	1 link	35	60	2	6	2.1	2.4	.5	Trace	1	21	.3	35	0	.10	.04	.5	—
	Salami:																		
205	Dry type, slice (12 per 4-oz pkg.).	1 slice	30	45	2	4	1.6	1.6	.1	Trace	1	28	.4	—	—	.04	.03	.5	—

338

Item No. (A)	Foods, approximate measures, units, and weight (edible part unless footnotes indicate otherwise) (B)		Water Per cent (C)	Food energy Kcalories (D)	Protein Grams (E)	Fat Grams (F)	Fatty Acids			Carbohydrate Grams (J)	Calcium Milligrams (K)	Phosphorus Milligrams (L)	Iron Milligrams (M)	Potassium Milligrams (N)	Vitamin A value International units (O)	Thiamin Milligrams (P)	Riboflavin Milligrams (Q)	Niacin Milligrams (R)	Ascorbic acid Milligrams (S)
							Saturated (total) Grams (G)	Unsaturated Oleic Grams (H)	Linoleic Grams (I)										
		Grams	Per cent	Kcalories	Grams	Grams	Grams	Grams	Grams	Grams	Milligrams	Milligrams	Milligrams	Milligrams	International units	Milligrams	Milligrams	Milligrams	Milligrams
206	Cooked type, slice (8 per 8-oz pkg.).	1 slice	28	51	90	5	7	3.1	3.0	.2	Trace	3	57	.7	—	—	.07	.07	1.2	—
207	Vienna sausage (7 per 4-oz can).	1 sausage	16	63	40	2	3	1.2	1.4	.2	Trace	1	24	.3	—	—	.01	.02	.4	—
	Veal, medium fat, cooked, bone removed:																			
208	Cutlet (4 1/8 by 2 1/4 by 1/2 in), braised or broiled.	3 oz	85	60	185	23	9	4.0	3.4	.4	0	9	196	2.7	258	—	.06	.21	4.6	—
209	Rib (2 pieces, 4 1/8 by 2 1/4 by 1/4 in), roasted.	3 oz	85	55	230	23	14	6.1	5.1	.6	0	10	211	2.9	259	—	.11	.26	6.6	—
	Poultry and poultry products:																			
	Chicken, cooked:																			
210	Breast, fried,[23] bones removed, 1/2 breast (3.3 oz with bones).	2.8 oz	79	58	160	26	5	1.4	1.8	1.1	1	9	218	1.3	—	70	.04	.17	11.6	—
211	Drumstick, fried,[23] bones removed (2 oz with bones).	1.3 oz	38	55	90	12	4	1.1	1.3	.9	Trace	6	89	.9	—	50	.03	.15	2.7	—
212	Half broiler, broiled, bones removed (10.4 oz with bones).	6.2 oz	176	71	240	42	7	2.2	2.5	1.3	0	16	355	3.0	483	160	.09	.34	15.5	—
213	Chicken, canned, boneless.	3 oz	85	65	170	18	10	3.2	3.8	2.0	0	18	210	1.3	117	200	.03	.11	3.7	3
214	Chicken a la king, cooked (home recipe).	1 cup	245	68	470	27	34	12.7	14.3	3.3	12	127	358	2.5	404	1,130	.10	.42	5.4	12
215	Chicken and noodles, cooked (home recipe).	1 cup	240	71	365	22	18	5.9	7.1	3.5	26	26	247	2.2	149	430	.05	.17	4.3	Trace
	Chicken chow mein:																			
216	Canned	1 cup	250	89	95	7	Trace	—	—	—	18	45	35	1.3	418	150	.05	.10	1.0	13
217	From home recipe	1 cup	250	78	255	31	10	2.4	3.4	3.1	10	58	293	2.5	473	280	.08	.23	4.3	10
218	Chicken potpie (home recipe), baked,19 piece (1/3 of 9-in diam. pie).	1 piece	232	57	545	23	31	11.3	10.9	5.6	42	70	232	3.0	343	3,090	.34	.31	5.5	5
	Turkey, roasted, flesh without skin:																			
219	Dark meat, piece, 2 1/2 by 1 5/8 by 1/4 in.	4 pieces	85	61	175	26	7	2.1	1.5	1.5	0	—	—	2.0	338	—	.03	.20	3.6	—
220	Light meat, piece, 4 by 2 by 1/4 in.	2 pieces	85	62	150	28	3	.9	.6	.7	0	—	—	1.0	349	—	.04	.12	9.4	—

[23]Vegetable shortening used.

NUTRIENTS IN INDICATED QUANTITY

Item No. (A)	Foods, approximate measures, units, and weight (edible part unless footnotes indicate otherwise) (B)		Water Per-cent (C)	Food energy Kcal-ories (D)	Pro-tein Grams (E)	Fat Grams (F)	Fatty Acids Satu-rated (total) Grams (G)	Unsatu-rated Oleic Grams (H)	Unsatu-rated Lino-leic Grams (I)	Carbo-hy-drate Grams (I)	Cal-cium Milli-grams (K)	Phos-pho-rus Milli-grams (L)	Iron Milli-grams (M)	Potas-sium Milli-grams (N)	Vita-min A value Inter-national units (O)	Thia-min Milli-grams (P)	Ribo-flavin Milli-grams (Q)	Nia-cin Milli-grams (R)	Ascor-bic acid Milli-grams (S)
	Light and dark meat:		Grams																
221	Chopped or diced	1 cup	140	265	44	9	2.5	1.7	1.8	0	11	351	2.5	514	—	.07	.25	10.8	—
222	Pieces (1 slice white meat, 4 by 2 by 1/4 in with 2 slices dark meat, 2 1/2 by 1 5/8 by 1/4 in).	3 pieces	85	160	27	5	1.5	1.0	1.1	0	7	213	1.5	312	—	.04	.15	6.5	—
	FRUITS AND FRUIT PRODUCTS																		
	Apples, raw, unpeeled, without cores:																		
223	2 3/4-in diam. (about 3 per lb with cores).	1 apple	138	84	80	Trace	1	—	—	—	20	10	14	.4	152	120	.04	.03	.1	6
224	3 1/4-in diam. (about 2 per lb with cores).	1 apple	212	84	125	Trace	1	—	—	—	31	15	21	.6	233	190	.06	.04	.2	8
225	Apple juice, bottled or canned[24]	1 cup	248	88	120	Trace	Trace	—	—	—	30	15	22	1.5	250	—	.02	.05	.2	25[2]
	Applesauce, canned:																		
226	Sweetened	1 cup	255	76	230	1	Trace	—	—	—	61	10	13	1.3	166	100	.05	.03	.1	25[3]
227	Unsweetened	1 cup	244	89	100	Trace	Trace	—	—	—	26	10	12	1.2	190	100	.05	.02	.1	25[2]
	Apricots:																		
228	Raw, without pits (about 12 per lb with pits).	3 apricots	107	85	55	1	Trace	—	—	—	14	18	25	.5	301	2,890	.03	.04	.6	11
229	Canned in heavy syrup (halves and syrup).	1 cup	258	77	220	2	Trace	—	—	—	57	28	39	.8	604	4,490	.05	.05	1.0	10
	Dried:																		
230	Uncooked (28 large or 37 medium halves per cup).	1 cup	130	25	340	7	1	—	—	—	86	87	140	7.2	1,273	14,170	.01	.21	4.3	16
231	Cooked, unsweetened, fruit and liquid.	1 cup	250	76	215	4	1	—	—	—	54	55	88	4.5	795	7,500	.01	.13	2.5	8
232	Apricot nectar, canned	1 cup	251	85	145	1	Trace	—	—	—	37	23	30	.5	379	2,380	.03	.03	.5	26[36]
	Avocados, raw, whole, without skins and seeds:																		
233	California, mid- and late-winter (with skin and seed, 3 1/8-in diam.; wt., 10 oz).	1 avocado	216	74	370	5	37	5.5	22.0	3.7	13	22	91	1.3	1,303	630	.24	.43	3.5	30

[24] Also applies to pasteurized apple cider.
[25] Applies to product without added ascorbic acid. For value of product with added ascorbic acid, refer to label.
[26] Based on product with label claim of 45% of U.S. RDA in 6 fl oz.

Item No. (A)	Foods, approximate measures, units, and weight (edible part unless footnotes indicate otherwise) (B)	Weight Grams	Water Per cent (C)	Food energy Kcalories (D)	Protein Grams (E)	Fat Grams (F)	Fatty Acids Saturated (total) Grams (G)	Unsaturated Oleic Grams (H)	Unsaturated Linoleic Grams (I)	Carbohydrate Grams (I)	Calcium Milligrams (K)	Phosphorus Milligrams (L)	Iron Milligrams (M)	Potassium Milligrams (N)	Vitamin A value International units (O)	Thiamin Milligrams (P)	Riboflavin Milligrams (Q)	Niacin Milligrams (R)	Ascorbic acid Milligrams (S)
234	Florida, late summer and fall (with skin and seed, 3 5/8-in diam.; wt., 1 lb). 1 avocado	304	78	390	4	33	6.7	15.7	5.3	27	30	128	1.8	1,836	880	.33	.61	4.9	43
235	Banana without peel (about 2.6 per lb with peel). 1 banana	119	76	100	1	Trace	—	—	—	26	10	31	.8	440	230	.06	.07	.8	12
236	Banana flakes. 1 tbsp	6	3	20	Trace	Trace				5	2	6	.2	92	50	.01	.01	.2	Trace
237	Blackberries, raw. 1 cup	144	85	85	2	1				19	46	27	1.3	245	290	.04	.06	.6	30
238	Blueberries, raw. 1 cup	145	83	90	1	1				22	22	19	1.5	117	150	.04	.09	.7	20
	Cantaloupe. See Muskmelons (item 271).																		
	Cherries:																		
239	Sour (tart), red, pitted, canned, water pack. 1 cup	244	88	105	2	Trace				26	37	32	.7	317	1,660	.07	.05	.5	12
240	Sweet, raw, without pits and stems. 10 cherries	68	80	45	1	Trace				12	15	13	.3	129	70	.03	.04	.3	7
241	Cranberry juice cocktail, bottled, sweetened. 1 cup	253	83	165	Trace	Trace				42	13	8	.8	25	Trace	.03	.03	.1	[27]81
242	Cranberry sauce, sweetened, canned, strained. 1 cup	277	62	405	Trace	1				104	17	11	.6	83	60	.03	.03	.1	6
	Dates:																		
243	Whole, without pits. 10 dates	80	23	220	2	Trace				58	47	50	2.4	518	40	.07	.08	1.8	0
244	Chopped. 1 cup	178	23	490	4	1				130	105	112	5.3	1,153	90	.16	.18	3.9	0
245	Fruit cocktail, canned, in heavy syrup. 1 cup	255	80	195	1	Trace				50	23	31	1.0	411	360	.05	.03	1.0	5
	Grapefruit: Raw, medium, 3 3/4-in diam. (about 1 lb 1 oz):																		
246	Pink or red. 1/2 grapefruit with peel[28]	241	89	50	1	Trace				13	20	20	.5	166	540	.05	.02	.2	44
247	White. 1/2 grapefruit with peel[28]	241	89	45	1	Trace				12	19	19	.5	159	10	.05	.02	.2	44
248	Canned, sections with syrup. 1 cup	254	81	180	2	Trace				45	33	36	.8	343	30	.08	.05	.5	76
	Grapefruit juice:																		
249	Raw, pink, red, or white. 1 cup	246	90	95	1	Trace				23	22	37	.5	399	(29)	.10	.05	.5	93
	Canned, white:																		
250	Unsweetened. 1 cup	247	89	100	1	Trace				24	20	35	1.0	400	20	.07	.05	.5	84
251	Sweetened. 1 cup	250	86	135	1	Trace				32	20	35	1.0	405	30	.08	.05	.5	78
	Frozen, concentrate, unsweetened:																		
252	Undiluted, 6-fl oz can. 1 can	207	62	300	4	1				72	70	124	.8	1,250	60	.29	.12	1.4	286

[27] Based on product with label claim of 100% of U.S. RDA in 6 fl oz.
[28] Weight includes peel and membranes between sections. Without these parts, the weight of the edible portion is 123 g for item 246 and 118 g for item 247.
[29] For white-fleshed varieties, value is about 20 International Units (I.U.) per cup; for red-fleshed varieties, 1,080 I.U.

Item No. (A)	Foods, approximate measures, units, and weight (edible part unless footnotes indicate otherwise) (B)	Weight Grams	Water Per cent (C)	Food energy Kcalories (D)	Protein Grams (E)	Fat Grams (F)	Saturated (total) Grams (G)	Oleic Grams (H)	Linoleic Grams (I)	Carbohydrate Grams (I)	Calcium Milligrams (K)	Phosphorus Milligrams (L)	Iron Milligrams (M)	Potassium Milligrams (N)	Vitamin A value International units (O)	Thiamin Milligrams (P)	Riboflavin Milligrams (Q)	Niacin Milligrams (R)	Ascorbic acid Milligrams (S)
253	Diluted with 3 parts water by volume. 1 cup	247	89	100	1	Trace	—	—	—	24	25	42	.2	420	20	.10	.04	.5	96
254	Dehydrated crystals, prepared with water (1 lb yields about 1 gal). 1 cup	247	90	100	1	Trace	—	—	—	24	22	40	.2	412	20	.10	.05	.5	91
	Grapes, European type (adherent skin), raw:																		
255	Thompson Seedless 10 grapes	50	81	35	Trace	Trace	—	—	—	9	6	10	.2	87	50	.03	.02	.2	2
256	Tokay and Emperor, seeded types 10 grapes[30]	60	81	40	Trace	Trace	—	—	—	10	7	11	.2	99	60	.03	.02	.2	2
	Grape juice:																		
257	Canned or bottled 1 cup	253	83	165	1	Trace	—	—	—	42	28	30	.8	293	—	.10	.05	.5	[25]Trace
	Frozen concentrate, sweetened:																		
258	Undiluted, 6-fl oz can 1 can	216	53	395	1	Trace	—	—	—	100	22	32	.9	255	40	.13	.22	1.5	[31][32]
259	Diluted with 3 parts water by volume. 1 cup	250	86	135	1	Trace	—	—	—	33	8	10	.3	85	10	.05	.08	.5	[31]10
260	Grape drink, canned 1 cup	250	86	135	Trace	Trace	—	—	—	35	8	10	.3	88	—	[32].03	[32].03	.3	[32]
261	Lemon, raw, size 165, without peel and seeds (about 4 per lb with peels and seeds). 1 lemon	74	90	20	1	Trace	—	—	—	6	19	12	.4	102	10	.03	.01	.1	39
	Lemon juice:																		
262	Raw 1 cup	244	91	60	1	Trace	—	—	—	20	17	24	.5	344	50	.07	.02	.2	112
263	Canned, or bottled unsweetened 1 cup	244	92	55	1	Trace	—	—	—	19	17	24	.5	344	50	.07	.02	.2	102
264	Frozen, single strength, unsweetened, 6-fl oz can. 1 can	183	92	40	1	Trace	—	—	—	13	13	16	.5	258	40	.05	.02	.2	81
	Lemonade concentrate, frozen:																		
265	Undiluted, 6-fl oz can 1 can	219	49	425	Trace	Trace	—	—	—	112	9	13	.4	153	40	.05	.06	.7	66
266	Diluted with 4 1/3 parts water by volume. 1 cup	248	89	105	Trace	Trace	—	—	—	28	2	3	.1	40	10	.01	.02	.2	17
	Limeade concentrate, frozen:																		
267	Undiluted, 6-fl oz can 1 can	218	50	410	Trace	Trace	—	—	—	108	11	13	0.2	129	Trace	.02	.02	.2	26
268	Diluted with 4 1/3 parts water by volume. 1 cup	247	89	100	Trace	Trace	—	—	—	27	3	3	Trace	32	Trace	Trace	Trace	Trace	6
	Limejuice:																		
269	Raw 1 cup	246	90	65	1	Trace	—	—	—	22	22	27	.5	256	20	.05	.02	.2	79

[30]Weight includes seeds. Without seeds, weight of the edible portion is 57 g.
[31]Applies to product without added ascorbic acid. With added ascorbic acid, based on claim that 6 fl oz of reconstituted juice contains 45% or 50% of the U.S. RDA, value in milligrams is 108 or 120 for a 6-fl oz can (item 258), 36 or 40 for 1 cup of diluted juice (item 259).
[32]For products with added thiamin and riboflavin but without added ascorbic acid, values in milligrams would be 0.60 for thiamin, 0.80 for riboflavin, and trace for ascorbic acid. For products with only ascorbic acid added, value varies with the brand. Consult the label.

NUTRIENTS IN INDICATED QUANTITY

Item No. (A)	Foods, approximate measures, units, and weight (edible part unless footnotes indicate otherwise) (B)		Water Per cent (C)	Food energy Kcal-ories (D)	Pro-tein (E)	Fat (F)	Fatty Acids Saturated (total) (G)	Unsaturated Oleic (H)	Unsaturated Lino-leic (I)	Carbo-hy-drate (J)	Cal-cium (K)	Phos-pho-rus (L)	Iron (M)	Potas-sium (N)	Vita-min A value (O)	Thia-min (P)	Ribo-flavin (Q)	Nia-cin (R)	Ascor-bic acid (S)
		Grams	Per-cent		Grams	Grams	Grams	Grams	Grams	Grams	Milli-grams	Milli-grams	Milli-grams	Milli-grams	Inter-national units	Milli-grams	Milli-grams	Milli-grams	Milli-grams
270	Canned, unsweetened	1 cup 246	90	65	1	Trace	—	—	—	22	22	27	.5	256	20	.05	.02	.2	52
	Muskmelons, raw, with rind, without seed cavity:																		
271	Cantaloupe, orange-fleshed 1/2 melon with rind[33] (with rind and seed cavity, 5-in diam., 2 1/3 lb).	477	91	80	2	Trace	—	—	—	20	38	44	1.1	682	9,240	.11	.08	1.6	90
272	Honeydew (with rind and seed cavity, 6 1/2-in diam., 5 1/4 lb). 1/10 melon with rind[33]	226	91	50	1	Trace	—	—	—	11	21	24	.6	374	60	.06	.04	.9	34
	Oranges, all commercial varieties, raw:																		
273	Whole, 2 5/8-in diam., without peel and seeds (about 2 1/2 per lb with peel and seeds). 1 orange	131	86	65	1	Trace	—	—	—	16	54	26	.5	263	260	.13	.05	.5	66
274	Sections without membranes 1 cup	180	86	90	2	Trace	—	—	—	22	74	36	.7	360	360	.18	.07	.7	90
	Orange juice:																		
275	Raw, all varieties 1 cup	248	88	110	2	Trace	—	—	—	26	27	42	.5	496	500	.22	.07	1.0	124
276	Canned, unsweetened 1 cup	249	87	120	2	Trace	—	—	—	28	25	45	1.0	496	500	.17	.05	.7	100
	Frozen concentrate:																		
277	Undiluted, 6-fl oz can	213	55	360	5	Trace	—	—	—	87	75	126	.9	1,500	1,620	.68	.11	2.8	360
278	Diluted with 3 parts water by volume. 1 cup	249	87	120	2	Trace	—	—	—	29	25	42	.2	503	540	.23	.03	.9	120
279	Dehydrated crystals, prepared with water (1 lb yields about 1 gal). 1 cup	248	88	115	1	Trace	—	—	—	27	25	40	.5	518	500	.20	.07	1.0	109
	Orange and grapefruit juice: Frozen concentrate:																		
280	Undiluted, 6-fl oz can	210	59	330	4	1	—	—	—	78	61	99	.8	1,308	800	.48	.06	2.3	302
281	Diluted with 3 parts water by volume. 1 cup	248	88	110	1	Trace	—	—	—	26	20	32	.2	439	270	.15	.02	.7	102
282	Papayas, raw, 1/2-in cubes 1 cup	140	89	55	1	Trace	—	—	—	14	28	22	.4	328	2,450	.06	.06	.4	78
	Peaches: Raw:																		
283	Whole, 2 1/2-in diam, peeled, pitted (about 4 per lb with peels and pits). 1 peach	100	89	40	1	Trace	—	—	—	10	9	19	.5	202	[34]1,300	.02	.05	1.0	7
284	Sliced 1 cup	170	89	65	1	Trace	—	—	—	16	15	32	.9	343	[34]2,260	.03	.09	1.7	12

[33] Weight includes rind. Without rind, the weight of the edible portion is 272 g for item 271 and 149 g for item 272.

[34] Represents yellow-fleshed varieties. For white-fleshed varieties, value is 50 International Units (I.U.) for 1 peach, 90 I.U. for 1 cup of slices.

Item No. (A)	Foods, approximate measures, units, and weight (edible part unless footnotes indicate otherwise) (B)		Water (C) Per cent	Food energy (D) Kcalories	Protein (E) Grams	Fat (F) Grams	Saturated (total) (G) Grams	Unsaturated Oleic (H) Grams	Unsaturated Linoleic (I) Grams	Carbohydrate (I) Grams	Calcium (K) Milligrams	Phosphorus (L) Milligrams	Iron (M) Milligrams	Potassium (N) Milligrams	Vitamin A value (O) International units	Thiamin (P) Milligrams	Riboflavin (Q) Milligrams	Niacin (R) Milligrams	Ascorbic acid (S) Milligrams
	Canned, yellow-fleshed, solids and liquid (halves or slices):	Grams																	
285	Syrup pack	1 cup	256 79	200	1	Trace	--	--	--	51	10	31	.8	333	1,100	.03	.05	1.5	8
286	Water pack	1 cup	244 91	75	1	Trace	--	--	--	20	10	32	.7	334	1,100	.02	.07	1.5	7
	Dried:																		
287	Uncooked	1 cup	160 25	420	5	1	--	--	--	109	77	187	9.6	1,520	6,240	.02	.30	8.5	29
288	Cooked, unsweetened, halves and juice.	1 cup	250 77	205	3	1	--	--	--	54	38	93	4.8	743	3,050	.01	.15	3.8	5
	Frozen, sliced, sweetened:																		
289	10-oz container		284 77	250	1	Trace	--	--	--	64	11	37	1.4	352	1,850	0.03	0.11	2.0	35,116
290	Cup		250 77	220	1	Trace	--	--	--	57	10	33	1.3	310	1,630	.03	.10	1.8	35,103
	Pears:																		
291	Raw, with skin, cored: Bartlett, 2 1/2-in diam. (about 2 1/2 per lb with cores and stems).	1 pear	164 83	100	1	1	--	--	--	25	13	18	.5	213	30	.03	.07	.2	7
292	Bosc, 2 1/2-in diam. (about 3 per lb with cores and stems).	1 pear	141 83	85	1	1	--	--	--	22	11	16	.4	83	30	.03	.06	.1	6
293	D'Anjou, 3-in diam. (about 2 per lb with cores and stems).	1 pear	200 83	120	1	1	--	--	--	31	16	22	.6	260	40	.04	.08	.2	8
294	Canned, solids and liquid, syrup pack, heavy (halves or slices).	1 cup	255 80	195	1	1	--	--	--	50	13	18	.5	214	10	.03	.05	.3	3
	Pineapple:																		
295	Raw, diced	1 cup	155 85	80	1	Trace	--	--	--	21	26	12	.8	226	110	.14	.05	.3	26
296	Canned, heavy syrup pack, solids and liquid: Crushed, chunks, tidbits	1 cup	255 80	190	1	Trace	--	--	--	49	28	13	.8	245	130	.20	.05	.5	18
	Slices and liquid:																		
297	Large	1 slice; 2 1/4 tbsp liquid.	105 80	80	Trace	Trace	--	--	--	20	12	5	.3	101	50	.08	.02	.2	7
298	Medium	1 slice; 1 1/4 tbsp liquid.	58 80	45	Trace	Trace	--	--	--	11	6	3	.2	56	30	.05	.01	.1	4
299	Pineapple juice, unsweetened, canned.	1 cup	250 86	140	1	Trace	--	--	--	34	38	23	.8	373	130	.13	.05	.5	27,80
	Plums:																		
300	Raw, without pits: Japanese and hybrid (2 1/8-in diam., about 6 1/2 per lb with pits).	1 plum	66 87	30	Trace	Trace	--	--	--	8	8	12	.3	112	160	.02	.02	.3	4
301	Prune-type (1 1/2-in diam., about 15 per lb with pits).	1 plum	28 79	20	Trace	Trace	--	--	--	6	3	5	.1	48	80	.01	.01	.1	1

[35] Value represents products without added ascorbic acid. For products with added ascorbic acid, value in milligrams is 116 for a 10-oz container, 103 for 1 cup.

Item No. (A)	Foods, approximate measures, units, and weight (edible part unless footnotes indicate otherwise) (B)		Water (C) Per cent	Food energy (D) Kcalories	Protein (E) Grams	Fat (F) Grams	Fatty Acids Saturated (total) (G) Grams	Unsaturated Oleic (H) Grams	Unsaturated Linoleic (I) Grams	Carbohydrate (J) Grams	Calcium (K) Milligrams	Phosphorus (L) Milligrams	Iron (M) Milligrams	Potassium (N) Milligrams	Vitamin A value (O) International units	Thiamin (P) Milligrams	Riboflavin (Q) Milligrams	Niacin (R) Milligrams	Ascorbic acid (S) Milligrams
	Canned, heavy syrup pack (Italian prunes), with pits and liquid:	Grams																	
302	Cup[36]	272	77	215	1	Trace	—	—	—	56	23	26	2.3	367	3,130	.05	.05	1.0	5
303	Portion 3 plums; 2 3/4 tbsp liquid.[36]	140	77	110	1	Trace	—	—	—	29	12	13	1.2	189	1,610	.03	.03	.5	3
	Prunes, dried, "softened," with pits:																		
304	Uncooked 4 extra large or 5 large prunes.[36]	49	28	110	1	Trace	—	—	—	29	22	34	1.7	298	690	.04	.07	.7	1
305	Cooked, unsweetened, all sizes, fruit and liquid. 1 cup[36]	250	66	255	2	1	—	—	—	67	51	79	3.8	695	1,590	.07	.15	1.5	2
306	Prune juice, canned or bottled 1 cup	256	80	195	1	Trace	—	—	—	49	36	51	1.8	602	—	.03	.03	1.0	5
	Raisins, seedless:																		
307	Cup, not pressed down 1 cup	145	18	420	4	Trace	—	—	—	112	90	146	5.1	1,106	30	.16	.12	.7	1
308	Packet, 1/2 oz (1 1/2 tbsp) 1 packet	14	18	40	Trace	Trace	—	—	—	11	9	14	.5	107	Trace	.02	.01	.1	Trace
	Raspberries, red:																		
309	Raw, capped, whole 1 cup	123	84	70	1	1	—	—	—	17	27	27	1.1	207	160	.04	.11	1.1	31
310	Frozen, sweetened, 10-oz container 1 container	284	74	280	2	1	—	—	—	70	37	48	1.7	284	200	.06	.17	1.7	60
	Rhubarb, cooked, added sugar:																		
311	From raw 1 cup	270	63	380	1	Trace	—	—	—	97	211	41	1.6	548	220	.05	.14	.8	16
312	From frozen, sweetened 1 cup	270	63	385	1	1	—	—	—	98	211	32	1.9	475	190	.05	.11	.5	16
	Strawberries:																		
313	Raw, whole berries, capped 1 cup	149	90	55	1	1	—	—	—	13	31	31	1.5	244	90	.04	.10	.9	88
	Frozen, sweetened:																		
314	Sliced, 10-oz container 1 container	284	71	310	1	1	—	—	—	79	40	48	2.0	318	90	.06	.17	1.4	151
315	Whole, 1-lb container (about 1 3/4 cups) 1 container	454	76	415	2	1	—	—	—	107	59	73	2.7	472	140	.09	.27	2.3	249
316	Tangerine, raw, 2 3/8-in diam., size 176, without peel (about 4 per lb with peels and seeds). 1 tangerine	86	87	40	1	Trace	—	—	—	10	34	15	.3	108	360	.05	.02	.1	27
317	Tangerine juice, canned, sweetened. 1 cup	249	87	125	1	Trace	—	—	—	30	44	35	.5	440	1,040	.15	.05	.2	54
318	Watermelon, raw, 4 by 8 in wedge with rind and seeds (1/16 of 32 2/3-lb melon, 10 by 16 in). 1 wedge with rind and seeds[37]	926	93	110	2	1	—	—	—	27	30	43	2.1	426	2,510	.13	.13	.9	30

[36] Weight includes pits. After removal of the pits, the weight of the edible portion is 258 g for item 302, 133 g for item 303, 43 g for item 304, and 213 g for item 305.
[37] Weight includes rind and seeds. Without rind and seeds, weight of the edible portion is 426 g.

Item No. (A)	Foods, approximate measures, units, and weight (edible part unless footnotes indicate otherwise) (B)	Water Per-cent (C)	Food energy Kcal-ories (D)	Pro-tein Grams (E)	Fat Grams (F)	Fatty Acids Satu-rated (total) Grams (G)	Unsaturated Oleic Grams (H)	Unsaturated Lino-leic Grams (I)	Carbo-hy-drate Grams (I)	Cal-cium Milli-grams (K)	Phos-pho-rus Milli-grams (L)	Iron Milli-grams (M)	Potas-sium Milli-grams (N)	Vita-min A value Inter-national units (O)	Thia-min Milli-grams (P)	Ribo-flavin Milli-grams (Q)	Nia-cin Milli-grams (R)	Ascor-bic acid Milli-grams (S)
	GRAIN PRODUCTS	Grams cent		Grams	Grams	Grams	Grams	Grams	Grams									
	Bagel, 3-in diam.:																	
319	Egg 1 bagel	55 32	165	6	2	0.5	0.9	0.8	28	9	43	1.2	41	30	.14	.10	1.2	0
320	Water 1 bagel	55 29	165	6	1	.2	.4	.6	30	8	41	1.2	42	0	.15	.11	1.4	0
321	Barley, pearled, light, uncooked 1 cup	200 11	700	16	2	.3	.2	.8	158	32	378	4.0	320	0	.24	.10	6.2	0
	Biscuits, baking powder, 2-in diam. (enriched flour, vegetable shortening):																	
322	From home recipe 1 biscuit	28 27	105	2	5	1.2	2.0	1.2	13	34	49	.4	33	Trace	.08	.08	.7	Trace
323	From mix 1 biscuit	28 29	90	2	3	.6	1.1	.7	15	19	65	.6	32	Trace	.09	.08	.8	Trace
	Breadcrumbs (enriched):[38]																	
324	Dry, grated 1 cup	100 7	390	13	5	1.0	1.6	1.4	73	122	141	3.6	152	Trace	.35	.35	4.8	Trace
	Soft. See White bread (items 349–350).																	
	Breads:																	
325	Boston brown bread canned, slice, 3 1/4 by 1/2 in.[38] 1 slice	45 45	95	2	1	.1	.2	.2	21	41	72	.9	131	[39]0	.06	.04	.7	0
	Cracked-wheat bread (3/4 enriched wheat flour, 1/4 cracked wheat):[38]																	
326	Loaf, 1 lb 1 loaf	454 35	1,195	39	10	2.2	3.0	3.9	236	399	581	9.5	608	Trace	1.52	1.13	14.4	Trace
327	Slice (18 per loaf) 1 slice	25 35	65	2	1	.1	.2	.2	13	22	32	.5	34	Trace	.08	.06	.8	Trace
	French or vienna bread, enriched:[38]																	
328	Loaf, 1 lb 1 loaf	454 31	1,315	41	14	3.2	4.7	4.6	251	195	386	10.0	408	Trace	1.80	1.10	15.0	Trace
	Slice:																	
329	French (5 by 2 1/2 by 1 in) 1 slice	35 31	100	3	1	.2	.4	.4	19	15	30	.8	32	Trace	.14	.08	1.2	Trace
330	Vienna (4 3/4 by 4 by 1/2 in) 1 slice	25 31	75	2	1	.2	.3	.3	14	11	21	.6	23	Trace	.10	.06	.8	Trace
	Italian bread, enriched:																	
331	Loaf, 1 lb 1 loaf	454 32	1,250	41	4	.6	.3	1.5	256	77	349	10.0	336	0	1.80	1.10	15.0	0
332	Slice, 4 1/2 by 3 1/4 by 3/4 in. 1 slice	30 32	85	3	Trace	Trace	Trace	.1	17	5	23	.7	22	0	.12	.07	1.0	0
	Raisin bread, enriched:[38]																	
333	Loaf, 1 lb 1 loaf	454 35	1,190	30	13	3.0	4.7	3.9	243	322	395	10.0	1,057	Trace	1.70	1.07	10.7	Trace
334	Slice (18 per loaf) 1 slice	25 35	65	2	1	.2	.3	.2	13	18	22	.6	58	Trace	.09	.06	.6	Trace

[38] Made with vegetable shortening.
[39] Applies to product made with white cornmeal. With yellow cornmeal, value is 30 International Units (I.U.).

Item No. (A)	Foods, approximate measures, units, and weight (edible part unless footnotes indicate otherwise) (B)		Water (C) Per cent	Food energy (D) Kcalories	Protein (E) Grams	Fat (F) Grams	Fatty Acids Saturated (total) (G) Grams	Unsaturated Oleic (H) Grams	Linoleic (I) Grams	Carbohydrate (I) Grams	Calcium (K) Milligrams	Phosphorus (L) Milligrams	Iron (M) Milligrams	Potassium (N) Milligrams	Vitamin A value (O) International units	Thiamin (P) Milligrams	Riboflavin (Q) Milligrams	Niacin (R) Milligrams	Ascorbic acid (S) Milligrams
		Grams	Per cent	Kcalories	Grams	Grams	Grams	Grams	Grams	Grams	Milligrams	Milligrams	Milligrams	Milligrams	International units	Milligrams	Milligrams	Milligrams	Milligrams
	Rye Bread:																		
	American, light (2/3 enriched wheat flour, 1/3 rye flour):																		
335	Loaf, 1 lb 1 loaf	454	36	1,100	41	5	.7	.5	2.2	236	340	667	9.1	658	0	1.35	.98	12.9	0
336	Slice (4 3/4 by 3 3/4 by 7/16 in.) 1 slice	25	36	60	2	Trace	Trace	Trace	.1	13	19	37	.5	36	0	.07	.05	.7	0
	Pumpernickel (2/3 rye flour, 1/3 enriched wheat flour):																		
337	Loaf, 1 lb 1 loaf	454	34	1,115	41	5	.7	.5	2.4	241	381	1,039	11.8	2,059	0	1.30	.93	8.5	0
338	Slice (5 by 4 by 3/8 in) 1 slice	32	34	80	3	Trace	.1	Trace	.2	17	27	73	.8	145	0	.09	.07	.6	0
	White bread, enriched:[38]																		
	Soft-crumb type:																		
339	Loaf, 1 lb 1 loaf	454	36	1,225	39	15	3.4	5.3	4.6	229	381	440	11.3	476	Trace	1.80	1.10	15.0	Trace
340	Slice (18 per loaf) 1 slice	25	36	70	2	1	.2	.3	.3	13	21	24	.6	26	Trace	.10	.06	.8	Trace
341	Slice, toasted 1 slice	22	25	70	2	1	.2	.3	.3	13	21	24	.6	26	Trace	.08	.06	.8	Trace
342	Slice (22 per loaf) 1 slice	20	36	55	2	1	.2	.2	.2	10	17	19	.5	21	Trace	.08	.05	.7	Trace
343	Slice, toasted 1 slice	17	25	55	2	1	.2	.2	.2	10	17	19	.5	21	Trace	.06	.05	.7	Trace
344	Loaf, 1 1/2 lb 1 loaf	680	36	1,835	59	22	5.2	7.9	6.9	343	571	660	17.0	714	Trace	2.70	1.65	22.5	Trace
345	Slice (24 per loaf) 1 slice	28	36	75	2	1	.2	.3	.3	14	24	27	.7	29	Trace	.11	.07	.9	Trace
346	Slice, toasted 1 slice	24	25	75	2	1	.2	.3	.3	14	24	27	.7	29	Trace	.09	.07	.9	Trace
347	Slice (28 per loaf) 1 slice	24	36	65	2	1	.2	.3	.2	12	20	23	.6	25	Trace	.10	.06	.8	Trace
348	Slice, toasted 1 slice	21	25	65	2	1	.2	.3	.3	12	20	23	.6	25	Trace	.08	.06	.8	Trace
349	Cubes 1 cup	30	36	80	3	1	.2	.3	.3	15	25	29	.8	32	Trace	.12	.07	1.0	Trace
350	Crumbs 1 cup	45	36	120	4	1	.3	.5	.5	23	38	44	1.1	47	Trace	.18	.11	1.5	Trace
	Firm-crumb type:																		
351	Loaf, 1 lb 1 loaf	454	35	1,245	41	17	3.9	5.9	5.2	228	435	463	11.3	549	Trace	1.80	1.10	15.0	Trace
352	Slice (20 per loaf) 1 slice	23	35	65	2	1	.2	.3	.3	12	22	23	.6	28	Trace	.09	.06	.8	Trace
353	Slice, toasted 1 slice	20	24	65	2	1	.2	.3	.3	12	22	23	.6	28	Trace	.07	.06	.8	Trace
354	Loaf, 2 lb 1 loaf	907	35	2,495	82	34	7.7	11.8	10.4	455	871	925	22.7	1,097	Trace	3.60	2.20	30.0	Trace
355	Slice (34 per loaf) 1 slice	27	35	75	2	1	.2	.3	.3	14	26	28	.7	33	Trace	.11	.06	.9	Trace
356	Slice, toasted 1 slice	23	24	75	2	1	.2	.3	.3	14	26	28	.7	33	Trace	.09	.06	.9	Trace
	Whole-wheat bread:																		
	Soft-crumb type:[38]																		
357	Loaf, 1 lb 1 loaf	454	36	1,095	41	12	2.2	2.9	4.2	224	381	1,152	13.6	1,161	Trace	1.37	.45	12.7	Trace
358	Slice (16 per loaf) 1 slice	28	36	65	3	1	.1	.2	.2	14	24	71	.8	72	Trace	.09	.03	.8	Trace
359	Slice, toasted 1 slice	24	24	65	3	1	.1	.2	.2	14	24	71	.8	72	Trace	.07	.03	.8	Trace
	Firm-crumb type:[38]																		
360	Loaf, 1 lb 1 loaf	454	36	1,100	48	14	2.5	3.3	4.9	216	449	1,034	13.6	1,238	Trace	1.17	.54	12.7	Trace
361	Slice (18 per loaf) 1 slice	25	36	60	3	1	.1	.2	.3	12	25	57	.8	68	Trace	.06	.03	.7	Trace
362	Slice, toasted 1 slice	21	24	60	3	1	.1	.2	.2	12	25	57	.8	68	Trace	.05	.03	.7	Trace

NUTRIENTS IN INDICATED QUANTITY

Item No. (A)	Foods, approximate measures, units, and weight (edible part unless footnotes indicate otherwise) (B)	Grams	Water Per cent (C)	Food energy Kcalories (D)	Protein Grams (E)	Fat Grams (F)	Fatty Acids Saturated (total) Grams (G)	Unsaturated Oleic Grams (H)	Unsaturated Linoleic Grams (I)	Carbohydrate Grams (I)	Calcium Milligrams (K)	Phosphorus Milligrams (L)	Iron Milligrams (M)	Potassium Milligrams (N)	Vitamin A value International units (O)	Thiamin Milligrams (P)	Riboflavin Milligrams (Q)	Niacin Milligrams (R)	Ascorbic acid Milligrams (S)
	Breakfast cereals:																		
	Hot type, cooked:																		
	Corn (hominy) grits, degermed:																		
363	Enriched 1 cup	245	87	125	3	Trace	Trace	Trace	.1	27	2	25	.7	27	[40]Trace	.10	.07	1.0	0
364	Unenriched 1 cup	245	87	125	3	Trace	Trace	Trace	.1	27	2	25	.2	27	[40]Trace	.05	.02	.5	0
365	Farina, quick-cooking, enriched. 1 cup	245	89	105	3	Trace	Trace	Trace	.1	22	147	[41]113	[42]	25	0	.12	.07	1.0	0
366	Oatmeal or rolled oats 1 cup	240	87	130	5	2	.4	.8	.9	23	22	137	1.4	146	0	.19	.05	.2	0
367	Wheat, rolled 1 cup	240	80	180	5	1	—	—	—	41	19	182	1.7	202	0	.17	.07	2.2	0
368	Wheat, whole-meal 1 cup	245	88	110	4	1	—	—	—	23	17	127	1.2	118	0	.15	.05	1.5	0
	Ready-to-eat:																		
369	Bran flakes (40% bran), added sugar, salt, iron, vitamins. 1 cup	35	3	105	4	1	—	—	—	28	19	125	5.6	137	1,540	.46	.52	6.2	0
370	Bran flakes with raisins, added sugar, salt, iron, vitamins. 1 cup	50	7	145	4	1	—	—	—	40	28	146	7.9	154	[43]2,200	[44]	[44]	[44]	0
	Corn flakes:																		
371	Plain, added sugar, salt, iron, vitamins. 1 cup	25	4	95	2	Trace	—	—	—	21	[44]	9	[44]	30	[44]	[44]	[44]	[44]	[45]13
372	Sugar-coated, added salt, iron, vitamins. 1 cup	40	2	155	2	Trace	—	—	—	37	1	10	[44]	27	1,760	.53	.60	7.1	[45]21
373	Corn, oat flour, puffed, added sugar, salt, iron, vitamins. 1 cup	20	4	80	2	1	—	—	—	16	4	18	5.7	—	880	.26	.30	3.5	11
374	Corn, shredded, added sugar, salt, iron, thiamin, niacin. 1 cup	25	3	95	2	Trace	—	—	—	22	1	10	.6	—	0	.33	.05	4.4	13
375	Oats, puffed, added sugar, salt, minerals, vitamins. 1 cup	25	3	100	3	1	—	—	—	19	44	102	4.0	—	1,100	.33	.38	4.4	13
	Rice, puffed:																		
376	Plain, added iron, thiamin, niacin. 1 cup	15	4	60	1	Trace	—	—	—	13	3	14	.3	15	0	.07	.01	.7	0
377	Presweetened, added salt, iron, vitamins. 1 cup	28	3	115	1	0	—	—	—	26	3	14	[44]	43	[45]1,240	[44]	[44]	[44]	[45]15

[40] Applies to white varieties. For yellow varieties, value is 150 International Units (I.U.).
[41] Applies to products that do not contain di-sodium phosphate. If di-sodium phosphate is an ingredient, value is 162 mg.
[42] Value may range from less than 1 mg to about 8 mg depending on the brand. Consult the label.
[43] Applies to product with added nutrient. Without added nutrient, value is trace.
[44] Value varies with the brand. Consult the label.
[45] Applies to product with added nutrient. Without added nutrient, value is trace.

Item No. (A)	Foods, approximate measures, units, and weight (edible part unless footnotes indicate otherwise) (B)		Grams	Water Per-cent (C)	Food energy Kcal-ories (D)	Protein Grams (E)	Fat Grams (F)	Fatty Acids Saturated (total) Grams (G)	Unsaturated Oleic Grams (H)	Unsaturated Linoleic Grams (I)	Carbo-hydrate Grams (J)	Calcium Milligrams (K)	Phosphorus Milligrams (L)	Iron Milligrams (M)	Potassium Milligrams (N)	Vitamin A value International units (O)	Thiamin Milligrams (P)	Riboflavin Milligrams (Q)	Niacin Milligrams (R)	Ascorbic acid Milligrams (S)
378	Wheat flakes, added sugar, salt, iron, vitamins.	1 cup	30	4	105	3	Trace	—	—	—	24	12	83	4.8	81	1,320	.40	.45	5.3	16
	Wheat, puffed:																			
379	Plain, added iron, thiamin, niacin.	1 cup	15	3	55	2	Trace	—	—	—	12	4	48	.6	51	0	.08	.03	1.2	0
380	Presweetened, added salt, iron, vitamins.	1 cup	38	3	140	3	Trace	—	—	—	33	7	52	(44)	63	1,680	.50	.57	6.7	45 20
381	Wheat, shredded, plain	1 oblong biscuit or 1/2 cup spoon-size biscuits.	25	7	90	2	1	—	—	—	20	11	97	.9	87	0	.06	.03	1.1	0
382	Wheat germ, without salt and sugar, toasted.	1 tbsp	6	4	25	2	1	—	—	—	3	3	70	.5	57	10	.11	.05	.3	1
383	Buckwheat flour, light, sifted.	1 cup	98	12	340	6	1	0.2	0.4	0.4	78	11	86	1.0	314	0	.08	.04	.4	0
384	Bulgur, canned, seasoned.	1 cup	135	56	245	8	4	—	—	—	44	27	263	1.9	151	0	.08	.05	4.1	0
	Cake icings. See Sugars and Sweets (items 532–536). Cakes made from cake mixes with enriched flour:46 Angelfood:																				
385	Whole cake (9 3/4-in diam. tube cake).	1 cake	635	34	1,645	36	1	—	—	—	377	603	756	2.5	381	0	.37	.95	3.6	0
386	Piece, 1/12 of cake.	1 piece	53	34	135	3	Trace	—	—	—	32	50	63	.2	32	0	.03	.08	.3	0
	Coffeecake:																				
387	Whole cake (7 3/4 by 5 5/8 by 1 1/4 in).	1 cake	430	30	1,385	27	41	11.7	16.3	8.8	225	262	748	6.9	469	690	.82	.91	7.7	1
388	Piece, 1/6 of cake	1 piece	72	30	230	5	7	2.0	2.7	1.5	38	44	125	1.2	78	120	.14	.15	1.3	Trace
	Cupcakes, made with egg, milk, 2 1/2-in diam.:																				
389	Without icing	1 cupcake	25	26	90	1	3	.8	1.2	.7	14	40	59	.3	21	40	.05	.05	.4	Trace
390	With chocolate icing	1 cupcake	36	22	130	2	5	2.0	1.6	.6	21	47	71	.4	42	60	.05	.06	.4	Trace
	Devil's food with chocolate icing:																				
391	Whole, 2 layer cake (8- or 9-in diam.).	1 cake	1,107	24	3,755	49	136	50.0	44.9	17.0	645	653	1,162	16.6	1,439	1,660	1.06	1.65	10.1	1
392	Piece, 1/16 of cake.	1 piece	69	24	235	3	8	3.1	2.8	1.1	40	41	72	1.0	90	100	.07	.10	.6	Trace
393	Cupcake, 2 1/2-in diam.	1 cupcake	35	24	120	2	4	1.6	1.4	.5	20	21	37	.5	46	50	.03	.05	.3	Trace
	Gingerbread:																				
394	Whole cake (8-in square)	1 cake	570	37	1,575	18	39	9.7	16.6	10.0	291	513	570	8.6	1,562	Trace	.84	1.00	7.4	Trace

46Excepting angelfood cake, cakes were made from mixes containing vegetable shortening; icings, with butter.

Item No. (A)	Foods, approximate measures, units, and weight (edible part unless footnotes indicate otherwise) (B)		Water Per-cent (C)	Food energy Kcal-ories (D)	Pro-tein (E)	Fat (F)	Satu-rated (total) (G)	Unsaturated Oleic (H)	Lino-leic (I)	Carbo-hy-drate (I)	Cal-cium (K)	Phos-pho-rus (L)	Iron (M)	Potas-sium (N)	Vita-min A value (O)	Thia-min (P)	Ribo-flavin (Q)	Nia-cin (R)	Ascor-bic acid (S)
			Per-cent		Grams	Grams	Grams	Grams	Grams	Grams	Milli-grams	Milli-grams	Milli-grams	Milli-grams	Inter-national units	Milli-grams	Milli-grams	Milli-grams	Milli-grams
		Grams																	
395	Piece, 1/9 of cake White, 2 layer with chocolate icing:	1 piece	63	37	175	2	4	1.1	1.8	1.1	32	57	63	.9	173	Trace	.09	.11	.8	Trace
396	Whole cake (8- or 9-in diam.)	1 cake	1,140	21	4,000	44	122	48.2	46.4	20.0	716	1,129	2,041	11.4	1,322	680	1.50	1.77	12.5	2
397	Piece, 1/16 of cake Yellow, 2 layer with chocolate icing:	1 piece	71	21	250	3	8	3.0	2.9	1.2	45	70	127	.7	82	40	.09	.11	.8	Trace
398	Whole cake (8- or 9-in diam.)	1 cake	1,108	26	3,735	45	125	47.8	47.8	20.3	638	1,008	2,017	12.2	1,208	1,550	1.24	1.67	10.6	2
399	Piece, 1/16 of cake	1 piece	69	26	235	3	8	3.0	3.0	1.3	40	63	126	.8	75	100	.08	.10	.7	Trace
	Cakes made from home recipes using enriched flour:[47] Boston cream pie with custard filling:																			
400	Whole cake (8-in diam.)	1 cake	825	35	2,490	41	78	23.0	30.1	15.2	412	553	833	8.2	[48]734	1,730	1.04	1.27	9.6	2
401	Piece, 1/12 of cake	1 piece	69	35	210	3	6	1.9	2.5	1.3	34	46	70	.7	[48]61	140	.09	.11	.8	Trace
	Fruitcake, dark:																			
402	Loaf, 1-lb (7 1/2 by 2 by 1 1/2 in),	1 loaf	454	18	1,720	22	69	14.4	33.5	14.8	271	327	513	11.8	2,250	540	.72	.73	4.9	2
403	Slice, 1/30 of loaf	1 slice	15	18	55	1	2	.5	1.1	.5	9	11	17	.4	74	20	.02	.02	.2	Trace
	Plain, sheet cake: Without icing:																			
404	Whole cake (9-in square)	1 cake	777	25	2,830	35	108	29.5	44.4	23.9	434	497	793	8.5	[48]614	1,320	1.21	1.40	10.2	2
405	Piece, 1/9 of cake	1 piece	86	25	315	4	12	3.3	4.9	2.6	48	55	88	.9	[48]68	150	.13	.15	1.1	Trace
	With uncooked white icing:																			
406	Whole cake (9-in square)	1 cake	1,096	21	4,020	37	129	42.2	49.5	24.4	694	548	822	8.2	[48]669	2,190	1.22	1.47	10.2	2
407	Piece, 1/9 of cake	1 piece	121	21	445	4	14	4.7	5.5	2.7	77	61	91	.8	[48]74	240	.14	.16	1.1	Trace
	Pound:[49]																			
408	Loaf, 8 1/2 by 3 1/2 by 3 1/4 in.	1 loaf	565	16	2,725	31	170	42.9	73.1	39.6	273	107	418	7.9	345	1,410	.90	.99	7.3	0
409	Slice, 1/17 of loaf	1 slice	33	16	160	2	10	2.5	4.3	2.3	16	6	24	.5	20	80	.05	.06	.4	0
	Spongecake:																			
410	Whole cake (9 3/4-in diam. tube cake).	1 cake	790	32	2,345	60	45	13.1	15.8	5.7	427	237	885	13.4	687	3,560	1.10	1.64	7.4	Trace

47 Excepting spongecake, vegetable shortening used for cake portion; butter, for icing. If butter or margarine used for cake portion, vitamin A values would be higher.
48 Applies to product made with a sodium aluminum-sulfate type baking powder. With a low-sodium type baking powder containing potassium, value would be about twice the amount shown.
49 Equal weights of flour, sugar, eggs, and vegetable shortening.

NUTRIENTS IN INDICATED QUANTITY

Item No. (A)	Foods, approximate measures, units, and weight (edible part unless footnotes indicate otherwise) (B)	Grams	Water Per-cent (C)	Food energy Kcalories (D)	Protein Grams (E)	Fat Grams (F)	Fatty Acids Saturated (total) Grams (G)	Unsaturated Oleic Grams (H)	Unsaturated Linoleic Grams (I)	Carbohydrate Grams (J)	Calcium Milligrams (K)	Phosphorus Milligrams (L)	Iron Milligrams (M)	Potassium Milligrams (N)	Vitamin A value International units (O)	Thiamin Milligrams (P)	Riboflavin Milligrams (Q)	Niacin Milligrams (R)	Ascorbic acid Milligrams (S)
411	Piece, 1/12 of cake	1 piece	66	32	195	5	4	1.1	1.3	.5	36	20	74	1.1	57	300	.09	.14	.6	Trace
	Cookies made with enriched flour:[50] [51]																			
	Brownies with nuts:																				
	Home-prepared, 1 3/4 by 1 3/4 by 7/8 in:																				
412	From home recipe, 1 brownie		20	10	95	1	6	1.5	3.0	1.2	10	8	30	.4	38	40	.04	.03	.2	Trace
413	From commercial recipe, 1 brownie		20	11	85	1	4	.9	1.4	1.3	13	9	27	.4	34	20	.03	.02	.2	Trace
414	Frozen, with chocolate icing,[52] 1 1/2 by 1 3/4 by 7/8 in.	1 brownie	25	13	105	1	5	2.0	2.2	.7	15	10	31	.4	44	50	.03	.03	.2	Trace
	Chocolate chip:																				
415	Commercial, 2 1/4-in diam., 3/8 in thick.	4 cookies	42	3	200	2	9	2.8	2.9	2.2	29	16	48	1.0	56	50	.10	.17	.9	Trace
416	From home recipe, 2 1/3-in diam.	4 cookies	40	3	205	2	12	3.5	4.5	2.9	24	14	40	.8	47	40	.06	.06	.5	Trace
417	Fig bars, square (1 5/8 by 1 5/8 by 3/8 in) or rectangular (1 1/2 by 1 3/4 by 1/2 in).	4 cookies	56	14	200	2	3	.8	1.2	.7	42	44	34	1.0	111	60	.04	.14	.9	Trace
418	Gingersnaps, 2-in diam., 1/4 in thick.	4 cookies	28	3	90	2	2	.7	1.0	.6	22	20	13	.7	129	20	.08	.06	.7	0
419	Macaroons, 2 3/4-in diam., 1/4 in thick.	2 cookies	38	4	180	2	9		—	—	25	10	32	.3	176	0	.02	.06	.2	0
420	Oatmeal with raisins, 2 5/8-in diam., 1/4 in thick.	4 cookies	52	3	235	3	8	2.0	3.3	2.0	38	11	53	1.4	192	30	.15	.10	1.0	Trace
421	Plain, prepared from commercial chilled dough, 2 1/2-in diam., 1/4 in thick.	4 cookies	48	5	240	2	12	3.0	5.2	2.9	31	17	35	.6	23	30	.10	.08	.9	0
422	Sandwich type (chocolate or vanilla), 1 3/4-in diam., 3/8 in thick.	4 cookies	40	2	200	2	9	2.2	3.9	2.2	28	10	96	.7	15	0	.06	.10	.7	0
423	Vanilla wafers, 1 3/4-in diam., 1/4 in thick.	10 cookies	40	3	185	2	6		—	—	30	16	25	.6	29	50	.10	.09	.8	0
	Cornmeal:																				
424	Whole-ground, unbolted, dry form.	1 cup	122	12	435	11	5	.5	1.0	2.5	90	24	312	2.9	346	620[53]	.46	.13	2.4	0

[50] Products are commercial unless otherwise specified.
[51] Made with enriched flour and vegetable shortening except for macaroons which do not contain flour or shortening.
[52] Icing made with butter.
[53] Applies to yellow varieties; white varieties contain only a trace.

NUTRIENTS IN INDICATED QUANTITY

Item No. (A)	Foods, approximate measures, units, and weight (edible part unless footnotes indicate otherwise) (B)		Grams (wt)	Water Percent (C)	Food energy Kcalories (D)	Protein Grams (E)	Fat Grams (F)	Fatty Acids Saturated (total) Grams (G)	Fatty Acids Unsaturated Oleic Grams (H)	Fatty Acids Unsaturated Linoleic Grams (I)	Carbohydrate Grams (J)	Calcium Milligrams (K)	Phosphorus Milligrams (L)	Iron Milligrams (M)	Potassium Milligrams (N)	Vitamin A value International units (O)	Thiamin Milligrams (P)	Riboflavin Milligrams (Q)	Niacin Milligrams (R)	Ascorbic acid Milligrams (S)
425	Bolted (nearly whole-grain), dry form.	1 cup	122	12	440	11	4	.5	.9	2.1	91	21	272	2.2	303	53590	.37	.10	2.3	0
	Degermed, enriched:																			
426	Dry form	1 cup	138	12	500	11	2	.2	.4	.9	108	8	137	4.0	166	53610	.61	.36	4.8	0
427	Cooked	1 cup	240	88	120	3	Trace	Trace	.1	.2	26	2	34	1.0	38	53140	.14	.10	1.2	0
	Degermed, unenriched:																			
428	Dry form	1 cup	138	12	500	11	2	.2	.4	.9	108	8	137	1.5	166	53610	.19	.07	1.4	0
429	Cooked	1 cup	240	88	120	3	Trace	Trace	.1	.2	26	2	34	.5	38	53140	.05	.02	.2	0
	Crackers:38																			
430	Graham, plain, 2 1/2-in square	2 crackers	14	6	55	1	1	.3	.5	.3	10	6	21	.5	55	0	.02	.08	.5	0
431	Rye wafers, whole-grain, 1 7/8 by 3 1/2 in.	2 wafers	13	6	45	2	Trace	—	—	—	10	7	50	.5	78	0	.04	.03	.2	0
432	Saltines, made with enriched flour.	4 crackers or 1 packet	11	4	50	1	1	.3	.5	.4	8	2	10	.5	13	0	.05	.05	.4	0
	Danish pastry (enriched flour), plain without fruit or nuts:54																			
433	Packaged ring, 12 oz.	1 ring	340	22	1,435	25	80	24.3	31.7	16.5	155	170	371	6.1	381	1,050	.97	1.01	8.6	Trace
434	Round piece, about 4 1/4-in diam. by 1 in.	1 pastry	65	22	275	5	15	4.7	6.1	3.2	30	33	71	1.2	73	200	.18	.19	1.7	Trace
435	Ounce.	1 oz	28	22	120	2	7	2.0	2.7	1.4	13	14	31	.5	32	90	.08	.08	.7	Trace
	Doughnuts, made with enriched flour:38																			
436	Cake type, plain, 2 1/2-in diam., 1 in. high.	1 doughnut	25	24	100	1	5	1.2	2.0	1.1	13	10	48	.4	23	20	.05	.05	.4	Trace
437	Yeast-leavened, glazed, 3 3/4-in diam., 1 1/4 in. high.	1 doughnut	50	26	205	3	11	3.3	5.8	3.3	22	16	33	.6	34	25	.10	.10	.8	0
	Macaroni, enriched, cooked (cut lengths, elbows, shells):																			
438	Firm stage (hot).	1 cup	130	64	190	7	1	—	—	—	39	14	85	1.4	103	0	.23	.13	1.8	0
	Tender stage:																			
439	Cold macaroni.	1 cup	105	73	115	4	Trace	—	—	—	24	8	53	.9	64	0	.15	.08	1.2	0
440	Hot macaroni.	1 cup	140	73	155	5	1	—	—	—	32	11	70	1.3	85	0	.20	.11	1.5	0
	Macaroni (enriched) and cheese:																			
441	Canned55	1 cup	240	80	230	9	10	4.2	3.1	1.4	26	199	182	1.0	139	260	.12	.24	1.0	Trace
442	From home recipe (served hot)56	1 cup	200	58	430	17	22	8.9	8.8	2.9	40	362	322	1.8	240	860	.20	.40	1.8	Trace

54 Contains vegetable shortening and butter.
55 Made with corn oil.
56 Made with regular margarine.

NUTRIENTS IN INDICATED QUANTITY

Item No. (A)	Foods, approximate measures, units, and weight (edible part unless footnotes indicate otherwise) (B)	(grams)	Water (C) Per cent	Food energy (D) Kcalories	Protein (E) Grams	Fat (F) Grams	Saturated (total) (G) Grams	Oleic (H) Grams	Linoleic (I) Grams	Carbohydrate (I) Grams	Calcium (K) Milligrams	Phosphorus (L) Milligrams	Iron (M) Milligrams	Potassium (N) Milligrams	Vitamin A value (O) International units	Thiamin (P) Milligrams	Riboflavin (Q) Milligrams	Niacin (R) Milligrams	Ascorbic acid (S) Milligrams
	Muffins made with enriched flour:38																		
	From home recipe:																		
443	Blueberry, 2 3/8-in diam., 1 1/2 in high. 1 muffin	40	39	110	3	4	1.1	1.4	.7	17	34	53	.6	46	90	.09	.10	.7	Trace
444	Bran 1 muffin	40	35	105	3	4	1.2	1.4	.8	17	57	162	1.5	172	90	.07	.10	1.7	Trace
445	Corn (enriched degermed corn meal and flour), 2 3/8-in diam., 1 1/2 in high. 1 muffin	40	33	125	3	4	1.2	1.6	.9	19	42	68	.7	54	57120	.10	.10	.7	Trace
446	Plain, 3-in diam., 1 1/2 in high. 1 muffin	40	38	120	3	4	1.0	1.7	1.0	17	42	60	0.6	50	40	.09	.12	.9	Trace
	From mix, egg, milk:																		
447	Corn, 2 3/8-in diam., 1 1/2 in high.58 1 muffin	40	30	130	3	4	1.2	1.7	.9	20	96	152	.6	44	57100	.08	.09	.7	Trace
448	Noodles (egg noodles), enriched, cooked. 1 cup	160	71	200	7	2	—	—	—	37	16	94	1.4	70	110	.22	.13	1.9	0
449	Noodles, chow mein, canned 1 cup	45	1	220	6	11	—	—	—	26	—	—	—	—	—	—	—	—	—
450	Pancakes, (4-in diam.).38 Buckwheat, made from mix (with buckwheat and enriched flours), egg and milk added. 1 cake	27	58	55	2	2	.8	.9	.4	6	59	91	.4	66	60	.04	.05	.2	Trace
	Plain:																		
451	Made from home recipe using enriched flour. 1 cake	27	50	60	2	2	.5	.8	.5	9	27	38	.4	33	30	.06	.07	.5	Trace
452	Made from mix with enriched flour, egg, and milk added. 1 cake	27	51	60	2	2	.7	.7	.3	9	58	70	.3	42	70	.04	.06	.2	Trace
	Pies, piecrust made with enriched flour, vegetable shortening (9-in diam.):																		
	Apple:																		
453	Whole 1 pie	945	48	2,420	21	105	27.0	44.5	25.2	360	76	208	6.6	756	280	1.06	.79	9.3	9
454	Sector, 1/7 of pie 1 sector	135	48	345	3	15	3.9	6.4	3.6	51	11	30	.9	108	40	.15	.11	1.3	2
	Banana cream:																		
455	Whole 1 pie	910	54	2,010	41	85	26.7	33.2	16.2	279	601	746	7.3	1,847	2,280	.77	1.51	7.0	9
456	Sector, 1/7 of pie 1 sector	130	54	285	6	12	3.8	4.7	2.3	40	86	107	1.0	264	330	.11	.22	1.0	1
	Blueberry:																		
457	Whole 1 pie	945	51	2,285	23	102	24.8	43.7	25.1	330	104	217	9.5	614	280	1.03	.80	10.0	28
458	Sector, 1/7 of pie 1 sector	135	51	325	3	15	3.5	6.2	3.6	47	15	31	1.4	88	40	.15	.11	1.4	4

57 Applies to product made with yellow cornmeal.
58 Made with enriched degermed cornmeal and enriched flour.

353

Item No. (A)	Foods, approximate measures, units, and weight (edible part unless footnotes indicate otherwise) (B)	Water Per-cent (C)	Food energy Kcal-ories (D)	Pro-tein (E)	Fat (F)	Fatty Acids Satu-rated (total) (G)	Unsaturated Oleic (H)	Lino-leic (I)	Carbo-hy-drate (J)	Cal-cium (K)	Phos-pho-rus (L)	Iron (M)	Potas-sium (N)	Vita-min A value (O)	Thia-min (P)	Ribo-flavin (Q)	Nia-cin (R)	Ascor-bic acid (S)
		Grams		Grams	Grams	Grams	Grams	Grams	Grams	Milli-grams	Milli-grams	Milli-grams	Milli-grams	Inter-national units	Milli-grams	Milli-grams	Milli-grams	Milli-grams
	Cherry:																	
459	Whole	945	2,465	25	107	28.2	45.0	25.3	363	132	236	6.6	992	4,160	1.09	.84	9.8	Trace
460	Sector, 1/7 of pie	135	350	4	15	4.0	6.4	3.6	52	19	34	.9	142	590	.16	.12	1.4	Trace
	Custard:																	
461	Whole	910	1,985	56	101	33.9	38.5	17.5	213	874	1,028	8.2	1,247	2,090	.79	1.92	5.6	0
462	Sector, 1/7 of pie	130	285	8	14	4.8	5.5	2.5	30	125	147	1.2	178	300	.11	.27	.8	0
	Lemon meringue:																	
463	Whole	840	2,140	31	86	26.1	33.8	16.4	317	118	412	6.7	420	1,430	.61	.84	5.2	25
464	Sector, 1/7 of pie	120	305	4	12	3.7	4.8	2.3	45	17	59	1.0	60	200	.09	.12	.7	4
	Mince:																	
465	Whole	945	2,560	24	109	28.0	45.9	25.2	389	265	359	13.3	1,682	20	.96	.86	9.8	9
466	Sector, 1/7 of pie	135	365	3	16	4.0	6.6	3.6	56	38	51	1.9	240	Trace	.14	.12	1.4	1
	Peach:																	
467	Whole	945	2,410	24	101	24.8	43.7	25.1	361	95	274	8.5	1,408	6,900	1.04	.97	14.0	28
468	Sector, 1/7 of pie	135	345	3	14	3.5	6.2	3.6	52	14	39	1.2	201	990	.15	.14	2.0	4
	Pecan:																	
469	Whole	825	3,450	42	189	27.8	101.0	44.2	423	388	850	25.6	1,015	1,320	1.80	.95	6.9	Trace
470	Sector, 1/7 of pie	118	495	6	27	4.0	14.4	6.3	61	55	122	3.7	145	190	.26	.14	1.0	Trace
	Pumpkin:																	
471	Whole	910	1,920	36	102	37.4	37.5	16.6	223	464	628	7.3	1,456	22,480	.78	1.27	7.0	Trace
472	Sector, 1/7 of pie	130	275	5	15	5.4	5.4	2.4	32	66	90	1.0	208	3,210	.11	.18	1.0	Trace
473	Piecrust (home recipe) made with enriched flour and vegetable short-ening, baked. 1 pie shell, 9-in diam.	180	900	11	60	14.8	26.1	14.9	79	25	90	3.1	89	0	.47	.40	5.0	0
474	Piecrust mix with en-riched flour and vege-table shortening, 10-oz pkg. prepared and baked. Piecrust for 2-crust pie, 9-in diam.	320	1,485	20	93	22.7	39.7	23.4	141	131	272	6.1	179	0	1.07	.79	9.9	0
475	Pizza (cheese) baked, 4 3/4-in sector; 1/8 of 12-in diam. pie.19 1 sector	60	145	6	4	1.7	1.5	.6	22	86	89	1.1	67	230	.16	.18	1.6	4
	Popcorn, popped:																	
476	Plain, large kernel 1 cup	6	25	1	Trace	Trace	.1	.2	5	1	17	.2	—	—	—	.01	.1	0
477	With oil (coconut) and salt added, large kernel. 1 cup	9	40	1	2	1.5	.2	.2	5	1	19	.2	—	—	—	.01	.2	0
478	Sugar coated 1 cup	35	135	2	1	.5	.2	.4	30	2	47	.5	—	—	—	.02	.4	0
	Pretzels, made with enriched flour:																	
479	Dutch, twisted, 2 3/4 by 2 5/8 in. 1 pretzel	16	60	2	1	—	—	—	12	4	21	.2	21	0	—	.04	.7	0
480	Thin, twisted, 3 1/4 by 2 1/4 by 1/4 in. 10 pretzels	60	235	6	3	—	—	—	46	13	79	.9	78	0	.20	.15	2.5	0

Item No. (A)	Foods, approximate measures, units, and weight (edible part unless footnotes indicate otherwise) (B)	Water Per-cent (C)	Food energy Kcal-ories (D)	Protein Grams (E)	Fat Grams (F)	Fatty Acids Saturated (total) (G) Grams	Unsaturated Oleic (H) Grams	Unsaturated Linoleic (I) Grams	Carbo-hydrate (J) Grams	Cal-cium (K) Milli-grams	Phos-phorus (L) Milli-grams	Iron (M) Milli-grams	Potas-sium (N) Milli-grams	Vita-min A value (O) Inter-national units	Thia-min (P) Milli-grams	Ribo-flavin (Q) Milli-grams	Nia-cin (R) Milli-grams	Ascor-bic acid (S) Milli-grams
481	Stick, 2 1/4 in long — 10 pretzels	3	10	Trace	Trace	–	–	–	2	1	4	Trace	4	0	.01	.01	.1	0
	Rice, white, enriched:																	
482	Instant, ready-to-serve, hot — 1 cup	73	180	4	Trace	Trace	Trace	Trace	40	5	31	1.3	–	0	.21	(59)	1.7	0
	Long grain:																	
483	Raw — 1 cup	12	670	12	1	.2	.2	.2	149	44	174	5.4	170	0	.81	.06	6.5	0
484	Cooked, served hot — 1 cup	73	225	4	Trace	.1	.1	.1	50	21	57	1.8	57	0	.23	.02	2.1	0
	Parboiled:																	
485	Raw — 1 cup	10	685	14	1	.2	.1	.2	150	111	370	5.4	278	0	.81	.07	6.5	0
486	Cooked, served hot — 1 cup	73	185	4	Trace	.1	.1	.1	41	33	100	1.4	75	0	.19	.02	2.1.	0
	Rolls, enriched:38																	
	Commercial:																	
487	Brown-and-serve (12 per 12-oz pkg.), browned. — 1 roll	27	85	2	2	.4	.7	.5	14	20	23	.5	25	Trace	.10	.06	.9	Trace
488	Cloverleaf or pan, 2 1/2-in diam., 2 in high. — 1 roll	31	85	2	2	.4	.6	.4	15	21	24	.5	27	Trace	.11	.07	.9	Trace
489	Frankfurter and hamburger (8 per 11 1/2-oz pkg.). — 1 roll	31	120	3	2	.5	.8	.6	21	30	34	.8	38	Trace	.16	.10	1.3	Trace
490	Hard, 3 3/4-in diam., 2 in high. — 1 roll	25	155	5	2	.4	.6	.5	30	24	46	1.2	49	Trace	.20	.12	1.7	Trace
491	Hoagie or submarine, 11 1/2 by 3 by 2 1/2 in. — 1 roll	31	390	12	4	.9	1.4	1.4	75	58	115	3.0	122	Trace	.54	.32	4.5	Trace
	From home recipe:																	
492	Cloverleaf, 2 1/2-in diam., 2 in high. — 1 roll	26	120	3	3	.8	1.1	.7	20	16	36	.7	41	30	.12	.12	1.2	Trace
	Spaghetti, enriched, cooked:																	
493	Firm stage, "al dente," served hot. — 1 cup	64	190	7	1	–	–	–	39	14	85	1.4	103	0	.23	.13	1.8	0
494	Tender stage, served hot — 1 cup	73	155	5	1	–	–	–	32	11	70	1.3	85	0	.20	.11	1.5	0
	Spaghetti (enriched) in tomato sauce with cheese:																	
495	From home recipe — 1 cup	77	260	9	9	2.0	5.4	.7	37	80	135	2.3	408	1,080	.25	.18	2.3	13
496	Canned — 1 cup	80	190	6	2	.5	.3	.4	39	40	88	2.8	303	930	.35	.28	4.5	10
	Spaghetti (enriched) with meat balls and tomato sauce:																	
497	From home recipe — 1 cup	70	330	19	12	3.3	6.3	.9	39	124	236	3.7	665	1,590	.25	.30	4.0	22

59 Product may or may not be enriched with riboflavin. Consult the label.

NUTRIENTS IN INDICATED QUANTITY

Item No. (A)	Foods, approximate measures, units, and weight (edible part unless footnotes indicate otherwise) (B)		Grams	Water Per cent (C)	Food energy Kcalories (D)	Protein Grams (E)	Fat Grams (F)	Fatty Acids Saturated (total) Grams (G)	Unsaturated Oleic Grams (H)	Linoleic Grams (I)	Carbohydrate Grams (I)	Calcium Milligrams (K)	Phosphorus Milligrams (L)	Iron Milligrams (M)	Potassium Milligrams (N)	Vitamin A value International units (O)	Thiamin Milligrams (P)	Riboflavin Milligrams (Q)	Niacin Milligrams (R)	Ascorbic acid Milligrams (S)
498	Canned	1 cup	250	78	260	12	10	2.2	3.3	3.9	29	53	113	3.3	245	1,000	.15	.18	2.3	5 (60)
499	Toaster pastries	1 pastry	50	12	200	3	6	—	—	—	36	54[60]	67[60]	1.9	74[60]	500	.16	.17	2.1	
	Waffles, made with enriched flour, 7-in diam.:38																			
500	From home recipe	1 waffle	75	41	210	7	7	2.3	2.8	1.4	28	85	130	1.3	109	250	.17	.23	1.4	Trace
501	From mix, egg and milk added	1 waffle	75	42	205	7	8	2.8	2.9	1.2	27	179	257	1.0	146	170	.14	.22	.9	Trace
	Wheat flours: All-purpose or family flour, enriched:																			
502	Sifted, spooned	1 cup	115	12	420	12	1	.2	.1	.5	88	18	100	3.3	109	0	.74	.46	6.1	0
503	Unsifted, spooned	1 cup	125	12	455	13	1	.2	.1	.5	95	20	109	3.6	119	0	.80	.50	6.6	0
504	Cake or pastry flour, enriched, sifted, spooned.	1 cup	96	12	350	7	1	.1	.1	.3	76	16	70	2.8	91	0	.61	.38	5.1	0
505	Self-rising, enriched, unsifted, spooned.	1 cup	125	12	440	12	1	.2	.1	.5	93	331	583	3.6	—	0	.80	.50	6.6	0
506	Whole-wheat, from hard wheats, stirred.	1 cup	120	12	400	16	2	.4	.2	1.0	85	49	446	4.0	444	0	.66	.14	5.2	0
	LEGUMES (DRY), NUTS, SEEDS; RELATED PRODUCTS																			
	Almonds, shelled:																			
507	Chopped (about 130 almonds)	1 cup	130	5	775	24	70	5.6	47.7	12.8	25	304	655	6.1	1,005	0	.31	1.20	4.6	Trace
508	Slivered, not pressed down (about 115 almonds).	1 cup	115	5	690	21	62	5.0	42.2	11.3	22	269	580	5.4	889	0	.28	1.06	4.0	Trace
	Beans, dry: Common varieties as Great Northern, navy, and others: Cooked, drained:																			
509	Great Northern	1 cup	180	69	210	14	1	—	—	—	38	90	266	4.9	749	0	.25	.13	1.3	0
510	Pea (navy)	1 cup	190	69	225	15	1	—	—	—	40	95	281	5.1	790	0	.27	.13	1.3	0
	Canned, solids and liquid: White with—																			
511	Frankfurters (sliced)	1 cup	255	71	365	19	18	—	—	—	32	94	303	4.8	668	330	.18	.15	3.3	Trace
512	Pork and tomato sauce	1 cup	255	71	310	16	7	2.4	2.8	.6	48	138	235	4.6	536	330	.20	.08	1.5	5

60 Value varies with the brand. Consult the label.

Item No. (A)	Foods, approximate measures, units, and weight (edible part unless footnotes indicate otherwise) (B)		Water Per cent (C)	Food energy Kcalories (D)	Protein Grams (E)	Fat Grams (F)	Fatty Acids Saturated (total) Grams (G)	Unsaturated Oleic Grams (H)	Unsaturated Linoleic Grams (I)	Carbohydrate Grams (J)	Calcium Milligrams (K)	Phosphorus Milligrams (L)	Iron Milligrams (M)	Potassium Milligrams (N)	Vitamin A value International units (O)	Thiamin Milligrams (P)	Riboflavin Milligrams (Q)	Niacin Milligrams (R)	Ascorbic acid Milligrams (S)
513	Pork and sweet sauce	1 cup	66	385	16	12	4.3	5.0	1.1	54	161	291	5.9	—	—	.15	.10	1.3	—
514	Red kidney	1 cup	76	230	15	1	—	—	—	42	74	278	4.6	673	10	.13	.10	1.5	—
515	Lima, cooked, drained	1 cup	64	260	16	1	—	—	—	49	55	293	5.9	1,163	—	.25	.11	1.3	—
516	Blackeye peas, dry, cooked (with residual cooking liquid).	1 cup	80	190	13	1	—	—	—	35	43	238	3.3	573	30	.40	.10	1.0	—
517	Brazil nuts, shelled (6–8 large kernels).	1 oz	5	185	4	19	4.8	6.2	7.1	3	53	196	1.0	203	Trace	.27	.03	.5	—
518	Cashew nuts, roasted in oil	1 cup	5	785	24	64	12.9	36.8	10.2	41	53	522	5.3	650	140	.60	.35	2.5	—
519	Coconut meat, fresh: Piece, about 2 by 2 by 1/2 in	1 piece	51	155	2	16	14.0	.9	.3	4	6	43	.8	115	0	.02	.01	.2	1
520	Shredded or grated, not pressed down.	1 cup	51	275	3	28	24.8	1.6	.5	8	10	76	1.4	205	0	.04	.02	.4	2
521	Filberts (hazelnuts), chopped (about 80 kernels).	1 cup	6	730	14	72	5.1	55.2	7.3	19	240	388	3.9	810	—	.53	—	1.0	Trace
522	Lentils, whole, cooked	1 cup	72	210	16	Trace	—	—	—	39	50	238	4.2	498	40	.14	.12	1.2	0
523	Peanuts, roasted in oil, salted (whole, halves, chopped).	1 cup	2	840	37	72	13.7	33.0	20.7	27	107	577	3.0	971	—	.46	.19	24.8	0
524	Peanut butter	1 tbsp	2	95	4	8	1.5	3.7	2.3	3	9	61	.3	100	—	.02	.02	2.4	0
525	Peas, split, dry, cooked	1 cup	70	230	16	1	—	—	—	42	22	178	3.4	592	80	.30	.18	1.8	—
526	Pecans, chopped or pieces (about 120 large halves).	1 cup	3	810	11	84	7.2	50.5	20.0	17	86	341	2.8	712	150	1.01	.15	1.1	2
527	Pumpkin and squash kernels, dry, hulled	1 cup	4	775	41	65	11.8	23.5	27.5	21	71	1,602	15.7	1,386	100	.34	.27	3.4	—
528	Sunflower seeds, dry, hulled	1 cup	5	810	35	69	8.2	13.7	43.2	29	174	1,214	10.3	1,334	70	2.84	.33	7.8	—
	Walnuts: Black:																		
529	Chopped or broken kernels	1 cup	3	785	26	74	6.3	13.3	45.7	19	Trace	713	7.5	575	380	.28	.14	.9	—
530	Ground (finely)	1 cup	3	500	16	47	4.0	8.5	29.2	12	Trace	456	4.8	368	240	.18	.09	.6	—
531	Persian or English, chopped (about 60 halves).	1 cup	4	780	18	77	8.4	11.8	42.2	19	119	456	3.7	540	40	.40	.16	1.1	2
	Cake icings: Boiled, white:																		
532	Plain	1 cup	18	295	1	0	0	0	0	75	2	2	Trace	17	0	Trace	.03	Trace	0
533	With coconut	1 cup	15	605	3	13	11.0	.9	Trace	124	10	50	.8	277	0	.02	.07	0.3	0
	Uncooked:																		
534	Chocolate made with milk and butter.	1 cup	14	1,035	9	38	23.4	11.7	1.0	185	165	305	3.3	536	580	.06	.28	.6	1

Item No. (A)	Foods, approximate measures, units, and weight (edible part unless footnotes indicate otherwise) (B)	Water (C) Per cent	Food energy (D) Kcalories	Protein (E) Grams	Fat (F) Grams	Fatty Acids Saturated (total) (G) Grams	Unsaturated Oleic (H) Grams	Unsaturated Linoleic (I) Grams	Carbohydrate (I) Grams	Calcium (K) Milligrams	Phosphorus (L) Milligrams	Iron (M) Milligrams	Potassium (N) Milligrams	Vitamin A value (O) International units	Thiamin (P) Milligrams	Riboflavin (Q) Milligrams	Niacin (R) Milligrams	Ascorbic acid (S) Milligrams
535	Creamy fudge from mix and water. 1 cup	245	830	7	16	5.1	6.7	3.1	183	96	218	2.7	238	Trace	.05	.20	.7	Trace
536	White. 1 cup	319	1,200	2	21	12.7	5.1	.5	260	48	38	Trace	57	860	Trace	.06	Trace	Trace
	Candy:																	
537	Caramels, plain or chocolate 1 oz	28	115	1	3	1.6	1.1	.1	22	42	35	.4	54	Trace	.01	.05	.1	Trace
	Chocolate:																	
538	Milk, plain 1 oz	28	145	2	9	5.5	3.0	.3	16	65	65	.3	109	80	.02	.10	.1	Trace
539	Semisweet, small pieces (60 per oz). 1 cup or 6-oz pkg	170	860	7	61	36.2	19.8	1.7	97	51	255	4.4	553	30	.02	.14	.9	0
540	Chocolate-coated peanuts 1 oz	28	160	5	12	4.0	4.7	2.1	11	33	84	.4	143	Trace	.10	.05	2.1	Trace
541	Fondant, uncoated (mints, candy corn, other). 1 oz	28	105	Trace	1	.1	.3	.1	25	4	2	.3	1	0	Trace	Trace	Trace	0
542	Fudge, chocolate, plain 1 oz	28	115	1	3	1.3	1.4	.6	21	22	24	.3	42	Trace	.01	.03	.1	Trace
543	Gum drops 1 oz	28	100	Trace	Trace	—	—	—	25	2	Trace	.1	1	0	0	Trace	Trace	0
544	Hard 1 oz	28	110	0	Trace	—	—	—	28	6	2	.5	1	0	0	0	0	0
545	Marshmallows 1 oz	28	90	1	Trace	—	—	—	23	5	2	.5	2	0	0	Trace	Trace	0
	Chocolate-flavored beverage powders (about 4 heaping tsp per oz):																	
546	With nonfat dry milk 1 oz	28	100	5	1	.5	.3	Trace	20	167	155	.5	227	10	.04	.21	.2	1
547	Without milk 1 oz	28	100	1	1	.4	.2	Trace	25	9	48	.6	142	—	.01	.03	.1	0
548	Honey, strained or extracted 1 tbsp	21	65	Trace	0	—	—	—	17	1	1	.1	11	0	Trace	.01	.1	Trace
549	Jams and preserves 1 tbsp	20	55	Trace	Trace	—	—	—	14	4	2	.2	18	Trace	Trace	.01	Trace	Trace
550	1 packet	14	40	Trace	Trace	—	—	—	10	3	1	.1	12	Trace	Trace	.01	Trace	Trace
551	Jellies 1 tbsp	18	50	Trace	Trace	—	—	—	13	4	1	.3	14	Trace	Trace	.01	Trace	1
552	1 packet	14	40	Trace	Trace	—	—	—	10	3	1	.2	11	Trace	Trace	Trace	Trace	1
	Syrups: Chocolate-flavored syrup or topping:																	
553	Thin type 1 fl oz or 2 tbsp	38	90	1	1	.5	.3	Trace	24	6	35	.6	106	Trace	.01	.03	.2	0
554	Fudge type 1 fl oz or 2 tbsp	38	125	2	5	3.1	1.6	.1	20	48	60	.5	107	60	.02	.08	.2	Trace
	Molasses, cane:																	
555	Light (first extraction) 1 tbsp	20	50	—	—	—	—	—	13	33	9	.9	183	—	.01	.01	Trace	—
556	Blackstrap (third extraction) 1 tbsp	20	45	—	—	—	—	—	11	137	17	3.2	585	—	.02	.04	.4	—
557	Sorghum 1 tbsp	21	55	—	—	—	—	—	14	35	5	2.6	—	—	—	.02	Trace	—
558	Table blends, chiefly corn, light and dark. 1 tbsp	21	60	0	0	—	—	—	15	9	3	.8	1	0	0	0	0	0
	Sugars:																	
559	Brown, pressed down 1 cup	220	820	0	0	0	0	0	212	187	42	7.5	757	0	.02	.07	.4	0
	White:																	
560	Granulated 1 cup	200	770	0	0	0	0	0	199	0	0	.2	6	0	0	0	0	0

Item No. (A)	Foods, approximate measures, units, and weight (edible part unless footnotes indicate otherwise) (B)	Weight Grams	Water Per cent (C)	Food energy Kcalories (D)	Protein Grams (E)	Fat Grams (F)	Fatty Acids Saturated (total) Grams (G)	Unsaturated Oleic Grams (H)	Unsaturated Linoleic Grams (I)	Carbohydrate Grams (I)	Calcium Milligrams (K)	Phosphorus Milligrams (L)	Iron Milligrams (M)	Potassium Milligrams (N)	Vitamin A value International units (O)	Thiamin Milligrams (P)	Riboflavin Milligrams (Q)	Niacin Milligrams (R)	Ascorbic acid Milligrams (S)
561	1 tbsp	12	1	45	0	0	0	0	0	12	0	0	0	Trace	0	0	0	0	0
562	1 packet	6	1	23	0	0	0	0	0	6	0	0	0	Trace	0	0	0	0	0
563	Powdered, sifted, spooned into cup. 1 cup	100	1	385	0	0	0	0	0	100	0	0	.1	3	0	0	0	0	0

VEGETABLE AND VEGETABLE PRODUCTS

Asparagus, green:
Cooked, drained:
Cuts and tips, 1 1/2- to 2-in lengths:

Item No. (A)	Foods (B)	Weight Grams	Water Per cent (C)	Food energy Kcalories (D)	Protein Grams (E)	Fat Grams (F)	Saturated (total) Grams (G)	Oleic Grams (H)	Linoleic Grams (I)	Carbohydrate Grams (I)	Calcium Milligrams (K)	Phosphorus Milligrams (L)	Iron Milligrams (M)	Potassium Milligrams (N)	Vitamin A value Int. units (O)	Thiamin Milligrams (P)	Riboflavin Milligrams (Q)	Niacin Milligrams (R)	Ascorbic acid Milligrams (S)
564	From raw — 1 cup	145	94	30	3	Trace	—	—	—	5	30	73	.9	265	1,310	.23	.26	2.0	38
565	From frozen — 1 cup	180	93	40	6	Trace	—	—	—	6	40	115	2.2	396	1,530	.25	.23	1.8	41
	Spears, 1/2-in diam. at base:																		
566	From raw — 4 spears	60	94	10	1	Trace	—	—	—	2	13	30	.4	110	540	.10	.11	.8	16
567	From frozen — 4 spears	60	92	15	2	Trace	—	—	—	2	13	40	.7	143	470	.10	.08	.7	16
568	Canned, spears, 1/2-in diam. at base — 4 spears	80	93	15	2	Trace	—	—	—	3	15	42	1.5	133	640	.05	.08	.6	12

Beans:
Lima, immature seeds, frozen, cooked, drained:

Item No. (A)	Foods (B)	Weight Grams	Water Per cent (C)	Food energy Kcalories (D)	Protein Grams (E)	Fat Grams (F)	Saturated (total) Grams (G)	Oleic Grams (H)	Linoleic Grams (I)	Carbohydrate Grams (I)	Calcium Milligrams (K)	Phosphorus Milligrams (L)	Iron Milligrams (M)	Potassium Milligrams (N)	Vitamin A value Int. units (O)	Thiamin Milligrams (P)	Riboflavin Milligrams (Q)	Niacin Milligrams (R)	Ascorbic acid Milligrams (S)
569	Thick-seeded types (Fordhooks) — 1 cup	170	74	170	10	Trace	—	—	—	32	34	153	2.9	724	390	.12	.09	1.7	29
570	Thin-seeded types (baby limas) — 1 cup	180	69	210	13	Trace	—	—	—	40	63	227	4.7	709	400	.16	.09	2.2	22

Snap:
Green:
Cooked, drained:

Item No. (A)	Foods (B)	Weight Grams	Water Per cent (C)	Food energy Kcalories (D)	Protein Grams (E)	Fat Grams (F)	Saturated (total) Grams (G)	Oleic Grams (H)	Linoleic Grams (I)	Carbohydrate Grams (I)	Calcium Milligrams (K)	Phosphorus Milligrams (L)	Iron Milligrams (M)	Potassium Milligrams (N)	Vitamin A value Int. units (O)	Thiamin Milligrams (P)	Riboflavin Milligrams (Q)	Niacin Milligrams (R)	Ascorbic acid Milligrams (S)
571	From raw (cuts and French style) — 1 cup	125	92	30	2	Trace	—	—	—	7	63	46	.8	189	680	.09	.11	.6	15
	From frozen:																		
572	Cuts — 1 cup	135	92	35	2	Trace	—	—	—	8	54	43	.9	205	780	.09	.12	.5	7
573	French style — 1 cup	130	92	35	2	Trace	—	—	—	8	49	39	1.2	177	690	.08	.10	.4	9
574	Canned, drained solids (cuts) — 1 cup	135	92	30	2	Trace	—	—	—	7	61	34	2.0	128	630	.04	.07	.4	5
	Yellow or wax: Cooked, drained:																		
575	From raw (cuts and French style) — 1 cup	125	93	30	2	Trace	—	—	—	6	63	46	.8	189	290	.09	.11	.6	16
576	From frozen (cuts) — 1 cup	135	92	35	2	Trace	—	—	—	8	47	42	.9	221	140	.09	.11	.5	8
577	Canned, drained solids (cuts) — 1 cup	135	92	30	2	Trace	—	—	—	7	61	34	2.0	128	140	.04	.07	.4	7

Beans, mature. See Beans, dry (items 509–515) and Blackeye peas, dry (item 516).

Item No. (A)	Foods, approximate measures, units, and weight (edible part unless footnotes indicate otherwise) (B)		Wa-ter Per-cent (C)	Food energy (D)	Pro-tein (E)	Fat (F)	Fatty Acids Satu-rated (total) (G)	Unsaturated Oleic (H)	Lino-leic (I)	Carbo-hy-drate (J)	Cal-cium (K)	Phos-pho-rus (L)	Iron (M)	Potas-sium (N)	Vita-min A value (O)	Thia-min (P)	Ribo-flavin (Q)	Nia-cin (R)	Ascor-bic acid (S)
			Grams, cent	Kcal-ories	Grams	Grams	Grams	Grams	Grams	Grams	Milli-grams	Milli-grams	Milli-grams	Milli-grams	Inter-national units	Milli-grams	Milli-grams	Milli-grams	Milli-grams
	Bean sprouts (mung):																		
578	Raw	1 cup	105 89	35	4	Trace	—	—	—	7	20	67	1.4	234	20	.14	.14	.8	20
579	Cooked, drained	1 cup	125 91	35	4	Trace	—	—	—	7	21	60	1.1	195	30	.11	.13	.9	8
	Beets:																		
	Cooked, drained, peeled:																		
580	Whole beets, 2-in diam.	2 beets	100 91	30	1	Trace	—	—	—	7	14	23	.5	208	20	.03	.04	.3	6
581	Diced or sliced	1 cup	170 91	55	2	Trace	—	—	—	12	24	39	.9	354	30	.05	.07	.5	10
	Canned, drained solids:																		
582	Whole beets, small	1 cup	160 89	60	2	Trace	—	—	—	14	30	29	1.1	267	30	.02	.05	.2	5
583	Diced or sliced	1 cup	170 89	65	2	Trace	—	—	—	15	32	31	1.2	284	30	.02	.05	.2	5
584	Beet greens, leaves and stems, cooked drained.	1 cup	145 94	25	2	Trace	—	—	—	5	144	36	2.8	481	7,400	.10	.22	.4	22
	Blackeye peas, immature seeds, cooked and drained:																		
585	From raw	1 cup	165 72	180	13	1	—	—	—	30	40	241	3.5	625	580	.50	.18	2.3	28
586	From frozen	1 cup	170 66	220	15	1	—	—	—	40	43	286	4.8	573	290	.68	.19	2.4	15
	Broccoli, cooked, drained:																		
	From raw:																		
587	Stalk, medium size	1 stalk	180 91	45	6	1	—	—	—	8	158	112	1.4	481	4,500	.16	.36	1.4	162
588	Stalks cut into 1/2-in pieces	1 cup	155 91	40	5	Trace	—	—	—	7	136	96	1.2	414	3,880	.14	.31	1.2	140
	From frozen:																		
589	Stalk, 4 1/2 to 5 in long	1 stalk	30 91	10	1	Trace	—	—	—	1	12	17	.2	66	570	.02	.03	.2	22
590	Chopped	1 cup	185 92	50	5	1	—	—	—	9	100	104	1.3	392	4,810	.11	.22	.9	105
591	Brussels sprouts, cooked, drained: From raw, 7–8 sprouts (1 1/4- to 1 1/2-in diam.).	1 cup	155 88	55	7	1	—	—	—	10	50	112	1.7	423	810	.12	.22	1.2	135
592	From frozen	1 cup	155 89	50	5	Trace	—	—	—	10	33	95	1.2	457	880	.12	.16	.9	126
	Cabbage:																		
	Common varieties:																		
	Raw:																		
593	Coarsely shredded or sliced	1 cup	70 92	15	1	Trace	—	—	—	4	34	20	.3	163	90	.04	.04	.2	33
594	Finely shredded or chopped	1 cup	90 92	20	1	Trace	—	—	—	5	44	26	.4	210	120	.05	.05	.3	42
595	Cooked, drained	1 cup	145 94	30	2	Trace	—	—	—	6	64	29	.4	236	190	.06	.06	.4	48
596	Red, raw, coarsely shredded or sliced	1 cup	70 90	20	1	Trace	—	—	—	5	29	25	.6	188	30	.06	.04	.3	43
597	Savoy, raw, coarsely shredded or sliced.	1 cup	70 92	15	2	Trace	—	—	—	3	47	38	.6	188	140	.04	.06	.2	39

Item No. (A)	Foods, approximate measures, units, and weight (edible part unless footnotes indicate otherwise) (B)		Water (C) Per cent	Food energy (D) Kcalories	Protein (E) Grams	Fat (F) Grams	Fatty Acids Saturated (total) (G) Grams	Unsaturated Oleic (H) Grams	Linoleic (I) Grams	Carbohydrate (I) Grams	Calcium (K) Milligrams	Phosphorus (L) Milligrams	Iron (M) Milligrams	Potassium (N) Milligrams	Vitamin A value (O) International units	Thiamin (P) Milligrams	Riboflavin (Q) Milligrams	Niacin (R) Milligrams	Ascorbic acid (S) Milligrams
		Grams																	
598	Cabbage, celery (also called pe-tsai or wongbok), raw, 1-in pieces.	1 cup	75	95	10	1	Trace	—	—	—	2	32	30	.5	190	110	.04	.03	.5	19
599	Cabbage, white mustard (also called bokchoy or pakchoy), cooked, drained.	1 cup	170	95	25	2	Trace	—	—	—	4	252	56	1.0	364	5,270	.07	.14	1.2	26
	Carrots: Raw, without crowns and tips, scraped:																			
600	Whole, 7 1/2 by 1 1/8 in, or strips, 2 1/2 to 3 in long.	1 carrot or 18 strips	72	88	30	1	Trace	—	—	—	7	27	26	.5	246	7,930	.04	.04	.4	6
601	Grated.	1 cup	110	88	45	1	Trace	—	—	—	11	41	40	.8	375	12,100	.07	.06	.7	9
602	Cooked (crosswise cuts), drained.	1 cup	155	91	50	1	Trace	—	—	—	11	51	48	.9	344	16,280	.08	.08	.8	9
	Canned:																			
603	Sliced, drained solids.	1 cup	155	91	45	1	Trace	—	—	—	10	47	34	1.1	186	23,250	.03	.05	.6	3
604	Strained or junior (baby food).	1 oz (1 3/4 to 2 tbsp)	28	92	10	Trace	Trace	—	—	—	2	7	6	.1	51	3,690	.01	.01	.1	1
	Cauliflower:																			
605	Raw, chopped.	1 cup	115	91	31	3	Trace	—	—	—	6	29	64	1.3	339	70	.13	.12	.8	90
606	Cooked, drained: From raw (flower buds).	1 cup	125	93	30	3	Trace	—	—	—	5	26	53	.9	258	80	.11	.10	.8	69
607	From frozen (flowerets).	1 cup	180	94	30	3	Trace	—	—	—	6	31	68	.9	373	50	.07	.09	.7	74
	Celery, Pascal type, raw:																			
608	Stalk, large outer, 8 by 1 1/2 in, at root end.	1 stalk	40	94	5	Trace	Trace	—	—	—	2	16	11	.1	136	110	.01	.01	.1	4
609	Pieces, diced.	1 cup	120	94	20	1	Trace	—	—	—	5	47	34	.4	409	320	.04	.04	.4	11
	Collards, cooked, drained:																			
610	From raw (leaves without stems).	1 cup	190	90	65	7	1	—	—	—	10	357	99	1.5	498	14,820	.21	.38	2.3	144
611	From frozen (chopped).	1 cup	170	90	50	5	1	—	—	—	10	299	87	1.7	401	11,560	.10	.24	1.0	56
	Corn, sweet: Cooked, drained:																			
612	From raw, ear 5 by 1 3/4 in.	1 ear[61]	140	74	70	2	1	—	—	—	16	2	69	.5	151	[62]310	.09	.08	1.1	7
	From frozen:																			
613	Ear, 5 in long.	1 ear[61]	229	73	120	4	1	—	—	—	27	4	121	1.0	291	[62]440	.18	.10	2.1	9

[61] Weight includes cob. Without cob, weight is 77 g for item 612, 126 g for item 613.
[62] Based on yellow varieties. For white varieties, value is trace.

361

Item No. (A)	Foods, approximate measures, units, and weight (edible part unless footnotes indicate otherwise) (B)		Water Per-cent (C)	Food energy Kcal-ories (D)	Protein (E)	Fat (F)	Fatty Acids Saturated (total) (G)	Unsaturated Oleic (H)	Unsaturated Linoleic (I)	Carbo-hydrate (I)	Calcium (K)	Phos-phorus (L)	Iron (M)	Potas-sium (N)	Vita-min A value (O)	Thia-min (P)	Ribo-flavin (Q)	Nia-cin (R)	Ascor-bic acid (S)
			Grams		Grams	Grams	Grams	Grams	Grams	Grams	Milli-grams	Milli-grams	Milli-grams	Milli-grams	Inter-national units	Milli-grams	Milli-grams	Milli-grams	Milli-grams
			Grams Per-cent																
614	Kernels	1 cup	165	77	130	5	1	—	—	—	31	5	120	1.3	304	62,580	.15	.10	2.5	8
	Canned:																		
615	Cream style	1 cup	256	76	210	5	2	—	—	—	51	8	143	1.5	248	62,840	.08	.13	2.6	13
	Whole kernel:																		
616	Vacuum pack	1 cup	210	76	175	5	1	—	—	—	43	6	153	1.1	204	62,740	.06	.13	2.3	11
617	Wet pack, drained solids	1 cup	165	76	140	4	1	—	—	—	33	8	81	.8	160	62,580	.05	.08	1.5	7
	Cowpeas. See Blackeye peas. (Items 585–586).																		
	Cucumber slices, 1/8 in thick (large, 2 1/8-in diam.; small, 1 3/4-in diam.):																		
618	With peel	6 large or 8 small slices	28	95	5	Trace	Trace	—	—	—	1	7	8	.3	45	70	.01	.01	.1	3
619	Without peel	6 1/2 large or 9 small pieces	28	96	5	Trace	Trace	—	—	—	1	5	5	.1	45	Trace	.01	.01	.1	3
620	Dandelion greens, cooked, drained	1 cup	105	90	35	2	1	—	—	—	7	147	44	1.9	244	12,290	.14	.17	—	19
621	Endive, curly (including escarole), raw, small pieces.	1 cup	50	93	10	1	Trace	—	—	—	2	41	27	.9	147	1,650	.04	.07	.3	5
	Kale, cooked, drained:																		
622	From raw (leaves without stems and midribs).	1 cup	110	88	45	5	1	—	—	—	7	206	64	1.8	243	9,130	.11	.20	1.8	102
623	From frozen (leaf style)	1 cup	130	91	40	4	1	—	—	—	7	157	62	1.3	251	10,660	.08	.20	.9	49
	Lettuce, raw: Butterhead, as Boston types:																		
624	Head, 5-in diam	1 head[63]	220	95	25	2	Trace	—	—	—	4	57	42	3.3	430	1,580	.10	.10	.5	13
625	Leaves	1 outer or 2 inner or 3 heart leaves.	15	95	Trace	Trace	Trace	—	—	—	Trace	5	4	.3	40	150	.01	.01	Trace	1
	Crisphead, as Iceberg:																		
626	Head, 6-in diam	1 head[64]	567	96	70	5	1	—	—	—	16	108	118	2.7	943	1,780	.32	.32	1.6	32
627	Wedge, 1/4 of head	1 wedge	135	96	20	1	Trace	—	—	—	4	27	30	.7	236	450	.08	.08	.4	8
628	Pieces, chopped or shredded	1 cup	55	96	5	Trace	Trace	—	—	—	2	11	12	.3	96	180	.03	.03	.2	3
629	Looseleaf (bunching varieties including romaine or cos), chopped or shredded pieces.	1 cup	55	94	10	1	Trace	—	—	—	2	37	14	.8	145	1,050	.03	.04	.2	10

[63]Weight includes refuse of outer leaves and core. Without these parts, weight is 163 g.
[64]Weight includes core. Without core, weight is 539 g.

Item No. (A)	Foods, approximate measures, units, and weight (edible part unless footnotes indicate otherwise) (B)		Grams	Water (C) Per cent	Food energy (D) Kcalories	Protein (E) Grams	Fat (F) Grams	Fatty Acids Saturated (total) (G) Grams	Unsaturated Oleic (H) Grams	Unsaturated Linoleic (I) Grams	Carbohydrate (I) Grams	Calcium (K) Milligrams	Phosphorus (L) Milligrams	Iron (M) Milligrams	Potassium (N) Milligrams	Vitamin A value (O) International units	Thiamin (P) Milligrams	Riboflavin (Q) Milligrams	Niacin (R) Milligrams	Ascorbic acid (S) Milligrams
630	Mushrooms, raw, sliced or chopped	1 cup	70	90	20	2	Trace	—	—	—	3	4	81	.6	290	Trace	.07	.32	2.9	2
631	Mustard greens, without stems and midribs, cooked, drained.	1 cup	140	93	30	3	1	—	—	—	6	193	45	2.5	308	8,120	.11	.20	.8	67
632	Okra pods, 3 by 5/8 in, cooked	10 pods	106	91	30	2	Trace	—	—	—	6	98	43	.5	184	520	.14	.19	1.0	21
	Onions: Mature: Raw:																			
633	Chopped	1 cup	170	89	65	3	Trace	—	—	—	15	46	61	.9	267	[65]Trace	.05	.07	.3	17
634	Sliced	1 cup	115	89	45	2	Trace	—	—	—	10	31	41	.6	181	[65]Trace	.03	.05	.2	12
635	Cooked (whole or sliced), drained.	1 cup	210	92	60	3	Trace	—	—	—	14	50	61	.8	231	[65]Trace	.06	.06	.4	15
636	Young green, bulb (3/8 in diam.) and white portion of top.	6 onions	30	88	15	Trace	Trace	—	—	—	3	12	12	.2	69	Trace	.02	.01	.1	8
637	Parsley, raw, chopped	1 tbsp	4	85	Trace	Trace	Trace	—	—	—	Trace	7	2	.2	25	300	Trace	.01	Trace	6
638	Parsnips, cooked (diced or 2-in lengths).	1 cup	155	82	100	2	1	—	—	—	23	70	96	.9	587	50	.11	.12	.2	16
	Peas, green: Canned:																			
639	Whole, drained solids	1 cup	170	77	150	8	1	—	—	—	29	44	129	3.2	163	1,170	.15	.10	1.4	14
640	Strained (baby food)	1 oz (1 3/4 to 2 tbsp)	28	86	15	1	Trace	—	—	—	3	3	18	.3	28	140	.02	.03	.3	3
641	Frozen, cooked, drained	1 cup	160	82	110	8	Trace	—	—	—	19	30	138	3.0	216	960	.43	.14	2.7	21
642	Peppers, hot, red, without seeds, dried (ground chili powder, added seasonings).	1 tbsp	2	9	5	Trace	Trace	—	—	—	1	5	4	.3	20	1,300	Trace	.02	.2	Trace
	Peppers, sweet (about 5 per lb, whole), stem and seeds removed:																			
643	Raw	1 pod	74	93	15	1	Trace	—	—	—	4	7	16	.5	157	310	.06	.06	.4	94
644	Cooked, boiled, drained	1 pod	73	95	15	1	Trace	—	—	—	3	7	12	.4	109	310	.05	.05	.4	70
	Potatoes, cooked:																			
645	Baked, peeled after baking (about 2 per lb, raw).	1 potato	156	75	145	4	Trace	—	—	—	33	14	101	1.1	782	Trace	.15	.07	2.7	31
	Boiled (about 3 per lb, raw):																			
646	Peeled after boiling	1 potato	137	80	105	3	Trace	—	—	—	23	10	72	.8	556	Trace	.12	.05	2.0	22
647	Peeled before boiling	1 potato	135	83	90	3	Trace	—	—	—	20	8	57	.7	385	Trace	.12	.05	1.6	22

[65]Value based on white-fleshed varieties. For yellow-fleshed varieties, value in International Units (I.U.) is 70 for item 633, 50 for item 634, and 80 for item 635.

Item No. (A)	Foods, approximate measures, units, and weight (edible part unless footnotes indicate otherwise) (B)		Grams	Water Per cent (C)	Food energy Kcalories (D)	Protein Grams (E)	Fat Grams (F)	Fatty Acids Saturated (total) (G) Grams	Unsaturated Oleic (H) Grams	Unsaturated Linoleic (I) Grams	Carbohydrate (J) Grams	Calcium Milligrams (K)	Phosphorus Milligrams (L)	Iron Milligrams (M)	Potassium Milligrams (N)	Vitamin A value International units (O)	Thiamin Milligrams (P)	Riboflavin Milligrams (Q)	Niacin Milligrams (R)	Ascorbic acid Milligrams (S)
	French-fried, strip, 2 to 3 1/2 in long:																			
648	Prepared from raw	10 strips	50	45	135	2	7	1.7	1.2	3.3	18	8	56	.7	427	Trace	.07	.04	1.6	11
649	Frozen, oven heated	10 strips	50	53	110	2	4	1.1	.8	2.1	17	5	43	.9	326	Trace	.07	.01	1.3	11
650	Hashed brown, prepared from frozen.	1 cup	155	56	345	3	18	4.6	3.2	9.0	45	28	78	1.9	439	Trace	.11	.03	1.6	12
	Mashed, prepared from—																			
	Raw:																			
651	Milk added	1 cup	210	83	135	4	2	.7	.4	Trace	27	50	103	.8	548	40	.17	.11	2.1	21
652	Milk and butter added	1 cup	210	80	195	4	9	5.6	2.3	.2	26	50	101	.8	525	360	.17	.11	2.1	19
653	Dehydrated flakes (without milk), water, milk, butter, and salt added.	1 cup	210	79	195	4	7	3.6	2.1	.2	30	65	99	.6	601	270	.08	.08	1.9	11
654	Potato chips, 1 3/4 by 2 1/2 in oval cross section.	10 chips	20	2	115	1	8	2.1	1.4	4.0	10	8	28	.4	226	Trace	.04	.01	1.0	3
655	Potato salad, made with cooked salad dressing.	1 cup	250	76	250	7	7	2.0	2.7	1.3	41	80	160	1.5	798	350	.20	.18	2.8	28
656	Pumpkin, canned	1 cup	245	90	80	2	1	—	—	—	19	61	64	1.0	588	15,680	.07	.12	1.5	12
657	Radishes, raw (prepackaged) stem ends, rootlets cut off.	4 radishes	18	95	5	Trace	Trace	—	—	—	1	5	6	.2	58	Trace	.01	.01	.1	5
658	Sauerkraut, canned, solids and liquid.	1 cup	235	93	40	2	Trace	—	—	—	9	85	42	1.2	329	120	.07	.09	.5	33
	Southern peas. See Blackeye peas (items 585–586).																			
	Spinach:																			
659	Raw, chopped	1 cup	55	91	15	2	Trace	—	—	—	2	51	28	1.7	259	4,460	.06	.11	.3	28
660	Cooked, drained: From raw	1 cup	180	92	40	5	1	—	—	—	6	167	68	4.0	583	14,580	.13	.25	.9	50
	From frozen:																			
661	Chopped	1 cup	205	92	45	6	1	—	—	—	8	232	90	4.3	683	16,200	.14	.31	.8	39
662	Leaf	1 cup	190	92	45	6	1	—	—	—	7	200	84	4.8	688	15,390	.15	.27	1.0	53
663	Canned, drained solids	1 cup	205	91	50	6	1	—	—	—	7	242	53	5.3	513	16,400	.04	.25	.6	29
	Squash, cooked:																			
664	Summer (all varieties), diced, drained.	1 cup	210	96	30	2	Trace	—	—	—	7	53	53	.8	296	820	.11	.17	1.7	21
665	Winter (all varieties), baked, mashed.	1 cup	205	81	130	4	1	—	—	—	32	57	98	1.6	945	8,610	.10	.27	1.4	27
	Sweetpotatoes:																			
	Cooked (raw, 5 by 2 in; about 2 1/2 per lb):																			
666	Baked in skin, peeled	1 potato	114	64	160	2	1	—	—	—	37	46	66	1.0	342	9,230	.10	.08	.8	25

NUTRIENTS IN INDICATED QUANTITY

Item No. (A)	Foods, approximate measures, units, and weight (edible part unless footnotes indicate otherwise) (B)	Weight Grams	Water (C) Per cent	Food energy (D) Kcalories	Protein (E) Grams	Fat (F) Grams	Saturated (total) (G) Grams	Unsaturated Oleic (H) Grams	Unsaturated Linoleic (I) Grams	Carbohydrate (J) Grams	Calcium (K) Milligrams	Phosphorus (L) Milligrams	Iron (M) Milligrams	Potassium (N) Milligrams	Vitamin A value (O) International units	Thiamin (P) Milligrams	Riboflavin (Q) Milligrams	Niacin (R) Milligrams	Ascorbic acid (S) Milligrams
667	Boiled in skin, peeled — 1 potato	151	71	170	3	1	—	—	—	40	48	71	1.1	367	11,940	.14	.09	.9	26
668	Candied, 2 1/2 by 2-in piece — 1 piece	105	60	175	1	3	2.0	.8	.1	36	39	45	.9	200	6,620	.06	.04	.4	11
	Canned:																		
669	Solid pack (mashed) — 1 cup	255	72	275	5	1	—	—	—	63	64	105	2.0	510	19,890	.13	.10	1.5	36
670	Vacuum pack, piece 2 3/4 by 1 in. — 1 piece	40	72	45	1	Trace	—	—	—	10	10	16	.3	80	3,120	.02	.02	.2	6
	Tomatoes:																		
671	Raw, 2 3/5-in diam. (3 per 12 oz pkg.) — 1 tomato[66]	135	94	25	1	Trace	—	—	—	6	16	33	.6	300	1,110	.07	.05	.9	[67]28
672	Canned, solids and liquid — 1 cup	241	94	50	2	Trace	—	—	—	10	[68]14	46	1.2	523	2,170	.12	.07	1.7	41
673	Tomato catsup — 1 cup	273	69	290	5	1	—	—	—	69	60	137	2.2	991	3,820	.25	.19	4.4	41
674	Tomato catsup — 1 tbsp	15	69	15	Trace	Trace	—	—	—	4	3	8	.1	54	210	.01	.01	.2	2
	Tomato juice, canned: Cup																		
675	Cup — 1 cup	243	94	45	2	Trace	—	—	—	10	17	44	2.2	552	1,940	.12	.07	1.9	39
676	Glass (6 fl oz) — 1 glass	182	94	35	2	Trace	—	—	—	8	13	33	1.6	413	1,460	.09	.05	1.5	29
677	Turnips, cooked, diced — 1 cup	155	94	35	1	Trace	—	—	—	8	54	37	.6	291	Trace	.06	.08	.5	34
	Turnip greens, cooked, drained:																		
678	From raw (leaves and stems) — 1 cup	145	94	30	3	Trace	—	—	—	5	252	49	1.5	—	8,270	.15	.33	.7	68
679	From frozen (chopped) — 1 cup	165	93	40	4	Trace	—	—	—	6	195	64	2.6	246	11,390	.08	.15	.7	31
680	Vegetables, mixed, frozen, cooked — 1 cup	182	83	115	6	1	—	—	—	24	46	115	2.4	348	9,010	.22	.13	2.0	15
	MISCELLANEOUS ITEMS																		
	Baking powders for home use: Sodium aluminum sulfate:																		
681	With monocalcium phosphate monohydrate — 1 tsp	3.0	2	5	Trace	Trace	0	0	0	1	58	87	—	5	0	0	0	0	0
682	With monocalcium phosphate monohydrate, calcium sulfate — 1 tsp	2.9	1	5	Trace	Trace	0	0	0	1	183	45	—	—	0	0	0	0	0
683	Straight phosphate — 1 tsp	3.8	2	5	Trace	Trace	0	0	0	1	239	359	—	6	0	0	0	0	0
684	Low sodium — 1 tsp	4.3	2	5	Trace	Trace	0	0	0	2	207	314	—	471	0	0	0	0	0

[66] Weight includes cores and stem ends. Without these parts, weight is 123 g.

[67] Based on year-round average. For tomatoes marketed from November through May, value is about 12 mg; from June through October, 32 mg.

[68] Applies to product without calcium salts added. Value for products with calcium salts added may be as much as 63 mg for whole tomatoes, 241 mg for cut forms.

NUTRIENTS IN INDICATED QUANTITY

Item No. (A)	Foods, approximate measures, units, and weight (edible part unless footnotes indicate otherwise) (B)		Water Per cent (C)	Food energy Kcalories (D)	Protein Grams (E)	Fat Grams (F)	Fatty Acids Saturated (total) Grams (G)	Unsaturated Oleic Grams (H)	Linoleic Grams (I)	Carbohydrate Grams (I)	Calcium Milligrams (K)	Phosphorus Milligrams (L)	Iron Milligrams (M)	Potassium Milligrams (N)	Vitamin A value International units (O)	Thiamin Milligrams (P)	Riboflavin Milligrams (Q)	Niacin Milligrams (R)	Ascorbic acid Milligrams (S)
		Grams																	
685	Barbecue sauce	1 cup	250 / 81	230	4	17	2.2	4.3	10.0	20	53	50	2.0	435	900	.03	.03	.8	13
686	Beverages, alcoholic:: Beer	12 fl oz	360 / 92	150	1	0	0	0	0	14	18	108	Trace	90	—	.01	.11	2.2	—
	Gin, rum, vodka, whisky:																		
687	80-proof	1 1/2-fl oz jigger	42 / 67	95	—	—	0	0	0	Trace	—	—	—	1	—	—	—	—	—
688	86-proof	1 1/2-fl oz jigger	42 / 64	105	—	—	0	0	0	Trace	—	—	—	1	—	—	—	—	—
689	90-proof	1 1/2-fl oz jigger	42 / 62	110	—	—	0	0	0	Trace	—	—	—	1	—	—	—	—	—
	Wines:																		
690	Dessert	3 1/2-fl oz glass	103 / 77	140	Trace	0	0	0	0	8	8	—	—	77	—	.01	.02	.2	—
691	Table	3 1/2-fl oz glass	102 / 86	85	Trace	0	0	0	0	4	9	10	.4	94	—	Trace	.01	.1	—
	Beverages, carbonated, sweetened, nonalcoholic:																		
692	Carbonated water	12 fl oz	366 / 92	115	0	0	0	0	0	29	—	—	—	—	0	0	0	0	0
693	Cola type	12 fl oz	369 / 90	145	0	0	0	0	0	37	—	—	—	—	0	0	0	0	0
694	Fruit-flavored sodas and Tom Collins mixer	12 fl oz	372 / 88	170	0	0	0	0	0	45	—	—	—	—	0	0	0	0	0
695	Ginger ale	12 fl oz	366 / 92	115	0	0	0	0	0	29	—	—	—	0	0	0	0	0	0
696	Root beer	12 fl oz	370 / 90	150	0	0	0	0	0	39	—	—	—	0	0	0	0	0	0
	Chili powder. See Peppers, hot, red (item 642).																		
	Chocolate:																		
697	Bitter or baking	1 oz	28 / 2	145	3	15	8.9	4.9	.4	8	22	109	1.9	235	20	.01	.07	.4	0
	Semisweet, see Candy, chocolate (item 539).																		
698	Gelatin, dry	1, 7-g envelope	7 / 13	25	6	Trace	0	0	0	0	—	—	—	—	—	—	—	—	—
699	Gelatin dessert prepared with gelatin dessert powder and water.	1 cup	240 / 84	140	4	0	0	0	0	34	—	—	—	—	—	—	—	—	—
710	Mustard, prepared, yellow	1 tsp or individual serving pouch or cup.	5 / 80	5	Trace	Trace	—	—	—	Trace	4	4	.1	7	—	—	—	—	—
	Olives, pickled, canned:																		
701	Green	4 medium or 3 extra large or 2 giant.[69]	16 / 78	15	Trace	2	.2	1.2	.1	Trace	8	2	.2	7	40	—	—	—	—
702	Ripe, Mission	3 small or 2 large[69]	10 / 73	15	Trace	2	.2	1.2	.1	Trace	9	1	.1	2	10	Trace	Trace	—	—
	Pickles, cucumber:																		
703	Dill, medium, whole, 3 3/4 in long, 1 1/4-in diam.	1 pickle	65 / 93	5	Trace	Trace	—	—	—	1	17	14	.7	130	70	Trace	.01	Trace	4
704	Fresh-pack, slices 1 1/2-in diam., 1/4 in thick.	2 slices	15 / 79	10	Trace	Trace	—	—	—	3	5	4	.3	—	20	Trace	Trace	Trace	1

[69]Weight includes pits. Without pits, weight is 13 g for item 701, 9 g for item 702.

366

NUTRIENTS IN INDICATED QUANTITY

Item No. (A)	Foods, approximate measures, units, and weight (edible part unless footnotes indicate otherwise) (B)	Grams	Water Per cent (C)	Food energy Kcal-ories (D)	Protein Grams (E)	Fat Grams (F)	Fatty Acids Saturated (total) Grams (G)	Unsaturated Oleic Grams (H)	Linoleic Grams (I)	Carbohydrate Grams (I)	Calcium Milligrams (K)	Phosphorus Milligrams (L)	Iron Milligrams (M)	Potassium Milligrams (N)	Vitamin A value International units (O)	Thiamin Milligrams (P)	Riboflavin Milligrams (Q)	Niacin Milligrams (R)	Ascorbic acid Milligrams (S)
705	Sweet, gherkin, small, whole, about 2 1/2 in long, 3/4-in diam. — 1 pickle	15	61	20	Trace	Trace	—	—	—	5	2	2	.2	—	10	Trace	Trace	Trace	1
706	Relish, finely chopped, sweet — 1 tbsp	15	63	20	Trace	Trace	—	—	—	5	3	2	.1	—	—	—	—	—	—
	Popcorn. See items 476–478.																		
707	Popsicle, 3-fl oz size — 1 popsicle	95	80	70	0	0	0	0	0	18	0	—	Trace	—	0	0	0	0	0
	Soups: Canned, condensed: Prepared with equal volume of milk:																		
708	Cream of chicken — 1 cup	245	85	180	7	10	4.2	3.6	1.3	15	172	152	.5	260	610	.05	.27	.7	2
709	Cream of mushroom — 1 cup	245	83	215	7	14	5.4	2.9	4.6	16	191	169	.5	279	250	.05	.34	.7	1
710	Tomato — 1 cup	250	84	175	7	7	3.4	1.7	1.0	23	168	155	.8	418	1,200	.10	.25	1.3	15
	Prepared with equal volume of water:																		
711	Bean with pork — 1 cup	250	84	170	8	6	1.2	1.8	2.4	22	63	128	2.3	395	650	.13	.08	1.0	3
712	Beef broth, bouillon, consomme — 1 cup	240	96	30	5	0	0	0	0	3	Trace	31	.5	130	Trace	Trace	.02	1.2	—
713	Beef noodle — 1 cup	240	93	65	4	3	.6	.7	.8	7	7	48	1.0	77	50	.05	.07	1.0	Trace
714	Clam chowder, Manhattan type (with tomatoes, without milk). — 1 cup	245	92	80	2	3	.5	.4	1.3	12	34	47	1.0	184	880	.02	.02	1.0	—
715	Cream of chicken — 1 cup	240	92	95	3	6	1.6	2.3	1.1	8	24	34	.5	79	410	.02	.05	.5	Trace
716	Cream of mushroom — 1 cup	240	90	135	2	10	2.6	1.7	4.5	10	41	50	.5	98	70	.02	.12	.7	Trace
717	Minestrone — 1 cup	245	90	105	5	3	.7	.9	1.3	14	37	59	1.0	314	2,350	.07	.05	1.0	—
718	Split pea — 1 cup	245	85	145	9	3	1.1	1.2	.4	21	29	149	1.5	270	440	.25	.15	1.5	1
719	Tomato — 1 cup	245	91	90	2	3	.5	.5	1.0	16	15	34	.7	230	1,000	.05	.05	1.2	12
720	Vegetable beef — 1 cup	245	92	80	5	2	—	—	—	10	12	49	.7	162	2,700	.05	.05	1.0	—
721	Vegetarian — 1 cup	245	92	80	2	2	—	—	—	13	20	39	1.0	172	2,940	.05	.05	1.0	—
	Dehydrated:																		
722	Bouillon cube, 1/2 in — 1 cube	4	4	5	1	Trace	—	—	—	Trace	—	—	—	4	—	—	—	—	—
	Mixes: Unprepared:																		
723	Onion — 1 1/2 oz pkg	43	3	150	6	5	1.1	2.3	1.0	23	42	49	.6	238	30	.05	.03	.3	6
	Prepared with water:																		
724	Chicken noodle — 1 cup	240	95	55	2	1	—	—	—	8	7	19	.2	19	50	.07	.05	.5	Trace
725	Onion — 1 cup	240	96	35	1	1	—	—	—	6	10	12	.2	58	Trace	Trace	Trace	Trace	2
726	Tomato vegetable with noodles. — 1 cup	240	93	65	1	1	—	—	—	12	7	19	.2	29	480	.05	.02	.5	5
727	Vinegar, cider — 1 tbsp	15	94	Trace	Trace	0	0	0	0	1	1	1	.1	15	—	—	—	—	—
728	White sauce, medium, with enriched flour. — 1 cup	250	73	405	10	31	19.3	7.8	.8	22	288	233	.5	348	1,150	.12	.43	.7	2

NUTRIENTS IN INDICATED QUANTITY

Item No. (A)	Foods, approximate measures, units, and weight (edible part unless footnotes indicate otherwise) (B)		Water (C)	Food energy (D)	Protein (E)	Fat (F)	Fatty Acids Saturated (total) (G)	Unsaturated Oleic (H)	Unsaturated Linoleic (I)	Carbohydrate (I)	Calcium (K)	Phosphorus (L)	Iron (M)	Potassium (N)	Vitamin A value (O)	Thiamin (P)	Riboflavin (Q)	Niacin (R)	Ascorbic acid (S)
		Grams	Per cent	Kcal-ories	Grams	Grams	Grams	Grams	Grams	Grams	Milli-grams	Milli-grams	Milli-grams	Milli-grams	Inter-national units	Milli-grams	Milli-grams	Milli-grams	Milli-grams
	Yeast:																		
729	Baker's, dry, active 1 pkg	7	5	20	3	Trace	—	—	—	3	[70]3	90	1.1	140	Trace	.16	.38	2.6	Trace
730	Brewer's, dry 1 tbsp	8	5	25	3	Trace	—	—	—	3	17	140	1.4	152	Trace	1.25	.34	3.0	Trace

[70]Value may vary from 6 to 60 mg.

Index

Page numbers in *italics* indicate page on which term is defined; numbers in **bold** indicate reference to an illustration.

Aangamik (*see* Pangamic acid)
Absorption
 factors affecting calcium,
  215–16
 iron and, 223
 mineral oil and, 184
 phosphorus and nutrients,
  218
 thermogenic effect, 150
Acetylcholine
 thiamin and, 191
Acid-base balance
 chloride and, 220
 electrolyte balance and,
  230–31
 mineral and, 214
 phosphorus and, 218
 protein as buffer, 120
Acidity (stomach), 215
 vitamin A and, 200–1
Acupuncture
 weight loss and, 170
Additives, 260–66 (*see also*
  Legislation; Preservaties)
 cancer and, 258
 coal tar dyes, 255
 color, *262*
  bans on, 258, 273
  Color Additive Amendment
   (1960), 258
  early 19th century, 256–57t
  pre-Civil War, 254
 common examples,
  264t–265t

Food Additives Amendment
 (1958), 255, 258
GRAS substances, *255*, 258
hazards of, 259, *263*, 266
hyperactivity and, 273–74
incidental, *260*, 274
intentional, 274
natural toxicants, 269
philosophy of the minimum,
 255
preservatives (19th century),
 256t–257t
prior sanctioned substances,
 255
risk vs. benefits, 263, 266,
 271–72, 274
safety of, 266
testing for safety, 255, 263
tolerance levels, 255
toxicity of, *263*
Adenosine triphosphate (*see*
 ATP)
Adipose tissue (*see* Fats, cells)
Adolescents
 caffeine intake of, 248
 calcium requirements, 216–17
 fat cell development, 157, 159
Adult onset obesity, 159
Adults
 caffeine intake of, 248–49
Adulterants (*see* Additives)
Advertising
 evaluating nutritional claims,
  3–8

Aerobic exercise (*see* Exercise)
Aflatoxin (a carcinogen), 282,
 284
Africa
 cancer rates in, 281
 fiber consumption, 68, 75
Age
 BMR and, 149
 hypertension and, 98
 pernicious anemia and, 194
 vitamin B-6 and, 192
 vitamin E and, 189, 203
 weight and, 153
Alcohol, *36–39*
 athletes and, 242
 cancer and, 284
 composition of beverages,
  36t
 as diuretic, 38
 drugs and, 39
 fetal alcohol syndrome, 38–39
 folacin and, 193
 health and, 38–39
 heart disease and, 102
 hypertension and, 97–99
 nutrients and, 37–38
 thiamin and, 191
Alcoholics
 deficiencies in, 191–93
 nutritional problems, 37–38
 vitamins and, 183
Allergies
 Yellow Dye No. 5 and, 273
Alpha-tocopherol, 188

thiamin sources, 191
vitamin B-6 source, 192
vitamin B-12 and, 194
Megadoses, 184 (*see also*
    Megavitamins; names of
    individual nutrients;
    Toxicity)
    controversy, 199–200
    iodine excess, 225
    iron excess, 224
    molybdenum excess, 227
    orthomolecular psychiatry
        and, 204–5
    pharmacological doses, 199
    physiological doses, 199
    potassium excess, 220
Megaloblastic anemia, 193 (*see
    also* Anemia)
Megavitamins (*see also*
    Megadoses; names of
    individual nutrients;
    Toxicity)
    orthomolecular psychiatry,
        204–5
    risks vs. benefits, 200–210
    therapy, 199–200
    toxicity
        niacin and, 205
        vitamin A, 201, **202**
        vitamin C, 205–8
        vitamin D, 202
        vitamin E, 204
Membranes
    electrolyte balance, 230–32
Menadione (synthetic vitamin
    K), 189
Menstruation
    anemia and, 224
    anorexia nervosa and, 180
    iron requirements of women
        athletes, 239–40
    obesity and, 157
Mental confusion (pellagra and),
    192
Mental performance (caffeine
    and), 249
Mental retardation
    from fetal alcohol syndrome,
        38
Mercury, 228, 229
Metabolic diseases
    fiber and, 73
    obesity and, 156
Metabolism (*see also* Basal
    metabolic rate; Liver
    (body organ); Thyroid)
    appetite suppressants and,
        170
    factors affecting, 149
    folacin and, 193
    riboflavin and, 191
Methionine (amino acid), 137
    choline and, 195

Methylxanthines, 247 (*see also*
    Caffeine)
Micronutrients, 11
Microorganisms
    vitamin B-12 and, 194
Milk (*see also* Anemia; Animal
    products; Dairy products)
    calcium in, 217
    carbohydrate source, 48
    sugar (lactose), 216
    tryptophan source, 192
    vitamin A and, 185, 186
    vitamin D and, 187
Miller Pesticide Amendment
    (1954), 255
Mineral oil (*see also* Laxatives)
    absorption and, 169
Mineral supplements
    recommended dosages, 209t
    who should take, 210
Minerals, 14–15, 213–14t, 229
    (*see also* Megadoses;
        names of individual
        nutrients; Toxicity)
    athletes and, 239–40
    body fluid balances and,
        230–32
    cancer and, 284
    as cofactors with enzymes, 14
    as components of tissues,
        14–15
    deficiencies
        fiber and, 66–67
        sugar and, 57
    essential to human nutrition,
        214t
    function of, 215
    oral contraceptive agents'
        effect on, 211
    present in large amounts,
        214–20
    water hardness and, 233
Minimum daily requirements
    (MDR), 35
Misinformation
    evaluation of nutritional
        claims, 3–8
    food faddism and, 2–3
    quackery, 2–3
Miso (vitamin B-12 source), 134
Molasses
    compared to table sugar, 52t
    iron source, 225
    niacin deficiency and, 192
Molybdenum, 227
Monosaccharides, 41–42, 43t
Monosodium glutamate
    ban on, 272
    as flavor enhancer, 262
    sodium intake and, 219
Monounsaturated fats (*see* Fats)
Monounsaturated fatty acids,
    79, **80** (*see also* Fatty acids)

Mormons (cancer and), 135–36
Morton, Dr. Richard, 180
Mucus (and vitamin A), 186
Multiple Risk Factor
    Intervention Study
    (MRFIT), 104
Muscles (*see also* Athletes;
    Exercise; Glycogen)
    athlete's protein needs,
        236–37
    contraction and minerals, 215,
        220
    cramps and thiamin, 191
    disorders and vitamin E, 203
    energy sources for, 240
    magnesium and, 218–19
    myoglobin and iron, 222
    potassium and, 220
Muslim(s)
    vitamin D deficiencies in, 187
Myocardial infarct, 90
Myoglobin
    athletes and, 236
    iron and, 222

Nails (fingernails)
    zinc and, 226
National Cancer Institute (NCI)
    artificial sweeteners and
        cancer, 58–59
Natto (B-12 source), 134
Natural foods (*see also*
    Additives)
    advertising and, 267
    claims for, 271
    controversy, 267–68, 271–72
Natural vitamins (vs. synthetic),
    209–10
Nausea
    alcoholics and, 37–38
Neoplasm, *279* (*see also* Cancer)
Nerves
    impulse transmission and
        minerals and, 214
    potassium and, 220
    thiamin and, 191
Nervous system
    vitamin B-6 and, 192
    vitamin B-12 and, 194
Nervousness
    caffeine and, 249
Net protein utilization (NPU),
    122
Niacin (vitamin B-3), 191–92 (*see
    also* B vitamins; Vitamins)
    absorption in alcoholic, 38
    enrichment and, 261
    in fast foods, 278t
    megadoses and, 204–5
    overdoses by alcoholics, 38
    vitamin B-6 and, 192
Niacinamide (*see* Nicotinamide)

Peptidases, 118
Periodontal disease
  sign of osteoporosis, 217
Peristalsis, 15
Pernicious anemia (Vitamin B-12
    deficiency), 194 (see also
    Anemia)
Personality (types)
  heart disease and, 101
Pesticides (see also Organic
    foods)
  cancer and, 282
  as hazard, 259
  lower residues in vegan
    mothers' milk, 135
  need for, 269
pH balance (see Acid-base
    balance)
Pharmacological doses (of
    vitamins), 199
Phenopropanolamine (appetite
    suppressant), 170
Phosphate
  electrolyte balance and,
    230–31t
  vitamin D and, 187
Phosphorus, 218 (see also
    Minerals)
  calcium absorption and,
    216–17
  in fast foods, 278t
Photosensitive pigment, 185
Photosynthesis, 144, **145**
Physical activity (see Exercise)
Physiological doses (of
    vitamins), 199
Physiological obesity (see
    Hypothalamic obesity)
Phytic acid
  calcium absorption and, 216,
    218
  iron absorption and, 223
  storage form of calcium, 218
  vegetarians and, 133
  zinc and, 226
Pica (clay eating), 226
Pill (see Oral contraceptive
    agents)
Placebo, 7
  effect in nutrition research, 7
Placenta (see also Pregnancy)
  alcohol absorption and, 38
  caffeine absorption and, 247
  vitamin E and, 188
Plants (see also Breads/cereals;
    Fruits; Grains; Legumes;
    Vegetables)
  fat synthesis and, 144
  photosynthesis in, 144
  vitamin A sources, 186–87
Plaque (atheroma), 90 (see also
    Atherosclerosis)
  illustrated, **91, 93**

Pollution (and vitamin E), 204
Polysaccharides, 43–44
  glucose chains and, **44**
Polyunsaturated fats (see also
    Fats)
  sources of, 109
  vitamin E and, 188–89
Polyunsaturated fatty acids, 85
    (see also Fatty acids)
Population studies
  diet and heart disease, 104
  vitamin A and, 201
Pork
  niacin deficiency and, 192
  thiamin and, 191
Potassium, 220 (see also
    Minerals)
  alcohol and, 38
  athletes loss of, 243
  deficiency
    Beverly Hills Diet and, 168
    fasting and, 170
    electrolyte balance and, 230
    sodium ions and, 219
Potatoes
  thiamin source, 191
  vitamin C source, 195
Poultry (see also Meats)
  riboflavin sources, 191
  thiamin source, 191
Poverty
  obesity and, 163
  riboflavin deficiency and, 191
  vitamin C deficiency and, 195
Precursors (provitamins), 184
  carotene and, 186–87
Pregame meal
  recommendations for athletes,
    241–42t
Pregnancy
  alcohol and, 38–39
  anemia and, 224
  caffeine consumption during,
    248–49
  calcium requirements, 216–17
  folacin and, 193
  iodine and cretinism, 225
  iron and, 223–24
  magnesium and, 219
  niacin and, 192
  riboflavin and, 191
  thiamin and, 191
  underweight and, 179
  vitamin C and, 208
  vitamin D and, 187
  vitamin E and, 189
Pregnant teenagers
  zinc and, 226
Prescription drugs
  (megavitamins as), 200
Preservatives (see also Additives)
  function of, 262
Prevention (magazine), 1

Prior sanctioned substances,
    255, 263 (see also
    Additives)
Pritikin diet, 106–7 (see also
    Diet(s))
Processed foods (see also
    Additives; Fast foods;
    Sweeteners)
  compared to natural foods,
    267–68
  criticisms of, 272
  high in sodium, 220
  sugar content of, 60t
  trace minerals and, 222
Prolamine, 170
Prolinn, 167
"Proof" number (of alcohol), 36
Prostaglandins, 12
Protein(s), 13–14 (see also Amino
    acids; Animal products;
    Meats)
  absorption in alcoholic, 37
  (acid-base) balance and, 120
  amino acids, 115
  animal, 124, 126
  athletes and, 236–37
  B vitamins and, 190
  biological value (BV), 122
  calcium absorption and, 216
  cancer and, 284
  cellular structures of, 13–14
  complementary, 136–37t
  complete vs. incomplete, 122
  component elements of, 13
  component of body tissues,
    119
  concentration in foods, 121t
  consumption of, 128
  conversion efficiency (animal
    vs. plant), 126
  costs of, 126, 127t
  deficiency (choline), 195
  denatured, 115
  digestion of, 118–**119**
  as energy source, 13, 120, 147
  fast foods and, 278t
  fluid balances and, 232
  food sources of, 124–25
  genetic coding of, 116
  intrinsic factor and vitamin
    B-12, 194
  limiting amino acid, 122, 124t
  low carbohydrate diet and,
    166
  meat substitutes and, 136–38
  needs by age, sex, 121t
  net protein utilization, 122
  niacin and, 191
  nitrogen balance studies, 122,
    124
  opsin, 185
  oral contraceptive agents and,
    211